SECOND EDITION

CLIENT EDUCATION

THEORY AND PRACTICE

Mary A. Miller, PhD, RN

Dean Emeritus

School of Nursing, Aurora University

Aurora, Illinois

Associate Dean Emeritus

School of Professional Studies, Metropolitan State College of Denver

Denver, Colorado

Pamella Rae Stoeckel, PhD, RN, CNE

Associate Professor

Loretta Heights School of Nursing

Regis University

Denver, Colorado

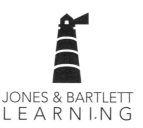

JONES & BARTLETT
LEARNING

World Headquarters
Jones & Bartlett Learning
5 Wall Street
Burlington, MA 01803
978-443-5000
info@jblearning.com
www.jblearning.com

Jones & Bartlett Learning books and products are available through most bookstores and online booksellers. To contact Jones & Bartlett Learning directly, call 800-832-0034, fax 978-443-8000, or visit our website, www.jblearning.com.

Substantial discounts on bulk quantities of Jones & Bartlett Learning publications are available to corporations, professional associations, and other qualified organizations. For details and specific discount information, contact the special sales department at Jones & Bartlett Learning via the above contact information or send an email to specialsales@jblearning.com.

The content, statements, views, and opinions herein are the sole expression of the respective authors and not that of Jones & Bartlett Learning, LLC. Reference herein to any specific commercial product, process, or service by trade name, trademark, manufacturer, or otherwise does not constitute or imply its endorsement or recommendation by Jones & Bartlett Learning, LLC and such reference shall not be used for advertising or product endorsement purposes. All trademarks displayed are the trademarks of the parties noted herein. *Client Education: Theory and Practice, Second Edition* is an independent publication and has not been authorized, sponsored, or otherwise approved by the owners of the trademarks or service marks referenced in this product.

There may be images in this book that feature models; these models do not necessarily endorse, represent, or participate in the activities represented in the images. Any screenshots in this product are for educational and instructive purposes only. Any individuals and scenarios featured in the case studies throughout this product may be real or fictitious, but are used for instructional purposes only.

The authors, editors, and publisher have made every effort to provide accurate information. However, they are not responsible for errors, omissions, or for any outcomes related to the use of the contents of this book and take no responsibility for the use of the products and procedures described. Treatments and side effects described in this book may not be applicable to all people; likewise, some people may require a dose or experience a side effect that is not described herein. Drugs and medical devices are discussed that may have limited availability controlled by the Food and Drug Administration (FDA) for use only in a research study or clinical trial. Research, clinical practice, and government regulations often change the accepted standard in this field. When consideration is being given to use of any drug in the clinical setting, the health care provider or reader is responsible for determining FDA status of the drug, reading the package insert, and reviewing prescribing information for the most up-to-date recommendations on dose, precautions, and contraindications, and determining the appropriate usage for the product. This is especially important in the case of drugs that are new or seldom used.

Production Credits
VP, Executive Publisher: David Cella
Executive Editor: Amanda Martin
Associate Acquisitions Editor: Rebecca Myrick
Production Editor: Amanda Clerkin
Senior Marketing Manager: Jennifer Stiles
Art Development Editor: Joanna Lundeen
Art Development Assistant: Shannon Sheehan

VP, Manufacturing and Inventory Control: Therese Connell
Composition: Cenveo® Publisher Services
Cover Design: Kristin E. Parker
Manager of Photo Research, Rights & Permissions: Lauren Miller
Cover Image: © ileana_bt/Shutterstock, Inc.
Printing and Binding: Edwards Brothers Malloy
Cover Printing: Edwards Brothers Malloy

To order this product, use ISBN: 978-1-284-08503-7

Library of Congress Cataloging-in-Publication Data
Miller, Mary A. (Mary Alice), author.
    Client education : theory and practice / Mary A. Miller and Pamella Rae Stoeckel. — Second edition.
    p.; cm.
Includes bibliographical references and index.
    ISBN 978-1-284-04828-5 (alk. paper)
    I. Stoeckel, Pamella Rae, author. II. Title.
    [DNLM: 1. Patient Education as Topic—Nurses' Instruction. 2. Nurse-Patient Relations—Nurses' Instruction. W 85]
    RT90
    615.5071–dc23
                                                                                    2014044039
    6048

Printed in the United States of America
19 18 17 16 15   10 9 8 7 6 5 4 3 2

To Benjamin, Diane, and the Taylor family
and to
The Stoeckel and Garhart families

and to

Our students,
Our clients,
Our colleagues:
Our teachers

CONTENTS

PREFACE

This text is written for nursing students and practicing health professionals who teach clients. We define clients to include not only patients, families, and communities, but also colleagues and other health team members. The text guides readers in the development of the knowledge, skills, and attitudes necessary to become effective client educators. While we are thorough in covering the broad expanse of health education, we have selected information that is most helpful to the reader.

This second edition explicates our evolving thoughts about client education, adds new information, and incorporates the suggestions we received from users of this text. The text represents the most current thinking about client education and its application to today's changing health delivery system. We focus on the practical application of information for students aspiring to become nurses and practicing health professionals. The usefulness of information is enhanced if readers see how it applies to professional practice. We have organized the text so health professionals with limited time can readily find the information they need.

Every chapter has been carefully reviewed and content enriched. We have added more emphasis on teaching health team members and clients throughout the text. In Chapters 2 and 3 we added clarifying content on thinking and learning theory. In Chapter 4 we expanded learner assessment to include new sections on assessing psychosocial vital signs and assessing background knowledge. In Chapter 6 we enhanced adult learning theory. We also added new sections on Working with Clients with Special Needs in Chapters 5 (Child Learners) and 7 (Older Learners). For older learners we provided recommendations for teaching that aligns with their changing physiologic situations. We reorganized Chapter 9 (Learning Objectives) to make it easier for readers to grasp the content. With the advancement of technology and the role it plays in client education, we have added information on Web-based delivery and e-Health interactive tutorials and how nurses can tap these resources (Chapters 10 and 11).

A significant change occurred as our thinking about client education evolved. We have revised the Client Education Outcomes component of the Miller–Stoeckel Client Education Model. The text now reflects the nature of both formative and summative evaluations as they apply to client education. The text has colorful, eye-pleasing slides in PowerPoint format that instructors and students can use to master the content.

Finally, we have carefully evaluated our writing to ensure the message is clearly communicated. We have removed ambiguity and aspired to be succinct. As with our first edition, we are fully responsible for the content of this text and our views on teaching, learning, and client education. We are grateful for our colleagues' contributions and continue to welcome your suggestions for improvement.

I

A Framework for Health Education

1

Overview of the Miller–Stoeckel Client Education Model

INTRODUCTION

This chapter introduces the Miller–Stoeckel Client Education Model as the conceptual framework around which this text is written. The **model** is supported by assumptions, concepts, and theories that are consistent with nursing as a practice discipline. We describe the model and its component parts and why it forms what we believe is the framework for **health** education in today's practice environment. We begin this discussion by examining the purposes and goals of health education and then move into a discussion of the Miller–Stoeckel Client Education Model itself. The four major components of the model are described and essential terms are defined to fully explain the meaning and scope of health education. We introduce the Stoeckel Wellness–Illness Functional Continuum to help **evaluate** clients' perceptions of their health and **illness** states. This continuum presents the status of individuals' health in positive and negative degrees of physical and mental health that can be described incrementally on a continuum. Each of us defines our own wellness based on our individual circumstances and perceptions. We use the Stoeckel Wellness–Illness Functional Continuum as an assessment tool to help determine clients' personal perceptions of health and illness and as a means of looking holistically at clients' health education needs. Finally, the chapter discusses the context for and the national importance of health education. Our premise is that client education improves the health status of individuals, families, and groups and communities and directs them toward healthful behavior changes. We begin by specifying the purposes and goals of health education.

PURPOSES AND GOALS OF HEALTH EDUCATION

We view *purpose* and *goal* as having essentially the same meaning (Webster's, 2013) and believe the overall purpose and goal of health education is to promote, retain, and restore health, which is a phrase you will see throughout this text. It involves the prevention, treatment, and management of illness and the preservation of clients' mental and physical well-being. Comprehensive client education includes maintenance and promotion of health, illness prevention, restoration of health, and coping with impaired **function**. This view of health care can be achieved only by shifting the emphasis away from illness and cure and integrating client education into a comprehensive approach to health maintenance, prevention, and promotion (Davidhizar & Cramer, 2002).

Health education promotes positive, informed changes in lifestyle and involves encouraging behaviors that prevent acute and chronic disease, decrease disability, and enhance wellness. Nurses as educators empower clients to strive for optimal health and well-being. Individuals learn to make informed decisions about personal and **family** health practices and use health services in the **community**. From a public health perspective, health education is intended not only to enhance individuals' abilities to make positive lifestyle changes, but also to support social and political actions that promote health and quality of life in communities. Hall (2001) notes that effective community education is essential as individuals, communities, and the nation shift focus to wellness and illness prevention. The concept of community empowerment is designed to help individuals and organizations use their abilities and resources in collective efforts to address their health priorities and needs. The ultimate goal of health education is for nurses as educators to help clients make changes in behavior that support healthy living.

THE MILLER–STOECKEL CLIENT EDUCATION MODEL

The Miller–Stoeckel Client Education Model provides the conceptual framework for understanding the essential, interrelated components of health education. The four major components of the model are Nurse as Educator, Client as Learner, Nurse–Client relationship, and Client Education Outcomes. The model assumptions are important to understand because they represent our fundamental beliefs about health education and its place in the context of today's healthcare delivery system. The model has widespread applications for **teaching** students how to teach clients and for practicing nurses to **implement** health education in their practice settings. In addition to the assumptions, each major component has supporting subcomponents that are essential to the delivery of competent and meaningful health education (**Figure 1-1**).

FIGURE 1-1

Overview of the Miller–Stoeckel Client Education Model

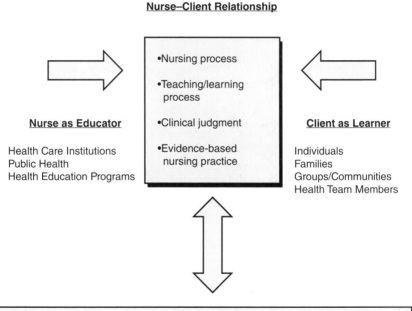

Nurse–Client Relationship

Nurse as Educator

Health Care Institutions
Public Health
Health Education Programs

- Nursing process
- Teaching/learning process
- Clinical judgment
- Evidence-based nursing practice

Client as Learner

Individuals
Families
Groups/Communities
Health Team Members

Client Education Outcomes	
Formative Evaluation	Summative Evaluation
• Evaluation of the teaching plan	• Evaluation of client learning
• Evaluation of the learning environment	• Evaluation of educational effectiveness
• Evaluation of the nurse–client interaction	• Evaluation of integration of learning into daily living

Model Assumptions

A model is a representation of something. Models are useful **learning** aids that conceptualize what is being represented through illustrations and figures rather than strictly textual information. They help **learners** grasp the larger picture and visualize relationships among component parts of something that would otherwise take many words to describe. For our purposes, models represent our view of client education in the context of professional nursing practice. Our assumptions and beliefs about the Miller–Stoeckel Client Education Model are as follows:

- Health status can be improved for most clients through health education.
- Nurses as Educators can help to promote, retain, and restore health.
- Health status is affected by a variety of factors, such as lifestyle, heredity, environment, and the availability of health care.
- Clients' motivation and perceptions affect learning about health.
- Clients can learn positive health behaviors.
- Teaching appropriate prevention strategies is effective in dealing with health problems.
- Clients are active participants in their health care, and they are responsible for choices under their control that affect their health.
- Nurses are responsible for health education in a variety of settings.
- A therapeutic Nurse–Client Relationship is essential to achieve positive health education outcomes.

Components of the Miller–Stoeckel Client Education Model

The Miller-Stoeckel Client Education Model provides a framework for viewing the essential components of health education. The four components of the model—Nurse as Educator, Client as Learner, the Nurse–Client Relationship, and Client Education Outcomes—provide the conceptual framework for this text. A discussion of the components is provided in the following sections.

NURSE AS EDUCATOR

Nurses are professionals who **plan**, organize, teach, and direct health education to promote, retain, and restore health in a variety of settings. The model shows that nurses work in public health, healthcare institutions, and health education programs. The model is not meant to limit nurses to those settings but to identify the most common places in which nurses are employed. Nurses as Educators are fortunate to be employed in many areas beyond what we have identified; we list these only as examples.

Nurses work with other healthcare professionals, civic groups, and community officials to identify health needs, develop desirable health education goals, and evaluate the availability of healthcare services. Nurses as Educators focus on promoting optimal health and preventing illness, but they also deal with social, cultural, behavioral, legal, and economic issues as they affect health.

Nurses' Role in Health Education

The teaching role of nurses has long been recognized as a function of nursing practice. It has been within the scope of nursing practice since the days of Florence Nightingale. In 1918 the National League of Nursing Education (NLNE), precursor to the present-day National League for Nursing (NLN), defined nursing as the prevention of illness and the promotion of health especially in public health, child welfare, schools, home visiting, industries, hospitals, and social services. Nurses were expected to be responsible for health teaching. Two decades later, in 1937, the NLNE stated that a nurse was essentially a teacher and an agent of health in whatever field nursing practice occurred. In 1998 the American Nurses Association (ANA) stated in the Standards of Clinical Nursing Practice that educating clients is a primary responsibility of nurses. The ANA continues its long-standing support for patient teaching as a primary component of nursing care. Today all state nurse practice acts in the United States include client teaching within the scope of nursing practice. Further support for the role of Nurses as Educators is found in the Patient's Bill of Rights, which was first adopted by the American Hospital Association (AHA) in 1973. The current bill was approved by the AHA board of trustees in 1992 and states that patients have the right to "relevant, current, and understandable information concerning diagnosis, treatment, and prognosis" (AHA, 1992, Right #2). The Joint Commission, the organization that accredits hospitals, revised their patient education standards to include follow-up treatment and services in 2009 (The Joint Commission, 2009). Many practicing nurses and nurse educators support client education as an essential role for nurses (Bastable & Alt, 2014; Pender, 2011; Redman, 2006).

Just as important as educating clients, nurses also have a professional responsibility to educate colleagues and **health team** members as necessary. Health care is rapidly changing and requires all colleagues and team members to stay current in their knowledge and skills. Nursing team members have differing levels of education and training that can vary from a few weeks to several years. They may also be new to the employing institution and need additional education. Because Nurses as Educators are in constant contact with colleagues and team members and are familiar with their knowledge and skills, they necessarily become the primary educator and resource for the team (Donner, Levonian, & Slutsky, 2005). Lifelong learning is essential for those in the healthcare professions and requires all providers to stay current with their knowledge and skills.

Nurses are in an essential position to coordinate client health education because they are the healthcare providers who have the most continuous contact with clients. Because nurses are with clients at teachable moments, they do most of the health education. As a nurse, your educational background in anatomy, physiology, nutrition, psychology, sociology, anthropology, and other social and physical sciences makes you a very appropriate health educator. Your education has taught you how the body can and should function and about the interplay among mind, body, and spirit. In addition, you have access to behavioral and evidence-based health research that can help people learn healthy behaviors and reduce unhealthy ones. This same body of research can be applied to help people change and maintain those changes in their health behaviors.

Firsthand knowledge about the consequences of various lifestyles will make you an authentic source of information. Nurses have earned the public's trust, and by modeling healthy habits they are more believable when they teach. Clients are entering the healthcare system better informed about health issues. This means they will be demanding more knowledgeable caregivers, and they expect to be provided with current and scientifically sound information. Many clients have done considerable reading about their particular health problem and consequently ask informed, sophisticated questions. Your credibility will be established by your answers.

CLIENT AS LEARNER

We chose the word *client* to describe the learner in this text because the client is the consumer of health education and is the focus of our teaching efforts. We define clients as individuals, families, groups and communities, and health team members, which covers the scope of humanity. Clients are everywhere and include everyone in need of health information. The word *client* connotes someone who is free to come and go from your presence; someone who is free to accept or refuse the services, counsel, and teaching that nurses offer. We view clients as responsible, thinking individuals who have the right to make choices about their health.

Contrast the view of the client with the view of the individual as a patient. When examined from this perspective, we think of someone who must depend on nurses for their care and sometimes for their very survival. The term *patient* conjures up an image of someone who is dependent and in need of physical or psychological assistance related to health. A patient is in your presence—on your nursing unit or in your service area—and needs the health education that nurses can deliver.

Clients bring their individual and collective perceptions of what optimal health is to the Nurse–Client Relationship. Perceptions are influenced by their expectations, emotions, and needs. Perceptions about health are determined individually, culturally, environmentally, and socially. Clients' perceptions may not always be the same as nurses' perceptions. In the client education context, we perceive clients as active participants in health education to the extent of their ability and choice.

NURSE–CLIENT RELATIONSHIP

Between the Nurse as Educator and Client as Learner is the Nurse–Client Relationship. This is the participants' point of contact where the relationship between them is created. Of the many nursing interventions that nurses offer to clients, one of the most important is health education. A positive, respectful, and thoughtful Nurse–Client Relationship is essential if we are to achieve the goal of promoting, retaining, and restoring the health of clients.

The Nurse as Educator brings a formal educational base to the Nurse–Client Relationship that is designed to promote, retain, and restore the health of clients. This includes preparation in the physical and social sciences, humanities, and nursing arts and science. Nurses use this base of knowledge to understand human behavior, engage in clear communication, and commit to standards of ethical behavior that are the foundation of the Nurse–Client Relationship.

The Nurse–Client Relationship is therapeutic, promoting a psychological climate that facilitates positive change and growth. This aspect of the model is drawn from Hildegard Peplau's interpersonal nursing theory (1952) that stressed the importance of the therapeutic interpersonal process. Therapeutic communication between the Nurse as Educator and the Client as Learner is collaborative and focuses on the achievement of health education goals. It focuses on the client achieving optimal personal growth and the highest level of wellness possible given the client's situation. An explicit time frame, a goal-directed approach, and the expectation of confidentiality are important to the relationship. The nurse establishes, directs, and takes responsibility for the interaction. In this relationship clients' needs take priority over nurses' needs.

Four goal-directed phases characterize the Nurse–Client Relationship. The preinteraction phase occurs before meeting the client and involves gathering all available client information. This gives the nurse time to anticipate health concerns and plan for the initial interaction. The orientation phase occurs when the Nurse as Educator meets the Client as Learner and they get to know one another. The working phase occurs when the Nurse as Educator engages in health teaching and works with the client to solve problems and accomplish goals. Last is the termination phase, which is the process of ending the relationship (Potter & Perry, 2009).

Within the Nurse–Client Relationship, we believe two processes—the exercise of judgment and the application of research—are integral to each component of the Nurse–Client Relationship. These components are the Nursing Process, the Teaching and Learning Process, Clinical Judgment, and Evidence-based Nursing Practice (EBNP). We describe each in order (**Figure 1-2**).

Nursing Process

The Nursing Process is the first component of the Nurse–Client Relationship. It is undoubtedly the most familiar to you as a student. It is the most common framework in nursing education and practice to conceptualize nursing practice and nurse–client interactions.

The Nursing Process is a variation of the scientific reasoning process that allows you to organize your thoughts and systematize nursing practice. Its focus is to address client problems in professional practice in a variety of clinical settings. Steps in the nursing process include assessment, analysis, planning, implementation, and evaluation. Applied to health education, the steps of the nursing process relate directly to the learning needs of clients that are designed to improve clients' health knowledge and promote, retain, and restore health.

FIGURE 1-2

Nurse–Client Relationship in the Miller–Stoeckel Client Education Model

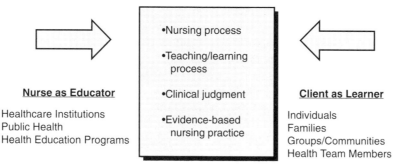

The steps of the Nursing Process are iterative because they may overlap or occur simultaneously. Reassessment, reordering of priorities, new goal setting, and revising the teaching plan continues as part of the process toward attainment of the health education goals. A discussion of the steps of the nursing process as they apply to health education follows.

Assessment

Assessment is gathering the essential information about the client to identify health education needs. As you **assess** the physiologic, psychological, sociocultural, developmental, and spiritual influences on each client, it helps to determine each individual's learning style and learning capacity. Assessment includes collecting subjective and objective client data, recording the data, and noting the data that affect learning. Subjective data include clients' perceptions of their condition and health status. How does the client view his or her situation? How does the client view his or her health? Is the client's situation conducive or obstructive to learning? Does the client show a readiness to learn? Do you have the requisite knowledge, skills, and attitudes to facilitate each client's learning in the situation at hand?

Analysis

The second step, analysis, is a careful examination and validation of the facts to identify the client's specific health education needs. When possible, you will collaborate with clients to diagnose their learning needs. A clear understanding of these needs becomes the basis for planning, implementing, and evaluating the teaching plan. This step includes analyzing both your perceptions and your clients' perceptions of the learning needs to validate them. Assessing and analyzing needs also includes determining the kind of learning clients want. For instance, in which domain are your clients deficient? Do they lack information? What do they want to know? Do they lack necessary skills? Is their developmental level a barrier to learning? Do they display attitudes that impair their optimum functioning?

When your client is a specific population, your assessment becomes complex. You may need to conduct a survey as part of the assessment. Another option is to form a focus group composed of individuals who are representative of the large group you are teaching. For smaller groups, interviewing selected members of the group may serve your purpose just as well. In all instances, it is important to avoid making assumptions about what clients need to learn. Ask them and be as thorough in your assessment and analysis as possible.

Another way to approach clients is from the perspective of potential growth. What information do they desire? What new skills do they wish to learn? What opportunities for growth are inherent in their developmental stages? What attitudes are they ready to exhibit? What attitudes do they already possess that could motivate further growth? What strengths of mind, body, and spirit do they manifest that can help them in the inevitable transitions of life?

A nursing diagnosis identifies the human response to the disease process. Standard classifications of nursing diagnosis used to identify dysfunctional patterns include North American Nursing Diagnosis Association (NANDA), Nursing Interventions Classification (NIC), and Nursing Outcomes Classification (NOC) (McFarland & McFarland, 1997). These diagnoses are applicable to health education.

Planning

Planning, the third step of the Nursing Process, is the development of the teaching plan. In this step you will outline the learning objectives based on the assessment and analysis of the findings. It involves identifying specific learning objectives and educational outcomes, establishing priorities, and selecting teaching strategies to achieve the outcomes. Planning is deciding what needs to be learned and what strategies and materials will most likely facilitate achievement of the learning objectives. Once these are selected, a written teaching plan is devised.

The planning step should involve clients and their families when appropriate. For example, if your client has Alzheimer's disease, then significant others, such as caregivers, a spouse, or family members, must be included in the formation of plans. It is important to get feedback during the planning process about what is to be learned and how this is to be accomplished to discover if you and the client are in accord.

Implementation

Implementing the plan involves acting to accomplish the learning objectives and educational outcomes. You and your clients will carry out the actions that are most likely to facilitate the desired learning. During this step you will need to elicit periodic feedback and stay attuned to behavioral clues that indicate clients' feelings of success or failure. You will use a variety of teaching strategies and instructional materials to facilitate client learning. Ongoing reassessment and continued analysis are part of implementation and involve adapting to feedback as you enact the plan. Note the client's responses to your teaching and modify your approach as needed. Last, it is important to document the health education that you provide.

Evaluation

The evaluation phase is the final step of the Nursing Process. This is where you and your clients evaluate teaching effectiveness. Did the clients learn what was expected? Is their behavior more conducive to good health? Has the client's level of wellness improved? Are the problems with which clients needed help diminished, or are they coping with their problems more effectively? Two-way communication with clients helps you to summarize and interpret results.

Although evaluation is presented as the final step of the Nursing Process, evaluation takes place throughout the Teaching and Learning Process. During the assessment phase, for instance, while identifying how clients perceive their problems, you will evaluate how well you communicated. Did you understand what the clients conveyed? To find out, repeat back your interpretation of what they said. Did clients indicate that they were understood correctly? Did clients indicate that your words and actions made sense to them? Such transactions are ongoing throughout each step of the Nursing Process. Evaluation involves determining the overall quality of health education.

Some suggest that the Nursing Process contributes to linear thinking. Chitty and Black state that "the nursing process can be taught, learned, and used in a rigid, mechanistic and linear manner" (2007, p. 194). However, we believe it can be used as a creative approach to health education by attending to feedback throughout the process. The Nursing Process used in health education is ongoing, with constant evaluation and reassessment to meet the ongoing learning needs of clients.

Teaching and Learning Process

The Teaching and Learning Process is the next component of the Nurse–Client Relationship. The process of teaching and learning means to engage with others to acquire new knowledge, behaviors, and skills. Nurses as Educators use "planned learning experiences based on sound theories that provide individuals, groups and communities the opportunity to acquire the information they need to make quality health decisions" (Wurzbach, 2004, p. 6). Learning is a process by which behavior changes as a result of experiences (Ormrod, 2012). In teaching, the Nurse as Educator chooses teaching strategies and selects instructional materials to assist the client as learner to make behavioral changes that promote, retain, and restore health.

Clients as Learner theories guide teaching practices. They are the foundation of the Teaching and Learning Process. Some learning theories are more applicable than others, depending on the teacher, the client, and the learning context. You will learn about behavioral, cognitive, and social theories of learning as they apply to learners at all ages. Learning theories are important and provide the foundation that guides you as you assume the role of educator. Together the Teaching and Learning Process and the Nursing Process provide a holistic approach to address clients' health education needs.

Clinical Judgment

The third component in the Nurse–Client Relationship is the exercise of sound Clinical Judgment during teaching and learning. Clinical Judgment in nursing is the outcome of clinical reasoning, often referred to as clinical decision making. It is a characteristic way of thinking in the nursing discipline. You exercise Clinical Judgment as you assess clients, develop teaching plans, select teaching strategies and instructional materials, and evaluate the success of your efforts. Your judgments and decisions impact the outcome of health education.

Some nursing educators believe that critical thinking is "the brain's tool for developing the expert nursing judgment needed to improve patient outcomes" (Scheffer & Rubenfeld, 2006, p. 195). Others believe that forming clinical judgments in the delivery of nursing care is distinct from general critical thinking skills (Tanner, 2005). Regardless, it is essential for nurses to exercise sound Clinical Judgment in the Teaching and Learning Process.

The Teaching and Learning and Nursing Processes provide the structural framework through which Clinical Judgment and clinical reasoning occur. Nurses engage in a variety of thinking patterns because no single pattern characterizes all situations. Tanner (2006) proposed a model with four aspects describing how nurses reason in the clinical area that is applicable to health education situations. The first aspect is noticing, whereby the nurse grasps the situation at hand. The second is interpreting, whereby the nurse develops an understanding of the situation. The third is responding, whereby the nurse decides on an appropriate course of action. The fourth is reflecting, whereby the nurse evaluates the effectiveness of the outcomes. These thinking and reasoning patterns occur within each step of the Teaching and Learning Process and Nursing Process to guide the nurse in the formation of Clinical Judgments related to health education.

Clinical Judgment in nursing develops as nurses gain experience and expertise in a practice area and expand their knowledge, moving from being a novice to being an expert. To become an expert in nursing, a beginning nurse passes through five levels of proficiency: novice, advanced beginner, competent, proficient, and expert (Benner, 1984). The novice has no experience in a situation, relies on rules, and is inflexible. The advanced beginner has more experience and has marginally acceptable performance. The competent nurse has 2 to 3 years of experience in similar situations and brings perspective, abstract, and analytic thinking to problem solving. The proficient nurse sees situations as wholes rather than specific aspects and has learned from past experience what to expect in situations and what to do when things do not go as expected. The expert nurse has a deep understanding and intuitive grasp of situations and no longer needs rules or guidelines. This nurse sees the totality of situations and quickly identifies the nature of the problem and how to solve it. These skill levels apply not only to the delivery of nursing care, but also to the delivery of health education.

Evidence-Based Nursing Practice

The last component of the Nurse–Client Relationship is EBNP as it relates to health education. EBNP is the use of current best practices in making decisions about patient care by using a problem-solving approach. This approach incorporates a systematic search for evidence, clinical expertise, and patient preferences and values (Melnyk & Fineout-Overholt, 2004). It is the act of applying current research findings to clinical practice. Applying research to health education is an integral part of the Miller–Stoeckel Client Education Model. It means using the best available and most pertinent research to make health education decisions.

The history of evidence-based research goes back to Dr. Archie Cochrane, an English physician who, in 1972, confronted healthcare professionals about the lack of randomized control studies to support medical practice decisions. Because of his influence, the first electronic database of clinical trials was established in 1988. First called the Oxford Database of Prenatal Trials, it later became The Cochrane Collaboration (Bliss-Holtz, 2007). The Cochrane Collaboration is now an international database that disseminates research worldwide.

The concept of evidence-based practice was embraced by nursing and other healthcare professions in the 1990s. The motivation behind this decision was the realization that many healthcare practices were based on intuition, experience, clinical skills, and guesswork rather than science. EBNP uses a research-based decision-making process to guide the delivery of holistic client-centered nursing care and health education. The specific steps involved in carrying out EBNP include defining the problem and searching for evidence, critically appraising the evidence, applying the findings to practice, taking into account the client–learner's values and preferences, and then evaluating outcomes.

Although EBNP is accepted as a means of promoting best practices, differences of opinion exist among nurses regarding what types of studies constitute the strongest evidence and what weight to give them. The terms *levels of evidence* and *strength of evidence* refer to systems for classifying the evidence in a body of literature through a hierarchy of scientific rigor and quality. Several dozen of these hierarchies exist (Agency for Healthcare Research and Quality, 2002). The reviewers must select the most relevant levels of evidence to meet their needs. The following concise definitions of terms are used in describing the levels of evidence.

- Meta-analysis is a statistical analysis of a collection of quantitative studies.
- Systematic review is a research summary that searches the literature and critically appraises individual quantitative studies to identify valid, applicable evidence.
- Randomized controlled trial is a study in which subjects are randomly assigned to groups; one receives the intervention, the other is a control group.
- Quasi-experimental design is a modification of an experimental design in which there may not be manipulation of the independent variable, random assignment, or control group.

- Observational study is a study in which researchers have no control; instead, they observe what happens to groups of people.
- Case study (case report, single case report) is an uncontrolled observational study involving an intervention and outcome in a single situation.
- Descriptive study is a statistical study to identify patterns or trends in a situation, but not cause and effect.
- Cohort study is a study that involves the selection of a large population of people who have the same condition, who receive a specific intervention, and who are followed over time and compared with a group that is not affected by the condition.
- Case-controlled study is a study that compares two groups of people: those with the condition, and a similar group without the condition. It is also called a retrospective study.
- Expert opinion is a judgment by people who have experience with a particular subject.
- Qualitative study is a study focused on subjective experiences in naturalistic settings rather than under experimental conditions. There are different types of qualitative studies.

A diagram of the hierarchy of research evidence is included in **Figure 1-3**. It illustrates a research hierarchy in which the lowest tier includes the descriptive studies, case studies, case

FIGURE 1-3

Levels of Evidence in Research

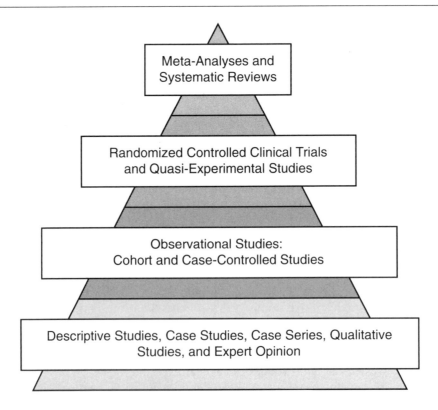

series, qualitative studies, and expert opinion. The highest tier includes meta-analyses and systematic reviews. Research at this tier has a greater chance of being generalized to a group of clients.

Nurses as Educators should rely on substantiated, critically **analyzed** research to ensure that the most current tested health education practices and teaching strategies are provided to clients. Nurses as Educators need a core foundation of health information that reflects quality care and best teaching practices supported by current research. Unfortunately, at this time there is a dearth of research studies that focus on health education. Research is needed on the effectiveness of various teaching strategies and instructional materials for different population groups. The absence of such research affects health education practices. In addition to using the best available evidence, nurses are called on to exercise their best judgment in clinical and health education situations. Clinical Judgment and expertise are very important and should never be minimized in providing health education.

Interrelatedness of Components in the Nurse–Client Relationship

The components in the Nurse–Client Relationship (Nursing Process, Teaching and Learning Process, Clinical Judgment, and EBNP) are interacting and interdependent. The components complement one another. During assessment and analysis the client's learning needs are assessed and analyzed to determine the extent of the client's need for health education. In this step the nurse grasps the client's situation. It may involve looking for applicable literature specific to the client's situation or a group's health education needs.

Planning involves developing individualized care plans drawn from EBNP and setting priorities and learning objectives based on client health education needs. The nurse develops sufficient understanding of the situation and responds by involving the client in designing the teaching plan.

Implementation is carrying out the teaching plan. The nurse takes action and responds based on EBNP where it exists, but it also reflects on client responses. Using judgment, the nurse is prepared to alter the teaching plan if necessary. The nurse uses judgment in selecting teaching strategies and instructional materials to meet the client's health education needs and preferences.

Evaluation reviews the successes and failures in meeting the learning objectives of the teaching plan. Teaching strategies may need to be modified to achieve the objectives. The nurse continually reviews the literature to update the teaching plan using current EBNP where available. The client's achievement of the learning objectives is measured and reinforced to help ensure continued success.

The interrelatedness of the Nursing Process, Teaching and Learning Process, Clinical Judgment, and EBNP components is illustrated in **Table 1-1**.

CLIENT EDUCATION OUTCOMES

Client Education Outcomes are achieved when health-promoting changes in knowledge, attitudes, and skills occur in clients. The last portion of the Miller–Stoeckel Client Education Model focuses on evaluation. To determine if health education efforts are successful, nurses

TABLE 1-1

Interrelatedness of the Nurse–Client Relationship Components

Nursing Process	*Teaching–Learning Process*	*Clinical Judgment*	*EBNP Process*
Assessment and analysis	Determine learning needs	Noticing	Define problem and search literature
Planning	Develop teaching plan	Interpreting	Appraise research findings
Implementation	Use teaching strategies	Responding	Apply to clinical situation
Evaluation	Determine behavior change	Reflecting	Assess the outcomes

must evaluate the results. Evaluation of client education outcomes is measuring the degree to which the learning objectives are met.

Evaluation is important to clients and educators because it informs them about their progress and the effectiveness of the Teaching and Learning Process. The Miller–Stoeckel Client Education Model addresses both Formative Evaluation and Summative Evaluation. Both are essential aspects of evaluation that provide a holistic picture of what was achieved (**Table 1-2**).

Formative Evaluation is ongoing during teaching and learning activities. It is important to know if the learning activities are meeting the learning objectives as teaching is progressing. If weaknesses are identified, they can be changed right away. Formative Evaluation addresses three areas: evaluation of the teaching plan, evaluation of the learning environment, and evaluation of the nurse–client interaction. The involvement of the Client as Learner and Nurse as Educator is essential to the process.

In formative evaluation, evaluation of the teaching plan is done by considering concept comprehension and client motivation. The learning environment is evaluated by assessing the effectiveness of the delivery format and the use of technology. The nurse–client interaction is evaluated by determining the level of client engagement and communication. These components of formative evaluation seek to answer the question, how are we doing?

Summative Evaluation occurs at the conclusion of the Teaching and Learning Process. It is directed toward measuring the degree to which the learning objectives and overall outcomes are met at the conclusion of the learning activity or program. It addresses three areas:

TABLE 1-2

Client Education Outcomes

Formative Evaluation	*Summative Evaluation*
Evaluation of the teaching plan	Evaluation of client learning
Evaluation of the learning environment	Evaluation of educational effectiveness
Evaluation of the nurse–client interaction	Evaluation of learning into daily living

evaluation of client learning, evaluation of educational effectiveness, and evaluation of integration of learning into daily living.

Measurement of learning occurs not only at the conclusion of individual learning activities and programs, but it also involves long-term follow-up of client learning. Results of systematically conducted long-term evaluations are important from an EBNP perspective. Findings from EBNP can serve to guide future health education practices. Summative Evaluation is directed toward outcomes that determine whether clients have learned and if the activities and programs are feasible to continue in the future. Determining feasibility includes examining the effectiveness of learning materials, the costs, the time requirements, the degree of client satisfaction, and the long-term benefits of programs. Basically, Summative Evaluation asks the question, how did we do?

DEFINITIONS

The following definitions support the Miller–Stoeckel Client Education Model and will broaden your understanding of health education. The most important terms to understand are health education, health, illness, Stoeckel Wellness–Illness Functional Continuum, and Health Belief and Health Promotion Models.

Health Education

Health education enhances the quality of life for people worldwide. It is defined broadly by Green and Kreuter (1991) as any combination of learning experiences designed to encourage voluntary actions that are beneficial to health. Health education is achieved through the use of learning theories combined with teaching strategies to help individuals, families, groups and communities, and health team members to promote, retain, and restore health. It not only involves providing relevant health information, but it also helps clients make appropriate health-related behavioral changes. The term *health education* also refers to the process of educating health team members to become more effective in their roles and responsibilities.

Health

Health, as defined by the World Health Organization in 1948, is "a state of complete physical, mental, and social well-being, not merely the absence of disease or infirmity" (2004). Health is a dynamic state in which individuals adapt to changes in the internal and external environments to maintain a state of well-being in all life dimensions. This is the most popular and comprehensive definition of health worldwide, and it is applicable to individuals, families, groups, and communities. Clients bring their own definitions and perceptions of health to clinical situations. Their perceptions of what is and is not normal health influence their willingness to accept health education teaching.

Illness

Illness is a subjective perception of not being well. It is a mismatch between an individual's needs and his or her ability to meet those needs. It signals that the present balance to maintain health is not working. During illness changes may occur in the structure and function of a person's body and mind. Illness has a classifiable set of signs and symptoms resulting from disturbed body functioning. These are associated with characteristic preclinical findings, course, and etiology.

Stoeckel Wellness–Illness Functional Continuum

An individual's level of health is a constantly changing state that moves along a continuum from optimal functioning to a state of total disability. The basic premise of the Stoeckel Wellness–Illness Functional Continuum is that wellness and illness involve a variety of factors: social, physiologic, environmental, emotional, activities of daily living, and health access. The factors in the model can either enhance or distract from the client's health. Disease and illness are a failure of an individual's adaptive mechanisms to adequately counteract changes in functional and structural disturbances. Factors are displayed along a continuum showing incremental increases or decreases in health functioning. Each factor is plotted on the continuum moving from the center (score of 5 is neutral) toward the right (highest score of 10 indicates highest level of wellness) or left (lowest score of 0 indicates lowest level of wellness) and shows changes in the state of health. High-level functioning or wellness involves increased ability to perform the activities of daily living. Low-level functioning is brought on by illness or disability, resulting in the decreased ability to perform activities of daily living.

This continuum is useful when working with clients to get a holistic picture of their functioning. Clients can place themselves on each factor's continuum to identify their strengths and weaknesses. Each person is unique, with different degrees of wellness and illness. Plotting the continuum for each factor helps the Nurse as Educator determine clients' health perceptions and needs. By using the Stoeckel Wellness–Illness Functional Continuum as an assessment tool when working with clients, you gain a more accurate picture of how the client perceives his or her state of health. The continuum can also be used to compare a client's previous level of health with the present level, but because of its subjective nature, it cannot be used to compare one client with another. The continuum illustrates the dynamic, ever changing state of health (**Figure 1-4**).

Health Belief and Health Promotion Models

The Health Belief Model (Rosenstock, 1974) was developed in the 1950s to explain why people did not use preventive health services such as immunizations. The model examines the relationship between a client's beliefs and behaviors, and it helps nurses understand these factors to plan teaching that effectively assists clients in promoting, retaining, and restoring health. An important assumption of this model is that the nurse collaborates with the client to reach mutually agreed-upon goals by understanding the factors that influence health beliefs. The Health Belief Model identifies the following factors that influence health beliefs:

■ Personal expectations regarding health and illness
■ Perception of the seriousness of the illness
■ Likelihood of following prescribed healthcare measures
■ Perceived barriers related to such factors as cost, inconvenience, or pain

A criticism of the Health Belief Model is that it is based on the Western cultural health belief system and does not allow for other influences and for the fact that clients do not always

FIGURE 1-4

Stoeckel Wellness-Illness Functional Continuum

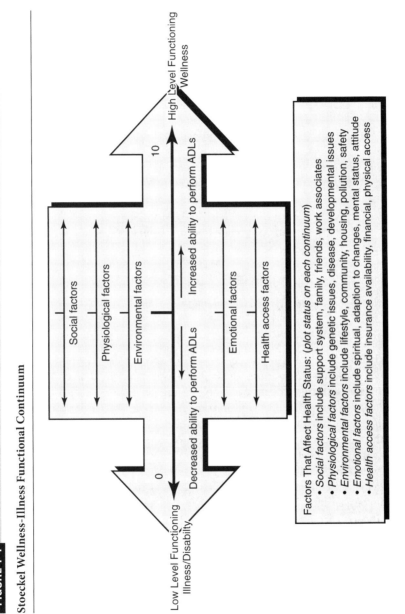

High Level Functioning
Wellness

10

Increased ability to perform ADLs

Social factors

Physiological factors

Environmental factors

Emotional factors

Health access factors

Decreased ability to perform ADLs

0

Low Level Functioning
Illness/Disability

Factors That Affect Health Status: (*plot status on each continuum*)
- *Social factors* include support system, family, friends, work associates
- *Physiological factors* include genetic issues, disease, developmental issues
- *Environmental factors* include lifestyle, community, housing, pollution, safety
- *Emotional factors* include spiritual, adaption to changes, mental status, attitude
- *Health access factors* include insurance availability, financial, physical access

TABLE 1-3

Health Belief Model: Perceptions

Client Perceptions	Nursing Application
Need for care	■ Clarifies client concerns and reasons for seeking treatment ■ Explores client experiences with health issues, past and present ■ Asks about family and cultural factors affecting client perceptions
Seriousness and consequences of condition	■ Clarifies client perceptions of harm that the condition can cause ■ Clarifies client perceptions of consequences without treatment ■ Answers questions and clarifies prognosis; describes experiences with similar problems ■ Explores common and different beliefs and values
Value of health intervention	■ Discusses treatment client is seeking ■ Describes treatment: medical treatment, behavior change (lifestyle), medication (side effects), costs, answers questions, and so forth ■ Clarifies client perceptions of treatment
Effectiveness, cost, and barriers of treatment	■ Prepares goals and timeline for client and nurse responsibilities ■ Sets ground rules and boundaries for nurse–client relationship ■ Outlines knowledge and skills for client and nurse ■ Suggests and provides resources for knowledge and skill development ■ Clarifies client understanding of proposed plan

Source: Adapted from Rankin, Stallings, and London (2005).

act on their belief system. Our approach, shown in **Table 1-3**, uses the basic format of the model, but it includes questions that address the cultural aspects of client teaching. Our approach is a starting point for examining client decision making concerning health education and can be used to develop teaching plans. It is important for the nurse to understand client perceptions about health and the likelihood of adhering to health recommendations. This involves examining beliefs through a cultural lens. Communication is targeted at clarifying the nurse's and the client's perceptions and beliefs. Based on this information, nurses use those strategies that are most effective to meet client health education needs.

Nora Pender's Health Promotion Model (2011) assists nurses in understanding the major determinants of health behaviors as a basis for behavioral counseling to promote healthy lifestyles. Her theory encourages health educators to look at variables that have been shown to impact health behavior. The model uses research findings from nursing, psychology, and public health to understand client health behaviors. This model can be used as a foundation to structure nursing protocols and interventions. This will be further discussed later in the text.

CONTEXT FOR HEALTH EDUCATION

Nurses play a vital role in improving health on a local, national, and global scale. Nurses, in partnership with other healthcare professionals, facilitate delivery of health education in different venues to achieve positive client education outcomes. In this section we address the importance of the wider scope of health education. Nurses should be aware that individual health affects the larger community and eventually affects global health.

National Importance of Health Education

The 1979 surgeon general's report, Healthy People, laid the foundation for a national prevention agenda. Every 10 years since that time, the U.S. Department of Health and Human Services has provided science-based, 10-year national objectives for promoting health and preventing disease. Healthy People 2000 and 2010 established national health objectives that serve as the basis for the development of state and community health initiatives. Currently Healthy People 2020 (U.S. Department of Health and Human Services, 2012) continues the tradition of improving the health of Americans by establishing benchmarks and monitoring progress over time to encourage collaboration across communities and sectors, empowering individuals toward making informed health decisions, and measuring the impact of prevention activities. Healthy People 2020 contains about 1,200 objectives in 42 topic areas designed to serve as this decade's framework for improving the health of all people in the United States (**Box 1-1**). This information is available at http:///www.healthypeople.gov/2020/about/default.aspx on a U.S. government website. Core objectives will remain centered on the prevention of illness and disease as the foundation of health.

Living in an Interactive and Interdependent Global Community

Maintaining health is a global concern. Health issues have global consequences that not only affect the people of developing nations, but also the world community. Healthy, productive citizens are essential for global economic growth and security. Stable populations reduce pressures on global economies and the environment. Stable populations also reduce the number and risk of humanitarian crises. Programs to control the spread of infectious diseases reduce the threat of epidemics. With healthcare services placing ever-greater pressures on state and federal health budgets, the economic burden of disease, and the burden to individuals and families, is a cause of great concern for governments and healthcare systems. Health education not only affects the immediate recipients, but also future generations that will benefit from improved health habits and efforts to prevent illness. Eventually improved health behavior will be ingrained when health education is widely available and an accepted part of health care. The prevention of

---

BOX 1-1

Healthy People 2020 Overarching Goals

- Attain high-quality, longer lives free of preventable disease, disability, injury, and premature death.
- Achieve health equality, eliminate disparities, and improve the health of all groups.
- Create social and physical environments that promote good health for all.
- Promote quality of life, healthy development, and healthy behaviors across all life stages.

illness and the promotion of health through the delivery of efficient and effective health education lie at the core of society's ability to affect health worldwide.

Future Challenges and Trends Facing Nurses as Educators

Future challenges in health care are difficult to predict, but current demographic and societal trends point to the increased need for Nurses as Educators. Demographic trends point to an increasing older population and a greater percentage of minority groups living in the United States that have unique health challenges. Societal trends show changes in social practices, such as cohabitation, acceptance of gay relationships, and more single-parent families. Other trends point to greater access to reliable information using technology, more reliance on alternative medicine, and more questioning of medical advice. Nurses as Educators must be aware of demographic and societal trends. They must adjust to these trends and incorporate the challenges they present into their health education practices.

It is important for nurses to expand their knowledge of health education, their leadership abilities, and their involvement in health policy development. More collaborative networks with other healthcare providers are needed that foster accountability. This collaboration should occur not only on the local level, but also within the global community. Basing health education practices on research, demanding adherence to ethical standards, and promoting social justice are escalating challenges and trends. Doing it more, doing it better, and doing it with less are the future challenges (Breckon, Harvey, & Lancaster, 1998).

SUMMARY

This chapter introduced the topic of health education by introducing the Miller–Stoeckel Client Education Model. The model serves as the conceptual framework around which this text is organized and written. The major components of Nurse as Educator, Client as Learner, Nurse–Client Relationship, and Client Education Outcomes were defined and explained. The role of the Nurse as Educator was clarified, described, and emphasized.

The nature of the Nurse–Client Relationship involves the Nursing Process, Teaching and Learning Process, Clinical Judgment, and EBNP. The model concludes with an examination of Client Education Outcomes to include Formative and Summative Evaluation. Finally the future challenges and trends facing Nurses as Educators were discussed. In this section we examined how health education can impact health, illness, and wellness in the local, national, and global health arenas. In the subsequent chapters of this book, we delve into greater depth about all of the components and aspects of providing health education.

EXERCISES

Exercise I: Philosophy of Health Education

Purpose: Develop a philosophy of health education.
Directions: Working with a small group of colleagues, write your philosophy of health education. This will take time, thought, and discussion. Your philosophy statement should be about two to three pages in length. Include your beliefs about the following:

1. The value of health education as an aspect of comprehensive health care
2. Teaching and what it means
3. Learning and its place in the human experience
4. The role of the Nurse as Educator
5. The role of the Client as Learner
6. The relationship that should exist between the educator and the learner
7. The value of Client Education Outcomes

Exercise II: Ways to Promote Client Education

Purposes:

- Promote creative thinking.
- Raise consciousness regarding client education.

Directions: Form small groups and discuss the following situation. Take notes and prepare a report to be shared with the rest of your peers.

While carrying heavy patient care assignments and responsibilities, some nurses are managing to teach their clients in mutually satisfactory ways. What client teaching have you observed by your clinical instructors, supervisors, primary nurses, or other nursing personnel? What are you doing to promote client teaching? If you are not yet in the clinical area, seek out nurses in your school, hospital, or neighborhood and ask them what they are doing to promote health teaching. Draw on your experiences as a patient, client, relative, or observer. Upon reflection, summarize the nurses' role in client education.

REFERENCES

Agency for Healthcare Research and Quality. (2002). Systems to rate the strength of scientific evidence. Summary, evidence report/technology assessment (No. 47, AHRQ Publication No. 02-E015). Rockville, MD: Author. Retrieved from http://www.thecre.com/pdf/ahrq-system-strength.pdf http://www.ahrq.gov/clinic/epcsums/strengthsum.htm

American Hospital Association. (1992). A patient's bill of rights. Retrieved from https://www.google.com/#q=american+hospital+association+patient+bill+of+rights+2011 http://www.patienttalk.info/AHA-Patient_Bill_of_Rights.htm

American Nurses Association. (1998). *Standards of clinical nursing practice* (2nd ed.). Washington, DC: Author.

Bastable, S. B., & Alt, M. F. (2014). Overview of education in health care. In S. B. Bastable (Ed.), *Nurse as educator: Principles of teaching and learning for nursing practice* (4th ed., pp. 3–30). Burlington, MA: Jones & Bartlett Learning.

Benner, P. (1984). *From novice to expert.* Menlo Park, CA: Addison-Wesley.

Bliss-Holtz, J. (2007). Evidence-based practice: A primer for action. *Issues in Comprehensive Pediatric Nursing, 30*(4), 165–182.

Breckon, D., Harvey, J., & Lancaster, R. (1998). *Community health education: Settings, roles, and skills for the 21st century.* Sudbury, MA: Jones and Bartlett.

Chitty, K. K., & Black, B. P. (2007). *Professional nursing: Concepts and challenges* (5th ed.). St. Louis, MO: Elsevier.

Davidhizar, R., & Cramer, C. (2002). "The best thing about the hospitalization was that the nurses kept me well informed": Issues and strategies of client education. *Accident and Emergency Nursing, 10,* 149–154.

Donner, C. L., Levonian, C., & Slutsky, P. (2005). Move to the head of the class: Developing staff nurses as teachers. *Journal for Nurses in Staff Development, 21*(6), 277–283.

Green, L. W., & Kreuter, M. (1991). *Health promotion planning: An educational and environmental approach.* Mountain View, CA: Mayfield.

Hall, A. (2001). Client education. In P. Potter & A. Perry (Eds.), *Fundamentals of nursing* (7th ed., pp. 328–347). St. Louis, MO: Mosby.

Healthy People 2020. (2009). US Department of Health, Education and Welfare, Public Health Service. Washington, DC: U.S. Government. Retrieved from http://www.healthypeople.gov/2020/default.aspx.htm

McFarland, G. K., & McFarland, E. A. (1997). *Nursing diagnoses and intervention, planning for patient care* (3rd ed.). St. Louis, MO: Mosby.

Melnyk, B. M., & Fineout-Overholt, E. (2004). *Evidence-based practice in nursing and healthcare: A guide to best practice.* Philadelphia, PA: Lippincott Williams & Wilkins.

National League of Nursing Education. (1918). *Standard curriculum for schools of nursing.* Baltimore, MD: Waverly Press.

National League of Nursing Education. (1937). *A curriculum guide for schools of nursing.* New York, NY: Author.

Ormrod, J. E. (2012). *Human learning* (6th ed.). Boston, MA: Pearson.

Pender, N. (2011). The health promotion manual. Retrieved from http://research2vrpractice.org/wp-content/uploads/2013/02/HEALTH_PROMOTION_MANUAL_Rev_5-2011.pdf

Peplau, H. E. (1952). *Interpersonal relations in nursing.* New York, NY: G. P. Putnam's Sons.

Potter, P., & Perry, A. (2009). *Fundamentals of nursing* (7th ed.). St. Louis, MO: Mosby.

Rankin, S. H., Stallings, K. D., & London, F. (2005). *Patient education in health and illness* (5th ed.). Philadelphia, PA: Lippincott Williams & Wilkins.

Redman, B. (2006). *The practice of patient education: A case study approach* (10th ed.). St. Louis, MO: Mosby Elsevier.

Rosenstock, I. (1974). Historical origins of the health belief model. *Health Education Monographs, 2*(4), 336–353.

Scheffer, B. K., & Rubenfeld, M. G. (2006). Critical thinking: A tool in search of a job. *Journal of Nursing Education, 45*(6), 195–196.

Tanner, C. (2005). What have we learned about critical thinking in nursing? *Journal of Nursing Education, 44*(2), 47–48.

Tanner, C. (2006). Thinking like a nurse: A research-based model of clinical judgment in nursing. *Journal of Nursing Education, 45*(6), 204–211.

The Joint Commission. (2009). Retrieved from http://www.jointcommission.org/assets/1/6/2009_CLASRelatedStandardsCAH.pdf

U.S. Department of Health and Human Services. (2012). *Healthy People 2020.* Washington, DC: Author. Retrieved from http://www.healthypeople.gov/2020/default.aspx

Webster's All-In-One Dictionary and Thesaurus (2nd ed.). (2013). Springfield, MA: Federal Street Press.

World Health Organization. (2004). About the World Health Organization. Retrieved from http://www.who.int/suggestions/faq/en/index.html

WHO (1948). Preamble to the Constitution of the World Health Organization as adopted by the International Health Conference, New York, 19-22 June 1946; signed on 22 July 1946 by the representatives of 61 States (Official Records of the World Health Organization, no. 2, p. 100) and entered into force on 7 April 1948.

Wurzbach, M. E. (2004). *Community health education and promotion: A guide to program design and evaluation* (2nd ed.). Sudbury, MA: Jones and Bartlett.

II

The Learning Process

2

Thinking and Learning

OBJECTIVES

Upon completion of this chapter, you will be able to do the following:

- Apply the concepts of thinking and learning to the Miller–Stoeckel Client Education Model.
- Analyze definitions of thinking and learning and formulate your own definition.
- Differentiate among cognitive, affective, and psychomotor domains of learning by giving an example of each.
- Give examples of how you have engaged in the following types of thinking in the context of health education: problem solving, nursing process, critical thinking, clinical judgment, creative thinking, intuition, reflection, fantasy, and reverie.
- Identify at least two ways to help clients as learners (individuals, families, groups and communities, and health team members) develop their thinking abilities.
- Describe the following styles and models of thinking and learning: Sternberg's thinking styles, Witkin and Goodenough's Cognitive-Style Dimensions, Kolb's Experiential Learning Model: Learning Cycle and Styles, and Gardner's Multiple Intelligences.
- Describe how to apply the thinking and learning styles to client education.

KEY TERMS

affective domain	fantasy	psychomotor domain
clinical judgment	intuition	reflection
cognitive domain	learning styles	reverie
creative thinking	nursing process	thinking
critical thinking	problem solving	thinking styles

INTRODUCTION

Thinking and learning form the basis for the teaching and learning process, which is part of the nurse–client relationship in the Miller–Stoeckel Client Education Model. This chapter makes the connection between thinking and learning and how they impact your approach to teaching clients. Thinking and learning are purposeful activities with the goal of bringing about a necessary change. The teaching and learning process encourages clients to engage in activities that are necessary to acquire new knowledge and new skills, and to incorporate new attitudes. Clients as learners do this by modifying and reorganizing knowledge that is already in place or by acquiring new knowledge. Clients as learners need specific, new information or assistance in learning how to use known information to their best advantage. The nurse also needs to engage in self-assessment of their individual thinking and learning styles (**Figure 2-1**).

This chapter introduces the broad domains of learning: cognitive, psychomotor, and affective. Next we examine thinking and the many ways thinking is categorized, including problem solving, nursing process, critical thinking, clinical judgment, creative thinking, intuition, and reflection. The chapter concludes by examining how thinking translates into various styles of learning and the implications this has for health education.

DOMAINS OF LEARNING

Clients learn as total beings, with all their senses. When they learn, they have thoughts about learning and they experience feelings about what they are doing, **thinking**, and learning. The doing, thinking, and feeling aspects of learning are clearly related, but they are not the same. When nurses help clients learn something, they select one or more domains in which clients need to focus most of their energy. The three domains that have received the most attention in educational literature are the cognitive, affective, and **psychomotor domains** (Bloom, Engelhart, Furst, Hill, & Krathwohl, 1956).

FIGURE 2-1

Nurse–Client Relationship in the Miller–Stoeckel Client Education Model

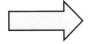
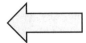

- Nursing process
- Teaching/learning process
- Clinical judgment
- Evidence-based nursing practice

Nurse as Educator

Healthcare Institutions
Public Health
Health Education Programs

Client as Learner

Individuals
Families
Groups/Communities
Health Team Members

FIGURE 2-2

The Interacting Domains of Learning: Cognitive (Think), Affective (Feel), and Psychomotor (Do) Maximize Learning

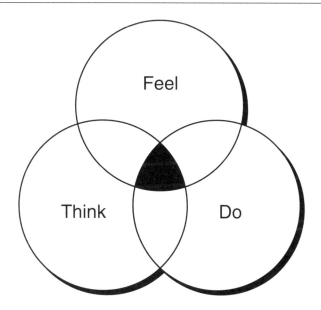

The learning domains have been separated for research and study purposes, but that separation is arbitrary. Human behavior includes components of each domain (Kretchmar, 2008). When you are providing health education to clients, the domains provide an organizational framework that is useful as you contemplate what clients need to learn and what should be taught. **Figure 2-2** illustrates the interactive, interdependent relationship among the three domains. The most effective learning occurs when all three domains are engaged in the learning process, as illustrated by the center triangle (Goulet & Owen-Smith, 2005).

Cognitive Domain

Cognitive learning is concerned with intellectual activities such as thinking, remembering, reasoning, and using language (Webster's, 2013). It involves judging, considering, believing, reflecting, and recalling. It also means using the mind to exercise judgment, draw inferences, arrive at conclusions, and make decisions (Miller & Babcock, 1996). The **cognitive domain** was the first domain developed by Bloom and colleagues in 1956. It has received the most attention in educational circles and enjoys the widest application to learning, in part because of the emphasis of Western cultures on reason over emotions (Kretchmar, 2008). Cognitive learning objectives are concrete and reflect this emphasis on reason. They are relatively easy to conceptualize, write, and measure.

Affective Domain

The **affective domain** deals with personal issues: attitudes, beliefs, behaviors, and emotions (Krathwohl, Bloom, & Masia, 1964). In the past educators believed that the affective domain was an area of learning that was too complex and fraught with conflicts. Research in this area, however, is changing that perception, and educators are realizing the importance of integrating the affective domain into their teaching. Because the affective domain deals with personal issues such as attitudes, beliefs, behaviors, and emotions, it is increasingly integral to the provision of a comprehensive program of health education. Educational research indicates that there is a relationship between emotional intelligence and general intelligence in academic achievement. This research has implications for health education. Learning objectives in the affective domain focus on influencing attitudes, motivating learners, developing respect, and clarifying values.

Attitudes are acquired by associating with others and participating in satisfying experiences. Clients are influenced by nurses' attitudes. Role modeling, for example, occurs when nurses work with clients. Nurses are constantly observed by clients, who are influenced by their behavior. Characteristics of kindness, fairness, compassion, honesty, punctuality, dependability, and competence are evident to clients as they observe nurses working. These characteristics help clients determine their perception of the quality of care they receive. Some examples of the way that nurses display their values are by treating clients with respect, such as providing privacy, adapting nursing interventions to their expressed concerns, and giving them undivided attention. It is important to include learning objectives in the affective domain as you provide health education for clients. Affective learning can also be facilitated by persuasion from other trusted authorities, such as parents, teachers, scientists, spiritual leaders, and valued colleagues with special expertise. Participating in group discussions and role playing also helps promote affective learning.

Psychomotor Domain

Psychomotor learning encompasses many physical procedures that individuals use in their activities of daily living and the complex physical activities required for work and recreation. It also includes learning physical skills and procedures applicable to healthcare delivery. Psychomotor learning requires that individuals acquire information and store it in memory. During the initial practice of a procedure, skills are shaped and learned until they become automatic (Marzano & Kendall, 2007). This type of learning is the most concrete, and it is the easiest to teach, observe, and measure. Clients form a mental image of how a skill is performed and then translate that image into external behavior. An example of psychomotor learning is performing an insulin injection. This type of learning is usually done best in a step-by-step fashion, from the simple to the complex. Nurses show clients how to perform the skill; then they guide them through return demonstrations. Nurses correct errors and reinforce correct responses. Practice is encouraged until both clients and nurses are satisfied with the clients' skills.

THINKING

Thinking is categorized in different ways. In this section we look at definitions of thinking and types of thinking engaged in by clients and nurses: problem solving, **critical thinking**, creative thinking, **intuition, reflection,** and other types of thinking. The **nursing process** and **clinical judgment** contribute to the nurse–client relationship. Each type of thinking has a distinct focus because they overlap, are complex, and cannot be confined to distinct categories. They are described separately for purposes of this discussion to highlight the particular focus of each type of thinking.

Definitions of Thinking

To think is an activity of the mind that is essential to living. It involves a myriad of processes such as observing, recalling, remembering, reasoning, drawing inferences, reflecting, and deciding. It also encompasses beliefs, opinions, and judgments. Thinking has a subjective quality in that all past experiences influence how we see the world. It includes our personal knowledge, our interpersonal relationships, and our role as nurses (Miller & Babcock, 1996).

Ruggiero defined thinking as "any mental activity that helps formulate or solve a problem, make a decision, or fulfill a desire to understand. It is a searching for answers, a reaching for meaning" (2012, p. 4). It also involves such mental activities as wondering, imagining, inquiring, interpreting, evaluating, and judging. Thinking can be concrete, referring to physical materials or objects (What instructional materials do I need to teach this information?), or abstract, referring to a quality of something (What value do instructional materials have in learning?). Thoughts can be about the past (What worked best yesterday in teaching Ms. Jones about diabetes?), the present (How shall I best present this material on smoking cessation?), or the future (How shall I use client feedback to improve my teaching?).

Thinking is complex, multifaceted, dynamic, and involves the creation of images (Halpern, 2003). For example, when you wonder if the intravenous solution is about to run out, you picture what the fluid level in the bottle looked like the last time you were in the room and you think about the amount of time that has passed. In this sense, thinking is imagery accompanied by silent, internal speech.

Thinking is described as directed or nondirected (Halpern, 2003). Directed thinking is a conscious mental focus on a problem or issue with a desired outcome. It is purposeful and goal directed. Directed thinking has an evaluation component that considers the effectiveness of thinking outcomes; that is, if the decisions were effective. For example, you might ask yourself, Did I make a good decision in this situation? In contrast, nondirected thinking occurs as a result of routine habits, such as getting up in the morning, going to work or school, and so forth. Many aspects of life involve nondirected thinking.

TYPES OF THINKING

Problem Solving

The most common type of thinking is problem solving. **Problem solving** is a process of developing, testing, and evaluating a method for overcoming an obstacle by identifying a problem and finding the best alternative to solve it. Problem solving consists of these steps: identifying the problem, analyzing aspects of the problem, collecting pertinent information, hypothesizing about its cause or causes, generating possible solutions, trying out one of the hypotheses, and evaluating the results.

In the process of problem solving, individuals use critical thinking skills to understand and solve a problem. Sometimes a situation requires considerable thought and contemplation (Should I attend school full or part time?), and at other times it is relatively simple (What shall I do this weekend?). Problem solving is conscious, focused thinking over which individuals exert control.

Problem solving requires being open to new ways of thinking, reflection, and clinical judgment. Nurses use problem solving most effectively in working with clients, assisting them to think through their health problems, and finding workable, realistic, and appropriate solutions.

Critical Thinking

Critical thinking is a specific type of thinking that emphasizes rational cognitive processes and certain attitudes and values. The word *critical* often connotes negativity, whereas the intended meaning of the word is *analytic*. Ideas about critical thinking that are applicable to all disciplines come from educators in the fields of philosophy and education (Brookfield, 2012; Browne & Keeley, 2012; McPeck, 1990; Paul, 1995; Ruggiero, 2012; Watson & Glaser, 1980). Common themes in definitions of critical thinking include conscious awareness of one's thinking processes, including acquiring knowledge and understanding. It involves examining assumptions and validating inferences, examining evidence, and searching for meaning and solutions through rational thinking processes. Attitudes and values include intellectual honesty, flexibility, and willingness to listen to other points of view. To be a critical thinker is to be analytic, reflect constructively, and evaluate fairly.

Nursing recognizes the importance of critical thinking in preparing practitioners (Kaddoura, 2013; Whiffin & Hasselder, 2013) and accepts critical thinking as an essential component of nursing education programs (Chan, 2013). However, the nursing profession continues to lack a widely accepted definition of critical thinking (Chan, 2013; Kaddoura, 2013; Victor-Chmil, 2013). Nurse educators accept rational, logical thinking as central features of critical thinking and recognize that critical thinking is different from clinical reasoning and clinical judgment. We agree with Victor-Chmil that these are distinct but interrelated concepts.

The most widely accepted definition of critical thinking comes from the research of Scheffer and Rubenfeld (2000). They conducted a study to define critical thinking in nursing with input from an international panel of nurse experts on critical thinking. They identified both cognitive and affective dimensions of critical thinking in nursing. Their consensus definition is as follows:

> Critical thinking in nursing is an essential component of professional accountability and quality nursing care. Critical thinkers in nursing exhibit these habits of the mind: confidence, contextual perspective, creativity, flexibility, inquisitiveness, intellectual integrity, intuition, open-mindedness, perseverance, and reflection. Critical thinkers in nursing practice the cognitive skills of analyzing, applying standards, discriminating, information seeking, logical reasoning, predicting and transforming knowledge. (p. 357)

Because of the research supporting this definition, we believe it best represents the meaning of critical thinking in nursing.

Creative Thinking

To create is to bring into being—to cause to exist (Webster's, 2013). It is the ability to go beyond current knowledge and think in a new way. **Creative thinking** has both a creative and a judgmental phase (Ruggiero, 2012). Individuals have creative thoughts and ideas and then proceed to judge them as they look for solutions to problems and answers to questions. This thinking moves back and forth between creating ideas and then judging them, the former being creative thinking and the latter being critical thinking. According to Halpern (2003), creative thinking has two aspects: novelty and quality, or appropriate and useful. Thus creative thinking and critical thinking are intertwined.

Creative thinkers are curious, adventurous, resourceful, undaunted by the prospect of failure, and independent in the sense that they are willing to speak freely and do not need a lot of approval from others (Ruggiero, 2012). Creative thinkers tolerate ambiguity and uncertainty, adjust easily to new and changing situations, and freely abandon old assumptions when confronted with new evidence. Creative thinkers are willing to be different, to think outside the box. In problem solving, creative thinkers propose multiple options to consider that are appropriate to the context rather than immediately focusing on one option.

Santrock (2014) described the creative process as a five-step sequence, the first of which is preparation. In this step, a problem or issue arouses interest and curiosity. The next step is incubation, whereby individuals think about the problem and mull over ideas. The third step is insight, that moment when the pieces of the puzzle seem to fit together. The fourth step is evaluation, when individuals bring their judgment to bear on a tentative solution to determine if it is workable and realistic. The final step is elaboration, the most difficult step requiring the most time. These steps move back and forth and do not follow a linear, sequential path. For example, insight and incubation can occur throughout each step, and evaluation is ongoing.

Intuition

Intuition is quick and ready insight, knowing things without conscious reasoning (Webster's, 2013). It is information that is not acquired by rational, analytic processes; rather, it occurs outside of conscious thought. Its source is from within the person and is based on life experiences and accumulated knowledge. It is the aha experience that occurs with sudden insight. For example, nurses sense something important about a client, often described as a gut feeling or a flash of insight, but they are unable to verbalize it or they verbalize it with difficulty. However, based on that insight, nurses adjust their teaching and care to be more suitable for the client.

Intuition was once thought to be characteristic of only expert nurses (Benner, 1984). However, intuition is now known to be used by nurses at all levels of expertise, including the novice (Ruth-Sahd & Hendy, 2005). The primary difference between novice and expert nurses is their knowledge, expertise, and years of experience. Those with greater knowledge, expertise, and experience bring more to assessment, intervention, and evaluation when working with clients (Faugier, 2005). Thus, intuition has somatic, affective, and cognitive components, but further research is needed to understand how these components are integrated (Hodgkinson, Langan-Fox, & Sadler-Smith, 2008). Your intuitive knowledge is important to take into consideration when making health education decisions. However, you should validate your intuitions through evidence-based research, because many psychologists have found that spontaneous, intuitive approaches to solving problems are frequently wrong (Halpern, 2003).

Reflection

Reflection results from meditation (Webster's, 2013) and is an important aspect of thinking. The word *reflective* comes from the Latin word *reflectere*, meaning bending back, casting back, introspecting, and deliberating. Reflection helps to clarify thoughts and values and how they affect problem solving and decision making. It is important to reflect on health education activities and consider what is and is not effective. If nurses fail to reflect, it reduces the self-correction that comes with evaluating teaching effectiveness.

Reflective skepticism is an important aspect of critical thinking. Reflective skepticism requires thinking about the universal truth of statements rather than immediately accepting or rejecting them. Rather than accepting or rejecting statements at face value, reflective critical thinkers ask questions, analyze responses, reflect, and evaluate the merits of statements. This process is not cynical or dismissive of new ideas; rather, it is a process of analyzing and determining what to believe. Reflective skepticism requires reflecting on beliefs, assumptions, and intuitive responses to clarify thinking (Browne & Keeley, 2012).

Reflection is described as an important parameter of clinical judgment (Tanner, 2006). Saylor (1990) describes reflective thinking as essential for self-evaluation and improving clinical performance. Reflection is viewed overall as a form of systematic inquiry that is used as a means to improve practice or as a way to make sense of learning, evaluation, and promotion of learning. Reflection may be a solitary process or involve collective reflection with colleagues, teachers, or interaction with theoretical literature.

Three different aspects of reflective practice are reflection before action, reflection in action, and reflection on action. Reflection before action is anticipatory reflection involving the careful consideration of what to do and why to do it before engaging in action. The nurse develops a rationale for actions, organizes and prioritizes a vision for future action, and examines core beliefs and values. Reflection before action gives the nurse an opportunity to deliberate about possible alternatives, decide on a course of action, develop plans, and anticipate what the experience will be like for the nurse and the client.

Reflection in action refers to reflective thinking as one is doing the action. Reflection in action in health education refers to the nurse's thinking about the teaching and learning process while directly engaged in teaching. Reflection is usually stimulated by a problem that the nurse is facing. The process of analysis includes asking questions, such as how the problem was perceived, what action was taken, and why this course of action was chosen. The nurse evaluates how the client is responding in the situation and then takes the opportunity to adjust the interventions based on that assessment. During reflection in action the problem is restructured and approached differently. This enables the nurse to reshape what he or she is doing while doing it.

Reflection on action occurs after the experience has taken place. The nurse looks back on experiences to analyze learning that occurred in light of the client outcomes. It means recalling the client's response and the evidence of client learning. It means assessing the client's satisfaction with the interaction. The act of reflecting on action enables the nurse to spend time exploring why he or she personally acted in a certain way and what was happening. In so doing, the nurse engages in self-questioning and considers ideas about how activities and practices could be done differently. Reflection on action may involve colleagues who observe, engage in critical conversations, and help the nurse become aware of aspects of practice he or she has not thought about. **Table 2-1** summarizes reflective practice questions.

TABLE 2-1

Reflective Practice Questions

Reflection-Before-Action	Reflection-in-Action	Reflection-on-Action
		Analysis of Past Actions and Rationale
Anticipatory Reflection	*Evaluation in Action and Revision*	
What do I want?	What is effective, and what needs to be different?	Why did I act as I did?
What outcome do I want?	What is the client's response?	What was the client outcome?
What is my plan?	What other options are available?	What actions did I take?
What is my rationale?	What is the plan revision?	Why did I respond as I did?

Other Ways of Thinking

Other ways of thinking include fantasy and reverie. **Fantasy** is the free play of creative imagination in the realm of the wild, visionary, or fancy (Webster's, 2013). It is a mental image, a capricious or whimsical idea or notion, a dramatic fiction characterized by highly fanciful or supernatural elements. Fantasy is useful in mentally working through difficult situations. For example, suppose you want to devote more time to teaching clients and anticipate that your supervisor will resist this idea. Fantasizing the supervisor's arguments helps you prepare to counter them.

Reverie, a synonym for daydream, is similar to fantasy and means dreamy thinking, imagining, or fanciful musing (Webster's, 2013). In general, reverie has a more meandering, less vivid quality to it than fantasy. An example of reverie occurs when a lecture is boring and learners' minds wander to something more engaging, like what they did last night or what they will do tonight. Fantasy, however, is more directed; for example, helping a client in labor to relax during contractions by focusing her mind on warm, soothing waves of water rushing over her body.

REFLECTING ON YOUR THINKING

Nurses are encouraged to become aware of their thinking processes. Thinking about thinking is called metacognition (Ruggiero, 2012). Nurses enhance their effectiveness when they reflect on the results of their thinking and decisions. For example, was a decision effective? Was there sufficient information on which to base good decisions? Were the inferences accurate? What were the underlying assumptions, and how did they affect problem solving? What influence did beliefs and values have on how the problem was framed and approached? Were the generalizations justified? When nurses internalize critical thinking skills, they are more effective in helping clients think more clearly.

How nurses think and go about their professional responsibilities are important insights. Although thinking per se is difficult to define, nurses will become skilled thinkers and increase their efficiency if they monitor their thought patterns. It is important to develop clear, analytic thinking habits. As nurses verbalize and critique their thoughts and practice clear thinking, they will develop confidence in their critical thinking skills (Miller & Babcock, 1996).

PROMOTING THINKING IN CLIENTS

The Miller–Stoeckel Client Education Model promotes thinking as an integral component of the teaching and learning process in the nurse–client relationship. Before nurses can promote critical thinking in clients, they need to be good listeners. Nurses in the educator role should listen to what clients say they want to learn. Frequently clients know what they need to learn and will verbalize it if they think the nurse is interested. Listen to how clients view their illness, what they think caused their health problem, and what home remedies they have taken to treat it. This will give you multiple clues for situation-appropriate health education. If the clients are team members, listen to what they already know and want to learn, then make teaching plans accordingly.

Just as important as listening is respecting clients and colleagues. Showing respect is fundamental for promoting critical thinking skills. Seeing life from the perspective of the other person creates a safe environment for that person to experiment with new thoughts and behaviors. As nurses go about their responsibilities, they serve as role models for critical thinking.

When assisting others in their thinking processes, nurses should note the client's frame of mind and readiness to entertain additional information and develop new insights. Remember that as an educator, nurses cannot completely change a client's thinking framework. Nurses can, however, promote small, incremental growth and expand clients' perceptions of their circumstances and options, and they can facilitate problem solving.

When clients share insightful information or engage in critical thinking, nurses should reinforce that behavior. Praise clients for their thinking processes and the decisions they make, when appropriate. Reinforce clients even when they question your procedure or teaching. Responses such as "I am glad you asked," "Let me think, that is a complex question," and "That is a good point" are ways to reinforce thinking.

When conversing with clients, it may be helpful to mirror their attitudes, rationalizations, and habitual ways of thinking and behaving. As you reflect your observations back to them, monitor their responses. Ask yourself how your comments are being received. Are your comments annoying clients? If you encounter resistance, stop your intervention and assess what is happening.

Nurses should ask questions as they teach. As clients answer, it tells you if your comments are understood. It also provides opportunities to stimulate thinking. For example, ask "If that is so, then how do you feel about …?" or "Will you explain …?" Another fruitful line of questioning that helps clients anticipate consequences is "What will you do if …?"

When teaching stress management, pain control, weight reduction, blood pressure control, and management of other stress-related diseases, make good use of the imaginative forms of thinking, fantasy, and reverie. Nurses who specialize in counseling and psychotherapy make use of these strategies. A nurse used fantasy to help a client who was under stress to relax.

The client found the sounds of surf soothing, so the nurse used this image and said, "Picture the waves of the ocean rolling over you. Flow with the waves. Listen to the surf. Smell the salty air. Feel the warm mist on your skin."

Role playing is based on recall and fantasy. It is an excellent diagnostic tool for discovering the client's way of thinking and approaching interpersonal problems. Role playing is also helpful to the client who is learning to be more assertive. When used by the nurse psychotherapist, role playing may take on more intensity, such as that encountered in gestalt exercises, sociodrama, and psychodrama.

The Socratic method uses creative questioning to enhance critical thinking skills. In Socratic teaching the focus is on asking questions, not giving answers. Nurses model what it means to have an inquiring mind by continually exploring a subject by asking questions. Socrates described a true teacher as one who is the midwife to another person's discovery of truth. Socratic learning is joining in discussions with others, asking questions, thinking and reasoning clearly, and discovering answers (Paul, 1995). Questions elicit new ideas and make connections with previous knowledge and experiences. Questions expose the truth and bring unconscious beliefs to the surface of self-awareness.

STYLES OF THINKING AND LEARNING

Learning styles refer to how individuals prefer to process information and learn. Styles develop from life experiences in the family, at school, and at work and result in preferred ways to learn. Consider how you learn best. Is it by reading a book, creating a mental image, watching a video, or hearing an explanation? Is it by working alone on a project or with a study group? Is it in a quiet environment or with music in the background?

While learning styles have been popular guides for teachers in education circles for many years, some question the validity of the research designs supporting the various learning styles. They point out that the concept of learning styles was embraced before sufficient research was conducted. Regardless, knowing about and attending to clients' learning preferences (styles) will enhance the effectiveness of your teaching.

In this section we examine several ways that thinking and learning styles are conceptualized. Styles are unique to each person and should be taken into consideration when providing health education. Keep in mind that one style is not better than another; styles are simply characteristics that individuals bring to the situation. Also keep in mind that individuals may change their style preference depending on the demands of the learning situation. They are not confined to only one style. The nature of the material will also lend itself to a particular learning style. For example, teaching self-injection of insulin is best taught with a syringe, sponge, and vial rather than through lecture alone. It will also be affected by the learner's past experiences, cultural background, and physical abilities.

Sternberg's Thinking Styles

Robert J. Sternberg (1997) distinguished between thinking ability and thinking style. Style refers to how an individual uses the abilities he or she possesses. Sternberg draws an analogy between how individuals think, which he called mental self-government, and civil government.

He uses the descriptive terms of the latter to describe his model of thinking styles. For example, legislative individuals are creative and prefer to decide for themselves what they will do and how they will do it. They like problems that are not already structured and prefer to create the framework themselves. They prefer to solve problems, apply rules to problems, apply lessons based on other people's work, and enforce rules. They tend to be nonconforming individuals.

Executive individuals like problems that have some structure so they can address problems within that structural framework. They like guidelines and prefer to follow directions. These individuals are usually successful as students and employees because they do as they are told and like being evaluated on that basis.

Judicial individuals like to oversee, analyze, and evaluate existing rules, procedures, and ideas. They like to critique, give opinions, and judge people and their work. These individuals prefer positions in which they can evaluate the effectiveness of programs, tasks, and human endeavors.

Sternberg distinguishes between global versus local individuals. Global thinkers see the forest rather than the trees; that is, they prefer to deal with relatively large and abstract issues, whereas local thinkers are more pragmatic, preferring to focus on details. Sternberg also distinguishes between the thinking of internal individuals—who tend to be introverted, task oriented, and prefer to work alone—and external individuals—who tend to be extroverted, outgoing, and people oriented. Individuals have a profile of thinking styles and may use more than one.

Witkin and Goodenough's Cognitive-Style Dimensions

Field preference is another way to conceptualize how individuals learn and process information. Developed by Herman Witkin and Donald Goodenough, it is a bipolar continuum with traits of field dependence and independence at opposite ends. Field refers to how individuals perceive their surroundings. It is important to view field dependence and independence as relative dimensions, not fixed ones. Although individuals favor a particular cognitive style, no one is exclusively one way or the other. The cognitive style dimensions are value neutral; each has qualities that are adaptive in particular circumstances (Witkin & Goodenough, 1981). Knowledge of these dimensions is useful for nurses as educators in planning health education activities.

Field dependent and independent individuals have different perceptual and intellectual qualities (Cassidy, 2004; Claxton & Murrell, 1987; Garity, 1985; Noble, Miller, & Heckman, 2008; Witkin & Goodenough, 1981). Individuals who are relatively field dependent rely on an external frame of reference rather than imposing their own. They see the whole situation and its context rather than focusing on the smaller aspects. They are sensitive to their surroundings and open to external sources of information. They show more social behaviors, which contribute to effective interpersonal relationships. They pay attention to social cues in the environment by looking at others' faces and listening to verbal messages to sense what others are thinking and feeling.

In a learning situation, field dependent learners prefer the spectator role and are influenced by authority figures. They like structure, guidance, and clearly defined learning goals provided by the educator. They are motivated by extrinsic rewards rather than intrinsic ones. They enjoy interaction with other learners and prefer to cooperate and collaborate. They are sensitive to

TABLE 2-2

Field Preference Characteristics

Field-Dependent Individuals	*Field-Independent Individuals*
External frame of reference	Internal frame of reference
See the whole situation	See both whole and parts of a situation
Sensitive to surroundings	Less sensitive to surroundings
Open to external sources of information	Strong sense of autonomy
Social and people oriented	Impersonal orientation to others
Attend to social cues	Less sensitive to social environment
Prefer the spectator role	Prefers active learner role; self-reliant
Influenced by authority figures	Analytic, tests opinions and ideas
Prefer structure and guidance	Enjoys abstract and theoretical concepts
Prefer clear learning objectives	Sets own learning goals
Motivated by extrinsic rewards	Structures own learning
Prefer group work and discussions	Intrinsically motivated
Sensitive to criticism	Less sensitive to criticism

criticism; when they talk they refer more to others and less to themselves. They are holistic in their approach to problem solving but are often unable to see the smaller components of larger problems, thereby making them less efficient.

Individuals who are relatively field independent are more autonomous and have a strong sense of self and differentiation from others. By having an internal frame of reference, they grasp the whole situation and its component parts. They are self-reliant, intrinsically motivated, and have their own learning goals. They are less sensitive to the social environment and less inclined to conform to group pressure.

In a learning situation, field-independent learners prefer to structure their own learning and study strategies. They are analytic, interested in abstract and theoretical concepts, and question opinions, ideas, and hypotheses. In learning situations they are able impose their own structure. They are less affected by criticism and make more I statements. They tend to be better at problem solving. **Table 2-2** summarizes these characteristics.

Kolb's Experiential Learning Model: Learning Cycle and Styles

Many educators believe that education, work, and personal development are closely linked in a process of learning called experiential learning. They believe that learning is an ongoing, continuous process that occurs as individuals adapt to their social and physical environment. The emphasis of experiential learning is on the learning process itself, rather than on the behavioral outcomes; it is grounded in experiences as the individual adapts to the world (Kolb, 1984).

FIGURE 2-3

The Experiential Learning Model

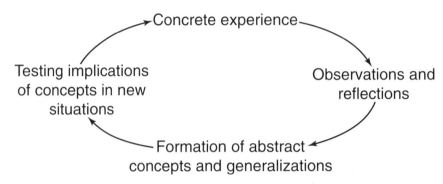

Source: Data from Friere, P. Pedagogy of the oppressed. New York: Continuum, 1970. Kolb, D. Experiential learning: Experience as the source of learning and development. Englewood Cliffs: Prentice-Hall, 1984.

Based on this philosophy, David Kolb (1981, 1984) proposed an experiential learning model that has a four-stage cycle with four adaptive learning modes: concrete experience, reflective observation, abstract conceptualization, and active experimentation (**Figure 2-3**).

The experiential learning model describes the learning cycle; that is, how experience translates into concepts that guide the choice of new experiences. Entry into the cycle begins with concrete experience (CE) followed by reflection and observation (RO). The third stage is abstract conceptualization (AC), which becomes the basis for ideas and theories that guide future behavior. In the fourth stage, active experimentation (AE), the individual tests the implications of new concepts and theories in different and more complex situations. By experimenting and applying new learning, individuals again engage in CEs, and so the cycle continues. As the knowledge base expands, the learning experiences become increasingly complex.Based on heredity, past experiences, and the demands of the present environment, individuals develop a unique, preferred style of learning. Based on his learning cycle, Kolb (1981) identified four learning styles: converger, which combines AC and AE; diverger, which combines CE and RO; assimilator, which combines AC and RO; and accommodator, which combines CE and AE. Their strengths are shown in **Table 2-3**.

Teaching strategies can be employed that are suitable for the different learning modes (Burris, Kitchel, Molina, Vincent, & Warner, 2008). For example, clients who favor CE benefit from small group discussion, specific examples, practical exercises, and role playing. Clients who favor reflective observation benefit from creative problem solving, personal journals, discussion groups, and thought questions. Clients who favor AC benefit from hearing lectures, analogies, and questioning. Clients who favor AE benefit from case studies, projects, and psychomotor activities.

Gardner's Multiple Intelligences

The study of intelligence originated when the French government commissioned Alfred Binet to develop a measure of intelligence. In 1904 Binet produced the first measure that assessed a

TABLE 2-3

Kolb's Learning Styles

Learning Style	Strength
Converger (AC and AE)	■ Applies practical application of ideas ■ Focuses on specific problems ■ Is relatively unemotional ■ Prefers dealing with things rather than people ■ Has a tendency to narrow interests ■ Specializes in physical sciences
Diverger (CE and RO)	■ Has good imaginative ability, generates ideas ■ Sees multiple perspectives ■ Is interested in people; emotional ■ Has broad cultural interests ■ Specializes in the arts and humanities
Assimilator (AC and RO)	■ Creates theoretical models ■ Reasons inductively, logically sound theories ■ Is interested in abstract concepts ■ Has less interest in people ■ Focuses less on practical use of theories ■ Specializes in basic sciences and math
Accommodators (CE and AE)	■ Likes to do things (plans, experiments, new experiences); willing to take risks ■ Adapts well to specific immediate circumstances ■ Solves problems intuitively, trial and error ■ Relies on others for information rather than self ■ Likes people; sometimes impatient ■ Specializes in technical or practical fields, such as business

Sources: Kolb (1981, 1984).

broad range of skills and performances. The findings were reduced to a single score, called the intelligence quotient or IQ (Slavin, 2012). IQ testing of school children was widely adopted in the United States. It is often used as a tool to place students in ability groups or tracks in the educational system.

Howard Gardner, professor of cognition and education at Harvard Graduate School of Education, is critical of quantifying actual or potential intelligence by using a single number expressed as the IQ score. In the early 1980s Gardner began looking for other ways to measure intelligence and developed the theory of multiple intelligences (Gardner, 1983). He has a pluralistic view of intelligence and believes that all humans possess these intelligences in varying degrees, with several of them working together. Where people differ is in the degree to which they possess the intelligences and the unique combinations in which they appear in each individual (Gardner, 2011).

Gardner defined intelligence as a biopsychological potential "to process certain kinds of information in certain kinds of ways" (2006, p. 64) and "the ability to solve problems, or to fashion products, that are valued in one or more cultural or community settings" (1993, p. 7). The phrase *fashion products* includes things such as writing a symphony, creating a painting, staging a play, building up and managing an organization, and carrying out an experiment.

Gardner's theory of multiple intelligences (2011), also called frames of mind, includes six autonomous intellectual competencies or strengths. He has attempted to capture those intelligences valued by human cultures and states that his list is neither fixed nor exhaustive. The intelligences are relatively independent of one another but are combined in a variety of ways by different individuals and cultures. Each type of intelligence is important and has equal status with the others. Because these intelligences are pertinent to health education, they are described here. The first two are highly valued in Western societies (linguistic and logical mathematical), because much academic testing and employment is based on verbal and mathematical skill. The next two intelligences are associated with the arts (spatial and musical). The next intelligence, bodily-kinesthetic, involves psychomotor skills and physical movement. The last intelligence (personal) combines two aspects: intrapersonal and interpersonal.

In most individuals the intelligences work together to solve problems. Most professions and vocations involve several intelligences working together to be successful. Most individuals possess several intelligences, although they may be able to process information better in one area than another. In terms of health education, a person may have difficulty learning in one area but be successful in another, so it is reasonable to try a variety of teaching strategies to help clients grasp the health information. A discussion of Gardner's multiple intelligences (2011) is provided in the following sections.

Linguistic Intelligence

People with this intelligence are sensitive to sounds, rhythms, and meanings of words, and they have a facility with words. They are interested in language and are sensitive to its different functions. They like to read, write, and tell stories. Linguistic intelligence is universal and constant across cultures. Poets, orators, and journalists possess this intelligence.

Logical Mathematical Intelligence

People with this intelligence have the ability to discern logical or numerical patterns and are skilled at handling long chains of reasoning. These people have a passion for abstraction and ideas that are characteristic of scientific thinking. In gifted individuals the process of problem solving is often rapid, and frequently a solution is found before it is articulated. Mathematicians and scientists possess this intelligence.

Spatial Intelligence

People with this intelligence rely on the sense of sight, whereas visually impaired people rely on tactile ability to achieve spatial understanding. These individuals have the ability to see things accurately in their environment. They are also able to create mental images, visualize objects, and re-create past visual experiences at will. They like to design and create things. Sculptors, architects, navigators, inventors, and land surveyors possess this intelligence.

Musical Intelligence

People with this intelligence can produce and appreciate rhythm, pitch, timbre, and the many forms of musical expression. Music is integral to life. This intelligence emerges earliest in life. Composers and musical artists possess this intelligence.

Bodily Kinesthetic Intelligence

People with this intelligence have the ability to control their bodily movements to express an emotion (dancer), play a game (athlete), or create a new product (inventor). They like physical activities and have the ability to skillfully use body cues and motions for expression, handling objects, and achieving goal-directed purposes. Athletes, actors, craftsmen, and surgeons possess this intelligence.

Personal Intelligences

This intelligence has two aspects: it looks inward toward the self (intrapersonal), and it looks outward to the relationship with others (interpersonal). Neither aspect can develop without the other, and they are characterized by the culture in which they develop. Intrapersonal intelligence involves knowing one's self and one's feelings and emotions. It is awareness of how this knowledge guides one's behavior. It is looking inward to the self. People with this intelligence focus inwardly on their feelings, talents, interests, and so forth. They are able to discriminate among their emotions, label them, and use them to understand and guide their behavior. It is the most private intelligence. They like to work alone and follow their interests. Persons with in-depth self-knowledge possess this intelligence.

Interpersonal intelligence involves one's relationship to others—one's interactions with family, colleagues, and community. It is the ability to observe the behavior of others in terms of their moods, feelings, motivations, and intentions. It is looking outward from the self. People with this intelligence have the ability to understand others through social interactions. They notice differences in moods, motivations, and intentions. This allows them to understand and work with others. They have many friends and like to talk to others. Helping professionals (nurses, doctors, therapists) and gifted salespersons possess this intelligence.

Multiple intelligences theory is a challenging view of learning because of the many ways that intelligence is expressed in different individuals. People learn differently and cannot be so easily assigned or confined to categories. **Table 2-4** offers some suggestions for how nurses as educators can work with clients who appear to fit this theory. To determine what kind of learners clients are, ask them how they best learn.

Sensory-Based Learning Styles

A common model for assessing learning styles is based on sensory input, such as auditory, visual, kinesthetic, and tactile. Visual learners prefer to see what needs to be learned in terms

TABLE 2-4

Multiple Intelligence and Teaching Strategies

Intelligence Type	Learns by	Teaching Strategies
Linguistic	Reading, writing, talking	Use handouts, pamphlets; encourage client to verbalize or write about experiences; encourage client to keep a journal if appropriate; discussion
Logical mathematical	Reasoning, computing, problem solving	Use case examples; ask questions; identify problems to solve ("how would you handle . . ."); encourage critical thinking in pondering solutions
Spatial	Forming mental images	Draw pictures, especially helpful with children; mind mapping, visualizations are helpful
Musical	Listening to music	Background music; comfortable learning environment; use rhythm or songs to aid memorization
Bodily kinesthetic	Touching, moving	Handle and manipulate equipment; develop skills
Personal	Sharing with others	Interpersonal individuals form groups to discuss common health problems or develop projects; group activities
	Working alone	Intrapersonal individuals use programmed instructional software; computer-assisted instruction; self-paced learning; individual learning projects

Source: Adapted from Holland, 2007; Miller and Babcock, 1996.

of pictures, movies, models, diagrams, and watching demonstrations. Auditory learners prefer to hear explanations from an instructor or from learning tools with audio, including MP3 players. Kinesthetic and tactile learners prefer physical involvement as a way to learn. This can be physical activity and movement, such as learning new exercises and proper body mechanics. It can also include hands-on activities, such as learning how to bathe a newborn or change a dressing. The final style is multisensory learners, who learn in all of these ways—for example, videos, slide shows with audio, and active participation in demonstrations. In reality, learning is rarely confined to one sensory mode. Individuals learn through all their senses even though they may favor one particular style over another (Reid, 1987; Veseghi, Ramezani, & Gholami, 2012).

Implications for Health Education

How does knowing about thinking and learning styles and models help nurses as educators? It is not possible to give clients a battery of tests to determine thinking and learning styles, so talk with clients and get a sense of how they learn. For example, do they become informed by reading, watching videos, talking with a professional, taking classes, or observing others performing (Chang & Kelly, 2007)? Ask if they have hobbies and what they enjoy doing in their spare time to gather clues to their thinking and learning styles. As you work with clients, be especially observant to note what is and is not effective in helping them learn. In working with clients in a nurse-managed center, Kessler and Alverson (2003) found that 82% of clients surveyed preferred hands-on instruction, 63% preferred reading, and 59% preferred listening.

Nurses also are learners with their own preferred style of thinking and learning. It adds to their effectiveness if nurses are aware of how they think and learn. Nurses in the educator role have a tendency to teach in ways that are consistent with how they themselves learn. When the clients' thinking and learning styles fit with the learning setting, the task at hand, and the teacher, clients thrive. When clients' thinking and learning styles do not fit with these factors, clients may have difficulty grasping the health message (Dunn, 1983; Sternberg, 1997).

Rassool and Rawaf (2007) found that undergraduate nursing students preferred the reflector learning style. Noble and colleagues (2008) found that nursing students were more field dependent than students in other health-related disciplines. When there is a mismatch between educator and learner, educators tend to attribute the problem to learners, assuming that they were not motivated or could not grasp the concepts. When that occurs, educators should consider that the problem may be with themselves and their failure to accurately assess clients. It is the responsibility of nurses as educators to evaluate the effectiveness of their teaching.

Nurses move beyond their concern with learning styles by creating a rich learning environment that provides many choices for clients (Moran, Kornhaber, & Gardner, 2006). Having abundant reading materials (books and pamphlets), pictures, videos, interactive instructional materials, demonstrations, and resource persons available are helpful. Multiple choices allow clients to select among the learning options that best suit their learning style.

SUMMARY

This chapter introduced thinking and learning processes as part of the nurse–client relationship of the Miller–Stoeckel Client Education Model. It stressed how that knowledge increases the effectiveness of nurses as educators in working with clients. The three domains of learning—cognitive, affective, and psychomotor—provide a framework for developing learning objectives. The cognitive domain involves intellectual activities; the affective domain deals with attitudes and values; and the psychomotor domain involves learning motor skills. Thinking underlies these domains, and a summary of types of thinking was discussed. These types include problem solving, nursing process, critical thinking, clinical judgment, creative thinking, intuition, reflection, fantasy, and reverie. It is important to understand your own thinking and how to promote thinking in clients.

This chapter also examined several styles and models of thinking and learning, including Sternberg's thinking styles, Witkin and Goodenough's Cognitive-Style Dimensions, Kolb's Experiential Learning Model, and Gardner's Multiple Intelligences. Each view of learning provides insight into the nurse–client relationship and how nurses as educators can best promote learning.

EXERCISES

Exercise I: Learning Domains

Purpose: Distinguish among cognitive, affective, and psychomotor learning domains.
Directions: Working alone, examine the learning objectives for the course you are taking. Place each objective into one of the learning domains. Then form small groups and compare your answers. Was each learning objective categorized correctly?

Exercise II: Affective Domain

Purpose: Examine the affective domain in teaching and learning.
Directions: Reflect on a client situation in which the client's attitudes and beliefs were different from your own. Journal about the following questions:

1. What was the difference between your attitudes and beliefs and those of the client?
2. Did the difference affect how you felt about the client?
3. How did you respond to the client when you became aware of the difference in attitudes and beliefs?
4. Do you think the client was aware that your attitudes and beliefs differed from theirs?
5. What effect did it have on the care you delivered?

Exercise III: Thinking

Purpose: Examine the various factors that influence your thinking.
Directions: Divide into small groups and discuss the following:

1. Identify factors that influence your present thinking. Consider your parents, siblings, close friends, schools attended, religion, music, and the media.
2. Under what circumstances do you do your best thinking? Consider factors such as noise level, time of day, and activity you may be engaged in, such as driving, gardening, sports, or watching TV. Why is this so?

Exercise IV: Types of Thinking

Purpose: Examine the types of thinking presented in this chapter.
Directions: Divide into small groups and discuss the following:

1. Share examples of how you have used these types of thinking: problem solving, nursing process, critical thinking, clinical judgment, creative thinking, intuition, reflection, fantasy, and reverie.
2. Share examples of observing these types of thinking in others (classmates and clients).
3. Identify ways you can stimulate thinking with your clients.

Exercise V: Critical Thinking

Purpose: Examine the impact of different frames of reference.

Directions: Divide into groups of four or five. Discuss the following situation and answer the questions. Then rejoin the larger group and compare your group's answers with the answers of other groups. How were your answers alike? Different? Discuss why the differences occurred.

A 23-year-old Hispanic woman had given birth to her second child and subsequently experienced kidney failure. On her 5th day of peritoneal dialysis, the client asked the nurse what the doctors left in her body that they were trying to wash out. She understood neither what the treatment was nor why it was necessary. Had she not asked the question, her misperceptions would never have been known. Pretend you are the nurse in this situation and answer the following questions:

1. Restate the problem from the client's perspective and from the nurse's perspective.
2. How is the nurse's frame of reference different from the client's?
3. What is the significance of this situation?
4. What is the nurse's goal in this situation? What is the nurse trying to achieve?
5. What assumptions has the client made? What assumptions has the nurse made?
6. What evidence does the client have? What evidence does the nurse have?
7. How has the client interpreted the evidence? How has the nurse interpreted the evidence?
8. What inference, or inferences, did the nurse make?
9. What value judgments did the nurse make?
10. What are the implications of this situation for the client? What are the implications of this situation for the nurse?

Exercise VI: Creative Thinking

Purpose: Conceptualize your creative thinking.
Directions: Divide into small groups and have each participant draw a picture of how he or she thinks.

1. Is your thinking scattered and free associating? Is your thinking goal directed and focused? Do ideas pop into your thinking when you are thinking about something else?
2. Compare your drawings with those of your group members. How similar and how different are they?
3. How did this exercise help you understand your thinking? Did it give you insight into how others think?

Exercise VII: Creative Thinking

Purpose: Generate creative solutions that are both novel and appropriate to the situation.
Directions: Divide into small groups of three to four. Have each participant describe a recent clinical situation with a client that required problem solving. Before stating how each problem was solved, have each group members describe how they would have handled the problem. Finally, share how the participant solved it. Discuss the following:

1. How were the solutions alike? How were the solutions different?
2. Which solution was the most novel?
3. Were the solutions appropriate (useful)? Were some more appropriate (useful) than others?

Exercise VIII: Intuition

Purpose: Examine intuition in teaching and learning.

Directions: A client was due to be discharged and needed instruction on how to change a dressing. When the nurse talked with the client, the client was distracted and busy collecting her possessions for discharge. The nurse had a hunch that the client was concerned about something else rather than learning how to change a dressing. How would you handle this situation? What is the appropriate use of intuition in this situation? Is there a difference between how you and others in your class would handle this situation?

Exercise IX: Learning Style

Purpose: Reflect on your partner's learning style in class.

Directions: Divide into groups of two and ask each other the following questions:

1. When you want to learn something, how do you go about it? Consider visual (movies, pictures, videos, TV), auditory (lectures, discussions, DVDs, MP3s), kinesthetic and tactile (hands-on, demonstrations, games, trips, experiments), and multisensory modalities.
2. Under what circumstance do you learn best (group, individual, structured, unstructured)?
3. What environmental conditions help or hinder your learning (quiet, music, lighting, study area, snacks)?
4. What types of information are easiest and most difficult for you to learn?
5. Which of the thinking and learning styles in this chapter apply to your responses?

REFERENCES

Benner, P. (1984). *From novice to expert.* Menlo Park, NY: Addison-Wesley.

Bloom, B. S., Engelhart, M. D., Furst, E. J., Hill, W. H., & Krathwohl, D. R. (Eds.). (1956). *Taxonomy of educational objectives: The classification of educational goals. Handbook I: Cognitive domain.* New York, NY: David McKay.

Brookfield, S. D. (2012). *Teaching for critical thinking: Tools and techniques to help students question their assumptions.* San Francisco, CA: Jossey-Bass.

Browne, M. N., & Keeley, S. M. (2012). *Asking the right questions: A guide to critical thinking* (10th ed.). Upper Saddle River, NJ: Prentice Hall.

Burris, S., Kitchel, T., Molina, Q., Vincent, S., & Warner, W. (2008). *The language of learning styles* (Research report). Alexandria, VA: Association for Career and Technical Education.

Cassidy, S. (2004). Learning styles: An overview of theories, models, and measures. *Educational Psychology, 24*(4), 419–444.

Chan, Z. C. Y. (2013). A systematic review of critical thinking in nursing education. *Nurse Education Today, 33*(3), 236–240.

Chang, M., & Kelly, A. E. (2007). Patient education: Addressing cultural diversity and health literacy issues. *Urological Nursing, 27*(5), 411–417.

Claxton, C. S., & Murrell, P. H. (1987). *Learning styles: Implications for improving educational practices* (ASHE-ERIC Higher Education Report No. 4). Washington, DC: Association for the Study of Higher Education.

Dunn, R. (1983). Can students identify their own learning styles? *Educational Leadership, 40*(5), 60–62.

Faugier, J. (2005). Basic instincts. *Nursing Standard, 19*(24), 14–15.

Gardner, H. (1983). *Frames of mind*. New York, NY: Basic Books.

Gardner, H. (1993). *Multiple intelligences: The theory in practice*. New York, NY: Basic Books.

Gardner, H. (2006). *Multiple intelligences: New horizons*. New York, NY: Basic Books.

Gardner, H. (2011). *Frames of mind: The theory of multiple intelligences*. New York, NY: Basic Books.

Garity, J. (1985). Learning styles basis for creative teaching and learning. *Nurse Educator, 10*(2), 12–16.

Goulet, C., & Owen-Smith, P. (2005). Cognitive-affective learning in physical therapy education: From implicit to explicit. *Journal of Physical Therapy Education, 19*(3), 67–72.

Halpern, D. F. (2003). *Thought and knowledge: An introduction to critical thinking* (4th ed.). Mahwah, NJ: Lawrence Erlbaum.

Hodgkinson, G. P., Langan-Fox, J., & Sadler-Smith, E. (2008). Intuition: A fundamental bridging construct in the behavioural sciences. *British Journal of Psychology, 99*, 1–27.

Holland, F. (2007). Bringing the body to life: Using multiple intelligence theory in the classroom. SportEX dynamics, *14*, 6–8.

Kaddoura, M. (2013). New graduate nurses' perceived definition of critical thinking during their first nursing experience. *Educational Research Quarterly, 36*(3), 3–21.

Kessler, T. A., & Alverson, E. (2003). Health concerns and learning styles of underserved and uninsured clients at a nurse managed center. *Journal of Community Health Nursing, 20*(2), 81–92.

Kolb, D. A. (1981). Learning styles and disciplinary differences. In A. W. Chickering & Associates (Eds.), *The modern American college* (pp. 232–255). San Francisco, CA: Jossey-Bass.

Kolb, D. A. (1984). *Experiential learning*. Englewood Cliffs, NJ: Prentice Hall.

Krathwohl, D. R., Bloom, B. S., & Masia, B. B. (1964). *Taxonomy of educational objectives: The classification of educational goals. Handbook II: Affective domain*. New York, NY: David McKay.

Kretchmar, J. (2008). *The affective domain*. EBSCO research starters. Ipswich, MA: EBSCO.

Marzano, R. J., & Kendall, J. S. (2007). *The new taxonomy of educational objectives* (2nd ed.). Thousand Oaks, CA: Corwin Press.

McPeck, J. (1990). *Teaching critical thinking*. New York, NY: Routledge.

Miller, M. A., & Babcock, D. E. (1996). *Critical thinking applied to nursing*. St. Louis, MO: Mosby.

Moran, S., Kornhaber, M., & Gardner, H. (2006). Orchestrating multiple intelligences. *Educational Leadership, 64*(1), 22–29.

Noble, K. A., Miller, S. M., & Heckman, J. (2008). The cognitive style of nursing students: Educational implications for teaching and learning. *Journal of Nursing Education, 47*(6), 245–253.

Paul, R. (1995). *Critical thinking: What every person needs to survive in a rapidly changing world*. Rohnert Park, CA: Foundation for Critical Thinking.

Rassool, G. H., & Rawaf, S. (2007). Learning style preferences of undergraduate nursing students. *Nursing Standard, 21*(32), 35–41.

Reid, M. J. (1987). The learning style preferences of ESL students. *TESO Quarterly, 21*(1), 87–111.

Ruggiero, V. R. (2012). *The art of thinking* (10th ed.). New York, NY: Pearson Education.

Ruth-Sahd, L., & Hendy, H. M. (2005). Predictors of novice nurses' use of intuition to guide patient care decisions. *Journal of Nursing Education, 44*(10), 450–458.

Santrock, J. W. (2014). *A topical approach to life-span development* (7th ed.). Boston, MA: McGraw-Hill.

Saylor, C. R. (1990). Reflection and professional education: Art, science, and competency. *Nurse Educator, 15*(2), 8–11.

Scheffer, B. K., & Rubenfeld, M. G. (2000). A consensus statement on critical thinking in nursing. *Journal of Nursing Education, 39*(8), 352–359.

Slavin, R. E. (2012). *Educational psychology theory and practice* (10th ed.). Englewood Cliffs, NJ: Pearson Education.

Sternberg, R. J. (1997). *Thinking styles*. Cambridge, United Kingdom: Cambridge University Press.

Tanner, C. A. (2006). Thinking like a nurse: A research-based model of clinical judgment in nursing. *Journal of Nursing Education, 45*(6), 204–211.

Vasegi, R., Ramezani, A. F., & Gholami, R. (2012). Language learning style preferences: A theoretical and empirical study. *Advances in Asian Social Science, 2*(2), 441–451.

Victor-Chmil, J. (2013). Critical thinking versus clinical reasoning versus clinical judgment: Differential diagnosis. *Nurse Educator, 39*(1), 34–36.

Watson, G., & Glaser, E. M. (1980). *Watson-Glaser critical thinking appraisal manual.* New York, NY: Harcourt Brace Jovanovich.

Webster's All-In-One Dictionary and Thesaurus (2nd ed.). (2013). Springfield, MA: Federal Street Press.

Whiffin, C. J., & Hasselder, A. (2013). Making the link between critical appraisal, thinking and analysis. *British Journal of Nursing, 22*(14), 831–834.

Witkin, H. A., & Goodenough, D. R. (1981). *Cognitive styles: Essence and origins.* New York, NY: International Universities Press.

3

Theories and Principles of Learning

OBJECTIVES

Upon completion of this chapter, you will be able to do the following:

- Apply the following learning theories to selected teaching–learning situations: behaviorism (stimulus–response and operant conditioning), cognitivism (gestalt and information processing), and social cognitive theory.
- Apply designated principles of learning in selected client education situations.
- Describe how theories and principles of learning enhance the teaching and learning process in the nurse–client relationship.

KEY TERMS

attention	long-term memory	stimulus–response
behaviorism	observational learning	theory
cognitive and cognitive	operant conditioning	vicarious punishment
field gestalt	retention	vicarious reinforcement
delayed modeling	role model	working memory
information processing	sensory register	

INTRODUCTION

The teaching and learning process as a component of the nurse–client relationship in the Miller–Stoeckel Client Education Model involves understanding theories and principles of learning and how they enhance client education (**Figure 3-1**). This chapter begins by introducing the

FIGURE 3-1

Nurse–Client Relationship in the Miller–Stoeckel Client Education Model

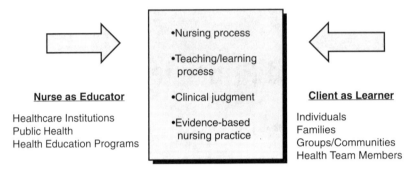

value of theory and how theories help us understand observations and experiences. We examine the learning theories of behaviorism, cognitivism, and social cognitive theory and how each conceptualizes how people learn.

For each theory you will learn how to apply theory to working with clients as learners in a health education context. We also consider learning principles that are applicable to client education. This knowledge is applied to situations in which nurses are the primary educators and clients are the primary learners.

VALUE OF THEORY

Theory is a way to explain some observed phenomenon. Expressed as abstract thoughts or general subject principles, theories help make sense of the world and research findings (Webster's, 2013). Theories provide the theoretical framework to view the process of learning, the progress of learners, and nurses' role as educators. Although theories help to understand learning, no single theory explains everything about a subject.

Nurses are pragmatic and eclectic thinkers. Nurses freely select ideas from diverse sources and conclude that something is good if it works. For example, when you observe something, you try to make sense of it by fitting it into your mental and experiential framework. This is most effective when you know something about what is observed and have had experience with it. When you observe things that are outside your framework—that is, things for which you have neither an explanation nor experience—you become curious and begin to seek answers. Current emphasis on using evidence-based research leads us to look to the current literature for studies that answer questions. This search for answers is the foundation of theory development. Theory helps make sense of what you observe; it is a way to view relationships among observed phenomena. **Box 3-1** identifies how theory is useful.

BOX 3-1	

Reasons for Theories

You need a theory when you:

- ▪ Confront a new situation and what you already know does not apply to that situation
- ▪ Want to increase your understanding of something relatively familiar
- ▪ Face a familiar situation, but what you already know does not work
- ▪ Wish to teach what you know to a colleague or client
- ▪ Question the validity of a cherished belief
- ▪ Explore new hypotheses
- ▪ Observe events for which you can find no explanation

THEORIES OF LEARNING

Learning theories provide the theoretical framework to understand how people learn. We want to know how people acquire new knowledge, develop skills, modify attitudes and values, and learn new behaviors. We know that learning is a dynamic, lifelong process that is unique to each individual.

In the context of health education, knowing about learning theories is a way to understand how people learn. Theory-based teaching is an effective way to organize your thinking and conceptualize what you want to convey to clients and team members. Clients experiencing health problems may need to learn new ways to maintain their health or deal with illness or disability. This is the time when clients are motivated to learn about their changing health status. Team members may also need to learn about new illnesses and new procedures. This need for continuing education falls under the nurse's purview as an educator.

There are various definitions of learning. Common to most definitions is the notion that a change occurs in the learner's behavior, attitudes, or skills (Merriam, Caffarella, & Baumgartner, 2007). The behavioral change is both observable and relatively permanent (Olson & Hergenhahn, 2013). Broadly speaking, learning theories fall into two camps: behaviorism and cognitivism (Ormrod, 2012). **Behaviorism** focuses on tangible, observable behaviors, such as learning to give an injection, changing dietary practices, and safely bathing an infant. Cognitivism focuses on the thought processes as humans learn; for example, seeing a relationship between food intake and blood glucose levels, using memory tricks to recall health instructions, and gaining insight into one's own behavior. Because there are many learning theories within these two camps and different ways to group them, for purposes of this discussion we will look at two theories of behaviorism (**stimulus–response** and operant conditioning), two theories of cognitivism (**gestalt** and **information processing**), and social cognitive theory.

BEHAVIORAL VIEWS OF LEARNING

Behavioral learning theories were among the first to be developed and were the first to be used in the U.S. educational system. They continue to be pervasive, and when the term *learning theory* is used, it usually refers to the body of knowledge accumulated by researchers in the field of behavioral psychology.

Behavioral theorists have generally accepted several basic assumptions in approaching their research (Ormrod, 2012):

- Humans and animals learn in the same way; consequently, early researchers studied rats and pigeons and applied that to human learning.
- Studying stimuli and response objectifies the learning processes.
- Internal processes, such as thoughts, motives, and emotions, are unimportant in understanding learning because they are not observable. Later behaviorists stated that motivation and the strength of the stimulus–response associations were important.
- Learning involves changing behavior.
- Organisms are born as blank slates and learning occurs after birth.
- Learning is largely the result of environmental events that condition behavior.
- The most useful theories explain behavior with as few learning principles as possible.

Learning for the behaviorist is focused on an observable change in the learner's behavior and is not concerned with the internal thought processes of the learner. The learner as a research subject is described as an organism rather than a person or human being. Behaviorists believe that the learner's behavior is shaped by elements in the environment that either precede the behavior (stimulus) or the consequences that follow it. These preceding events can precipitate the behavior, and the events that follow can have positive or negative consequences on the behavior. These events must occur closely in time so that a bond is formed, which is called the principle of contiguity (Olson & Hergenhahn, 2013). An example of a preceding event is a nurse approaching a child with a clearly visible syringe, and the nurse intends to vaccinate him. The sight of the syringe frightens the child, who anticipates pain, starts crying, and clings to his mother for protection. Thereafter the child may be frightened of syringes until he matures and learns differently. An example of a reinforcing event is a smile and hug from the child's mother that assures him he is safe and well. The child knows he can find solace and protection from his mother and will seek her out in future frightening situations.

Behavioral theories today encompass a number of individual theories and continue to be widely applied in understanding how people learn. We review the stimulus–response theories of Pavlov, Thorndike, and Guthrie, as well as Skinner's operant conditioning.

Stimulus–Response

Stimulus–response theories have their origins in the 19th century with Ivan Pavlov (1849–1936) and Edward Lee Thorndike (1874–1949), who studied how animals and humans learn. Pavlov was a Russian physiologist who is famous for discovering the principle of classical conditioning in his work with a hungry dog. He discovered that when meat powder was placed in a dog's mouth, the dog automatically salivated (unconditioned stimulus). When a bell was sounded simultaneously with the offering of meat powder, the bell (conditioned stimulus) became paired with the dog's salivation. Eventually the bell by itself stimulated the dog to salivate. If the bell was presented often enough without the accompanying meat powder, the dog eventually stopped salivating. This phenomenon was called *extinction*. Pavlov's experiment is commonly known as classical conditioning (Ormrod, 2012).

Thorndike did extensive pioneering research in learning, and his work is considered the first modern theory of learning. He noted that the most characteristic method of learning for both animals and humans was trial and error, also called connectionism or the stimulus–response theory of learning. The organism confronts a problem and selects a response most likely to lead to the goal. Much random behavior occurs until the goal is met. On each successive trial the random behavior decreases and the goal-directed behavior increases. This forms the basis for the principle of positive reinforcement that Thorndike called the Law of Effect. It means that the organism remembers responses that had satisfying effects, which strengthens the connection. If the responses were unsatisfying, the strength of the connection decreases. Thorndike formulated two other laws, the Law of Exercise and the Law of Readiness. The Law of Exercise states that repeated use of meaningful connections results in substantial learning, whereas lack of connections inhibits learning. The Law of Readiness states that learning is enhanced when the organism is ready for the connection; otherwise it is inhibited (Olson & Hergenhahn, 2013).

Edwin Ray Guthrie (1886–1959) built on the work of Thorndike and Pavlov. Guthrie felt that the rules they proposed were unnecessarily complicated; he proposed one law of learning, the Law of Contiguity (Olson & Hergenhahn, 2013). He wrote, "A combination of stimuli which has accompanied a movement will on its recurrence tend to be followed by that movement" (Guthrie, 1935, 1952, p. 23). In other words, events that occur together in time tend to be paired. If, for example, a person did something in a given situation, he or she tends to repeat the action when faced with that situation again. Guthrie proclaimed, as do behaviorists today, that a science of psychology must be based on a study of what is observable: behaviors, bodily changes, or data that can be detected by an observer or a measuring device. All data are admissible except introspection, which can be reported only by the client. Later Guthrie revised his theory to recognize the many stimuli to which the organism is exposed and that associations cannot be formed with all of them. The organism responds selectively to only a small number of stimuli, and those are the ones that become associated with the response. What captures the organism's **attention** becomes important along with the association that is formed.

Operant Conditioning

Burrhus Frederic Skinner (1904–1990) is probably the most familiar of the behaviorists in the United States. He is famous for his Skinner box, an experimenter-controlled cage in which the behavior of animals (rats and pigeons) was studied. Skinner acknowledges two kinds of learning. The first is respondent behavior, which occurs in response to a known stimulus, such as a knee jerk in response to an examiner's hammer. The second type of learning, which Skinner believes is more important in human behavior, is an operant response, which refers to the consequences of behavior. When a response is reinforced, whether random or planned, the behavior tends to be repeated; when the consequences are unpleasant, the behavior tends to be suppressed (Slavin, 2012). This statement is a simple way to explain operant learning. Most human behavior is the result of operant learning, according to Skinner.

Propositions of Behavioral Theory

The propositions of behavioral theory as they are understood today are as follows (Olson & Hergenhahn, 2013; Slavin, 2012):

1. Behavior that is followed by reinforcement tends to strengthen the behavior. After being taught how to transfer from a bed to a chair, a client is given smiles and verbal encouragement from the nurse. Praise reinforces the client's behavior and increases the likelihood of further attempts to transfer.

2. Behavior followed by punishment tends to be suppressed. For example, a young man is compliant with his father's commands because he knows that his father will react negatively to his behavior. The son complies because he has learned that rebellion or questioning will result in punishment.

3. Behavior followed by the removal of a negative stimulus tends to increase in strength. Deep breathing relieves tension during an asthma attack and thus decreases the severity of the attack. When clients experience how proper breathing makes a difference, they are motivated to continue this type of breathing.

4. Behavior that tends to recur is in some way being reinforced or is reinforcing itself. An infant crawls and gets into things because it is fun and satisfies the infant's curiosity. Overeating under stressful conditions is reinforcing when it relieves anxiety.

5. A behavior may serve to reinforce or strengthen another behavior. Some individuals can be persuaded to act appropriately for something they value. For example, a client can be given something in exchange for sitting quietly.

6. Irregular and inconsistent reinforcement of a behavior strengthens the continuance of that behavior. Parents who try to resist an uncooperative child's demands but who eventually give in are inadvertently strengthening the behavior with the most powerful method known: intermittent reinforcement.

7. Immediate and consistent reinforcement of a behavior strengthens that behavior most rapidly. A breastfeeding baby soon learns that sucking satisfies hunger.

8. Rewards that are specific to and desired by the learner are more powerful than general or routine rewards. A teenage client may respond well to compliments from the nurse, whereas another client may respond better to matching wits with the nurse.

9. Rewards and punishments that are clearly connected to the behavior are more powerful than vague or inconsistent responses. A client who moves in certain ways after surgery quickly learns that certain motions produce pain, so those movements are avoided. This principle helps explain why eating disorders are so difficult to change. The pleasure or relief that the overeater experiences outweighs the hazards because the pleasure is more immediate and the hazards are more remote. The effects of overeating do not show up on the body or the scale for days, and the health hazards may not become evident for many years. The connection between overeating and health issues is vague and inconsistent because other variables, such as genetics and exercise, are thought to add to or reduce the health risks.

10. Behavior that receives no response and meets no biologic need tends to extinguish. Children bring home new words that they hear while playing. Some of the words may include language the family does not sanction. Children who experience no response when they try out the new vocabulary tend to lose interest in those words.

FIGURE 3-2

Stimulus-Behavior-Consequences. **To change a behavior you can change the stimulus that elicits it and/or the consequences that follow it.**

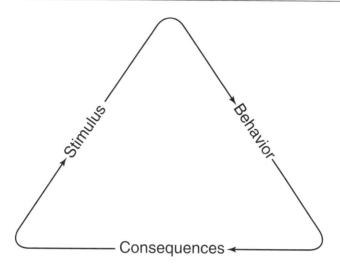

Behavior modification is the application of learning theory to modify a behavior by changing the stimulus that elicits it or by changing the consequences that follow it. Classical conditioning emphasizes that whatever came before a behavior (antecedent event) influences that behavior (responding behavior). **Operant conditioning** stresses that a behavior is influenced by the response that follows. A behavior that is followed by a negative response or no response at all will diminish, whereas a behavior followed by a positive consequence will increase. When both of these theories are applied together, behavior is seen as a result of an antecedent event, and that behavior is further influenced by the consequences that follow it. This is illustrated in **Figure 3-2**.

Implications for Health Education

Decreasing an undesirable behavior involves eliminating or changing the antecedent event that evoked the behavior. Another option is to punish the behavior after it occurs. To increase a desirable behavior, the educator changes the antecedent event to one that is more likely to evoke the desired behavior or reinforces the desired behavior when it occurs or does both actions. An example of controlling antecedent behavior is to advise a client who is learning weight control to shop on a full stomach and use a shopping list. The antecedent event of a full stomach and a shopping list prepared in advance influences shoppers' behavior in the desired direction: wise shopping for wholesome food.

Using behavioral principles, the nurse identifies a client's desired behavior and then creates an environment that stimulates the client to comply by producing this desired response. When the desired behavior occurs, the nurse reinforces it. Immediate reinforcement increases the likelihood that the behavior will recur. Over time the nurse moves from reinforcing the behavior every time it occurs to an intermittent reinforcement schedule. This gives the new behavior more stability.

Educators have discovered that punishment is not a long-term solution to undesirable behavior. Punishment may indeed suppress it, but if the behavior is meeting some need, that behavior is likely to return as soon as the threat is removed. Another possible consequence of punishment is erratic and unpredictable response. The most effective way to eliminate an undesirable behavior is to find out what need the behavior is meeting and reinforce a more desirable method of meeting that need. The example used previously was an uncooperative child. It could be applied just as easily to an uncooperative client of any age. Solutions to this problem include frequent, pleasant, and predictable attention by nurses along with encouragement and assistance.

COGNITIVE VIEWS OF LEARNING

Cognitivism (also known as cognitive psychology) is the predominant theoretical perspective for studying human learning today. Its focus is on the cognitive processes; that is, "how people perceive, interpret, remember and in other ways think about environmental events" (Ormrod, 2012, p. 141). Cognitive theorists study humans, believing that some human learning is unique and differs from how animals learn. Whereas behaviorism focuses on observable behavioral changes, cognitivism expands the understanding of learning to include internal mental processes unique to each person, such as perception, insight, and meaning (Olson & Hergenhahn, 2013; Ormrod, 2012). Cognitive views of learning encompass several perspectives; in this section we focus on Gestalt psychology and information processing theory.

Gestalt or Cognitive Field View of Learning

Three German psychologists, Max Wertheimer (1880–1943), Wolfgang Köhler (1887–1967), and Kurt Koffka (1886–1941), departed from behaviorism and are considered the founders of Gestalt psychology. Later another German Gestalt psychologist, Kurt Lewin (1890–1947), developed a field theory of human learning. These psychologists insisted that behavior was much more than a conditioned response and that perception and memory can be studied by introspection in addition to external observation. Further, they posit that humans selectively perceive and react to complex patterns of stimuli as wholes, not as disconnected parts. It is the total pattern of stimuli that determines what a person perceives and learns (Olson & Hergenhahn, 2013; Ormrod, 2012).

Gestalt is a German word that means "the configuration or pattern" (Olson & Hergenhahn, 2013, p. 240), the whole or totality. In the field of Gestalt psychology the concept means that the whole is more than merely the sum of its parts. Gestalt psychologists hold that psychological phenomena are irreducible wholes that cannot be derived just from analysis of their parts. If the totality of a particular perception is dissected, the meaning is lost.

Perception refers to the act of becoming aware of something by the use of any of the senses. To perceive means to take notice of, observe, detect, become aware of in one's mind, achieve understanding of, or apprehend. Perception refers to the portion of the world that is grasped mentally through sight, hearing, touch, taste, and smell (Webster's, 2013). Perception can vary among individuals and may be different from the reality of the situation.

Our perception of any object is affected by the context in which we become aware of it. Clients who are in a strange hospital and in pain will perceive your messages differently than clients who greet you in their homes. Team members who just heard about another reduction in work force and feel overloaded with responsibilities will perceive your messages differently than those who feel in control of their circumstances. Our perceptions of events are affected by life experiences and interests.

Gestalt and cognitive field theories of learning take into account both the learner and the learning context and all of the individual's experiences and perceptions. In many circumstances individuals' perceptions are dissimilar, and other possible perceptions are not easily seen. Even individuals who experience the same event at the same time may have different perceptions of that event. Because of the tendency to assume that others perceive events the same way you do, you may not be aware that clients may see events differently.

It is possible that you and others may not perceive the same events the same way. An equally important factor to consider is that you may not even be aware of your perceptual differences. It is important to look for clues to these differences and address them. Review the example of the 23-year-old Hispanic woman from a previous chapter who had given birth to her second child and subsequently experienced kidney failure. On her fifth day of undergoing peritoneal dialysis, the client asked what the doctor had left in her body that the nurses were trying to wash out. She understood neither the treatment nor the reason it was necessary. Had she not asked the question, her misunderstanding would never have been known. This supports how important it is to listen carefully and assess client perceptions.

Lewin stated that each individual exists in an environment known as a field or life space, affected by many forces. Life space is a psychological field unique to each individual and includes things to which the person reacts; for example, material objects, people, private thoughts, tensions, and goals. He proposed that behavior is the interplay of these forces in the life space at the moment in which the behavior occurs. Analysis begins with examining the environment as a whole. Lewin made it clear that the environment as interpreted by the individual did not necessarily correspond with reality. Learning occurs as a result of a change in individual psychological interpretations or changes in the internal needs or motivations of the individual (Knowles, Holton, & Swanson, 2005; Olson & Hergenhahn, 2013).

Jean Piaget (1896–1980), a Swiss psychologist, focused his detailed studies on the thinking process of children (1972). He conducted one-on-one interactions during which he presented various stimuli to infants and children. He then observed and recorded their responses. The responses led him to believe that thinking and learning are active processes, not merely passive or trial-and-error responses to stimuli as behaviorists believe. As the children grew old enough to speak, Piaget spoke with the children as he conducted the experiments. He concluded that intellectual development is a gradual process that evolves over time.

Learning is a transactional process in which individuals gain further understanding, new insights, or more developed cognitive structures through interaction. Two ways of learning that Piaget identified were assimilation and accommodation. Assimilation is a way of learning in which new ideas are incorporated by association with known ideas, concepts, and memories. Individuals may assimilate new ideas into their current beliefs. If the knowledge is different from what they already know, they may respond with the intellectual process known as

FIGURE 3-3

Assimilation and Accommodation

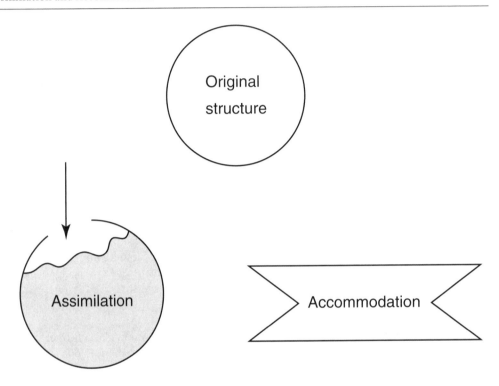

Original structure

Assimilation

Accommodation

Incorporating the new learning into the present structure

Changing the existing structure to accommodate the new learning

accommodation, which is more difficult than assimilation. When accommodating new ideas, individuals give up former beliefs or substantially change their frame of reference, or they do both. Accommodation may also occur after a person has assimilated so many new concepts that the concepts can no longer be contained in the person's old cognitive structure. A paradigm shift occurs in the aftermath of an accumulation process (Olson & Hergenhahn, 2013). **Figure 3-3** illustrates assimilation and accommodation.

Implications for Health Education

Nurses frequently deal with clients who are undergoing life transitions, such as birth, death, parenthood, or divorce. They also deal with clients who experience alterations in personal integrity, such as physical assault, accidental loss of sight or limb, loss of a way of life, or surgical removal of an organ. Such transitions can force clients into reconstructing and reorganizing their perceptions of themselves and reality (Edelman, Kudzma, & Mandle, 2014; Selder, 1989). When clients struggle with questions such as Who am I? and What is life about? they are going through the process of accommodation.

The following is an example of the use of Gestalt psychology in teaching children. The nurse involved with doing preoperative teaching of young children arranges for the children and their parents to come to the day surgery area for a visit. While the children are in the unit, they see a video portraying surgery from a child's perspective. The video tells them the following:

> You wear green pajamas with a hat and socks to match. You get a shot (ouch) that makes you sleepy, and you ride on a table with wheels. The ceiling and people look funny when you ride flat. When you wake up, you will be sore, but you will get more shots that will make the soreness go away.

After the video the children are led to a room with pieces of equipment, drapes, and surgical clothing that they are invited to play with. Dolls set up with various kinds of medical equipment (without real needles) are also within reach so that children can handle and play "operation." The nurse observes the children and listens to their conversations, using their responses as clues to what further teaching might be needed.

The main goal of the Gestalt psychology perspective is to promote understanding and insight. Nurses as educators assess the client's perceptions and design a learning situation that will stimulate interest and understanding. Nurses organize the learning situation to fit the client's developmental stage, previous experiences, and learning ability.

Information Processing View of Learning

Another view of human learning is a sophisticated form of information processing. This view of learning was inspired by advances in computer science by theorists who hypothesized that human minds perform mental operations like computers. Slavin (2012) described a model of information processing proposed by Atkinson and Shiffrin as a model of information processing with three components focusing on how individuals register sensory information taken in from the environment (**sensory register**), how they process information in short-term memory (working or short-term memory), and how that information is stored and retrieved (**long-term memory**) (Slavin, 2012).

The first component of the information processing model is the sensory register, which receives large amounts of information from the five senses: sight, hearing, touch, smell, and taste. This component decides whether or not to notice or register an external sensory bit of information, such as an odor, flavor, touch, sound, or visual stimulus. It also decides whether or not to register sensory information that is internal; for example, an itch, a chill, a peristaltic wave, a headache, or a memory. Individuals' interpretation of sensory information is influenced by many factors, such as past experiences, knowledge, motivation, culture, gender, and so forth. The information is quickly lost if it is given no further attention. Individuals must pay attention to the sensory information if it is to be retained. Individuals often describe stimuli that they did not notice if they are asked to do so immediately after the stimulus. However, they are unable to do this after a few seconds have passed. In addition, people retain less if they are bombarded with too many diverse stimuli at one time (Slavin, 2012).

The second component of the information processing model is short-term memory, also called **working memory**. Here the individual pays attention to sensory information. Short-term memory holds thoughts a person is conscious of having at any given moment. The storage capacity of short-term memory appears limited in most individuals and holds approximately five to seven thoughts. As if they were bowling pins, ideas in the mind can be crowded out by the introduction of more items. These thoughts can be related to what the person is feeling, doing, or thinking at the moment, or they can be related to thoughts retrieved from storage in long-term memory that are associated with current stimuli. In this component the mind processes the information by organizing it for storage, or associating it with other information, or discarding it. When the person stops thinking about the sensory information, it disappears from short-term memory.

For example, a nurse admits a small child for surgery who is tightly clutching a teddy bear. While observing the child's color, breathing ability, alertness, and the parent–child interaction, the nurse remembers a teddy bear from years ago, or that of a daughter or son. Such recollections make the nurse more sensitive to the child at hand. If too many memories impinge on the nurse's consciousness, the memories may detract from the nurse's ability to note and track client data. Another example is a charge nurse giving instructions to a health team member at the change of shift. The team member is struggling with personal issues, including a paraplegic husband at home without a caretaker. Her personal concerns are crowding the space that might store the instructions she is receiving from the charge nurse.

The third component of the information processing model is long-term memory, in which an infinite amount of information is stored for a prolonged period of time. Long-term memory is thought to have a large capacity provided that it has not been damaged by pathology. Stored in long-term memory are images and thoughts about past experiences (episodic memory); facts, knowledge, general information that we have learned, and problem-solving and learning strategies (semantic memory); and procedural knowledge, such as how to do things like giving an injection, riding a bike, and general living skills (procedural memory) (Squire, Knowlton, & Musen, 1993).

Implications for Health Education

The nurse's job as an educator, from an information processing point of view, is to program the client with new information. It is important to divide learning into steps that are compatible with the client's health, intelligence, and previous learning experiences. The nurse assists the client in acknowledging current beliefs that enhance or inhibit learning. The new information is then translated into a message that the client is able to process. This involves capturing the client's attention through teaching strategies and teaching materials. Selecting attractive, colorful materials with sufficient emphasis on fonts and type size helps clients attend to the message.

The information processing model is particularly useful for teaching skills online, such as procedures that must be done in an ordered sequence. As educators, nurses assess educational needs and choose online resources to facilitate learning. This is a useful teaching strategy for individuals who are self-directed, visual, and experienced with computers. Nurses give feedback through discussion forums, email, or phone calls.

In using the information processing model, it is important for nurses to avoid overloading clients with too much information, especially if the information is new. If a lot of information must be communicated in a short period of time, try grouping the information in categories that make sense. For example, if you are teaching a client who has been newly diagnosed with diabetes, it would be helpful to create groupings of information to aid the client's memory. Grouping information for diabetic clients includes dietary information, exercise routine, injection procedure and supplies, and signs and symptoms of hyperglycemia and hypoglycemia. Having printed information about each group also facilitates learning. Clients who have concerns should be given written instructions to read at home that serve as memory aids. Booklets with illustrations are helpful.

If the client in the preceding example had diabetes for many years and was well informed about the disease, your approach would be different. Assess where the client has gaps in knowledge and provide appropriate instruction. The goal is to complement what the client already knows and facilitate learning where it is needed.

SOCIAL COGNITIVE VIEW OF LEARNING

Albert Bandura developed the social cognitive theory of learning. Born in 1925, he is currently an emeritus professor of social science in psychology at Stanford University. His theory is an outgrowth of the behavioral theories of learning that resulted from his belief that these theories lack a complete explanation for learning. He incorporated many contributions from cognitive theorists into what is now referred to as **observational learning**. Bandura believes that people are neither driven by inner forces nor automatically shaped by external forces; rather, they are creative, active participants in shaping their lives. In other words, people are proactive rather than reactive; they have some control over how they live their lives (Bandura, 1986, 2001).

Bandura's social cognitive theory states that people learn from observing others in a social setting. By observing others, people acquire knowledge and skills, learn social rules and norms, and develop beliefs and attitudes. They observe which behaviors are useful, appropriate, and valued by society and which are not. Social cognitive theory posits that people learn most efficiently from observing others' behavior and less from the consequences of behavior (Skinner's view). In other words, this theory states that people learn primarily by observing the successes and failures of others (Santrock, 2014; Slavin, 2012). It is important to distinguish between learning by observation and the act of imitation. Learning may or may not include imitating the observed behavior.

Bandura's theory of observation learning involves four phases: attention, **retention,** reproduction, and motivation (1986). In the first phase, attention, the client must focus on the behavior of the model. In the second phase, retention, the client must have an opportunity to practice imitating the behavior of the model. In the third phase, reproduction, the client tries to match the behavior of the model. In the fourth phase, motivation, the client finds satisfying reasons to imitate the behavior of the model. The teacher's smile and verbal reinforcement are important here. The model is especially useful in teaching and learning situations that involve demonstration and return demonstration activities.

Models and modeling behavior are important concepts. A model can be anything that conveys information; for example, a person, film, television program, picture, or instructions. Models convey messages about behavior. Bandura believes that behavior is the result of the bidirectional interaction of three classes of behavioral determinants: cognitive and personal

FIGURE 3-4

Reciprocal Determinism. Behavior is the result of the bidirectional interaction of three classes of behavioral determinants: cognitive and personal factors (P), environmental events (E), and behavior (B), called reciprocal determinism.

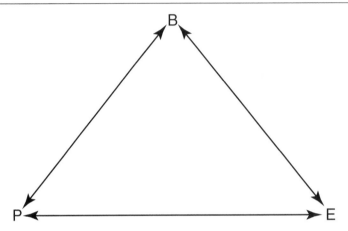

Source: Data from Bandura, A. (1986). Social Foundations of Thought and Action: A Social Cognitive Theory. Englewood Cliffs, NJ: Prentice-Hall.

factors, environmental events, and behavior. The interaction is reciprocal in that each operates interactively as determinants of the other. Behavior is a result of the interacting determinants and cannot be understood by viewing them in isolation. The strength of the influence of each determinant on behavior varies according to the situation. **Figure 3-4** illustrates this reciprocal relationship, which Bandura calls reciprocal determinism (Bandura, 1986; Olson & Hergenhahn, 2013).

The nurse as educator wittingly or unwittingly teaches clients and health team members by his or her behavior. This example helps to explain some cognitive factors in social learning. Emily, a new nurse, observes Nurse X assisting a physician during a diagnostic procedure. Nurse X is poorly prepared to assist the physician and does not have knowledge of the procedure or the physician's requirements and needs. Consequently, both Nurse X and the physician are unhappy at the conclusion of the procedure. The next day Emily observes Nurse Y assist a physician with the same procedure. Nurse Y is prepared, organized, and familiar with the physician's requirements and needs. The outcome is better, and the physician thanks Nurse Y for her preparedness and efficiency. Later Emily seeks out her supervisor and together they discuss both situations. They identify what was effective and what was ineffective behavior of each nurse's performance. In this example Emily observes both positive and negative modeling and is able to see the differences. Emily verbally rehearses her responsibilities with her supervisor. Six months later, Emily is assigned to assist a physician with the same diagnostic procedure. She mentally rehearses her role and responsibilities. The procedure goes smoothly, and the participants are satisfied. This shows how modeling can produce successful performance. From this example, the following components of social cognitive learning theory are illustrated (Bandura, 1986; Ormrod, 2012):

■ Emily's learning was a mental activity; she learned by observing. She paid attention to what each nurse was doing and made a mental note of what was ineffective (Nurse X) and what was effective (Nurse Y). She learned by observing each nurse and mentally rehearsing effective behavior (vicarious learning).

■ Although Emily did not have an opportunity to immediately imitate Nurse Y's behavior, her learning was verbal when she discussed her observations with her supervisor. Together they reviewed what she learned through observation.

■ Emily had no opportunity to immediately imitate the desired assisting behavior; however, 6 months later she remembered what she learned and was able to imitate the behavior (**delayed modeling**).

■ Emily was aware of how unhappy both Nurse X and the physician were at the conclusion of the procedure. Observing their unhappiness, Emily experienced **vicarious punishment** (response–punishment contingency) and did not want to experience the same outcome.

■ Emily was aware of how pleased Nurse Y and the physician were at the conclusion of the procedure. Observing their satisfaction and the physician's compliments with her supervisor's positive input, Emily experienced **vicarious reinforcement** (response–reinforcement contingency), and she desired that outcome for herself.

■ Emily felt confident and believed in her ability to successfully perform the behavior (self-efficacy expectation). Subsequently when she was in the assisting role again, she fulfilled her expectations of herself and rewarded herself with a mental pat on the back.

Bandura identified four processes that influence observational learning (Bandura, 1986; Olson & Hergenhahn, 2013): attentional processes, retentional processes, behavioral production processes, and motivational processes. Attentional processes occur when the learner actively pays attention to what is observed. Models that are similar to the observer in terms of age and gender and who are respected, competent, powerful, attractive, and have high status are attended to more often. Heroes in various age groups act as models for people of their age groups. Retentional processes mean that, for observational learning to be useful, what is learned must be remembered for future use. Learning can be stored verbally in words or in the form of mental pictures or images of modeled behaviors (imagined). When needed, learning is retrieved, rehearsed, and used long after it is observed. Behavioral production processes refer to the person's ability to actually perform what has been learned. Some individuals may be unable to perform or retain information that was learned because of age-related developmental immaturity, illness, or injury. Motivational processes include two aspects: (1) it refers to the expectation that acting like the model in certain situations will result in reinforcement similar to that received by the model; and (2) it serves to motivate a person to use (perform) what has been learned.

Implications for Health Education

Role modeling is a form of observational learning. Nurses learn by observing their professional colleagues. In the same way, clients learn by observing nurses. Clients observe nurses and other healthcare providers and regard them as experts. If they model good health practices, that behavior sends an important message to clients; the converse is also true. Nurses who are overweight or smoke have little credibility when it comes to teaching clients about

TABLE 3-1

Views Regarding Thinking, Learning, Teacher, and Learner

Views of	*Thinking*	*Learning*	*Teacher*	*Learner*
Behaviorist	Covert trial and error	Change in behavior	Directs	Complies
Gestaltist	Knows, perceives	Understands, gains insight	Designs	Participates
Processor	Processes information	Registers, retains, recalls	Programs	Inputs, outputs
Social cognitivist	Observes, mentally processes	Attends, retains, performs	Models	Imitates

weight reduction or smoking cessation. The old adage is true: what we do is a stronger message than what we say, regardless of how sincerely we present the message. If nurses are to be effective educators, they must model good health practices and behaviors (Rush, Kee, & Rice, 2005; Spencer, 2007).

Bandura's modeling phases and processes are important when teaching clients by demonstrating a desired action and having them return the demonstration. By observing you performing, clients and health team members can mimic your performance while they are under your supervision. This gives you an opportunity to guide, correct, and provide positive reinforcement as indicated.

Table 3-1 summarizes the views of learning discussed in this chapter. Each view has advantages and disadvantages, depending on the type of intended learning and on the learner and teacher interaction. When selecting a view, ask yourself the following questions: What is the purpose of the learning? Who initiates the learning? Who evaluates whether or not the learning has been effective?

Educator responsibilities vary, depending on the learning view used. In each view the teacher's role is that of director (behaviorism); designer (gestaltism); programmer (information processing); or model (social cognitive). The main goal of the learner in each view is to change behavior (behaviorism); understand (gestaltism); register, retain, and recall information (information processing); and observe and imitate (social cognitive). Table 3-1 compares these concepts.

PRINCIPLES OF LEARNING

Principles are the foundation or general laws of teaching and learning derived from research based on consistently observed phenomena. Learning principles are formulations that are generally true and stable over multiple learning situations (Ormrod, 2012). These principles, summarized in **Box 3-2**, are derived from research (Slavin, 2012) and informal feedback from more than 800 registered nurses over 15 years who were taught clinical teaching methods in a baccalaureate registered nurse program by authors Babcock and Miller (1994). These principles of learning are applicable to health education.

BOX 3-2

Principles of Learning

- Focusing
- Repetition
- Learner control
- Active participation
- Individual styles
- Organization
- Association
- Imitation
- Motivation
- Spacing
- Recency
- Primacy
- Arousal
- Accurate and prompt feedback
- Application
- Personal history

Focusing Intensifies Learning

Individuals vary in ways that help them learn. Some learners depend on eye contact with the teacher; they focus on the teacher's verbalizations and body language. Others make images in their mind of what is being presented. Kinesthetic learners are people who learn through the awareness of body position. Some learners write images on paper or write notes to stay actively involved.

While studying, some learners listen to music to help them concentrate. Others want minimal auditory and visual distractions. Some learners have rituals that help them focus. Examples of rituals include meditation, organizing materials, and preparing a snack. Most learners enhance their ability to retain and recall information by developing a pattern that provides for physical comfort, a heightened level of arousal, and a clear mind.

Repetition Enhances Learning

This approach is where learners repeat the information until they are able to produce it from memory. Sustained practice enforces learning. This is true for memorizing facts and mastering psychomotor skills.

Learner Control Increases Learning

Learners do better when they feel in control of the learning process, and they are more likely to choose learning methods that worked for them in the past. Past experience demonstrates that nurses are successful adult learners who can verbalize what they need to master new information and skills. Most nurses take responsibility for their learning and do better when educators acknowledge this in both actions and words. This same principle applies to learners of any age. Older learners generally need more time to absorb new information. They are successful when they are in control of both the pace and the increments of learning.

Active Participation Is Necessary for Learning

Learning is an active process. Most people find that the more they are able to involve themselves in learning, the more they are able to learn. Participation in learning means having input into the learning process, including the time, place, pace, and increments of learning.

Learning Styles Vary

Some learners find it easier to comprehend verbal discourse, while others comprehend visual cues more easily. Still others seek hands-on experience to grasp the meaning of learning concepts. Many find that a combination of verbal, visual, auditory, and kinesthetic experiences is most effective. Be aware of your preferred learning style because it is the style you are most likely to use when you teach. Assess your clients' learning styles so you can plan an approach to enhance learning. The skill in facilitating learning is to find an effective match between the clients' learning styles and your teaching approach.

Organization Promotes Learning

Learners often highlight readings, summarize paragraphs, explain their assignments to others, and ask questions. These are ways of actively organizing learning materials. This personal intellectual activity makes the information meaningful and easier to retain. Methods of organization vary, but to be most effective, materials should be organized in a way that fits both the content and the learner. A cognitive task, such as learning historical facts, is facilitated by using chronology. Learning psychomotor skills is enhanced by teaching from the simple to the complex. Affective learning frequently is best organized around the principle of low- to high-risk behaviors from the learner's point of view.

Association Is Necessary to Learning

To retain any new information or skill, learners must be able to associate the new learning with phenomena that are already within their repertoire of experience. Association provides relevance to learners.

Imitation Is a Method of Learning

Imitating is particularly useful for mastering psychomotor skills, but attitudes and beliefs can also be incorporated if learners observe a respected role model.

Motivation Strengthens Learning

It is easier for learners to grasp facts, learn new skills, and change attitudes when they anticipate gaining benefits from the effort. Past success and the expectation of future success are powerful motivating forces. Educators should perform a needs assessment to understand what motivates clients and use this knowledge to create an atmosphere that sustains motivation and builds confidence.

Spacing New Material Facilitates Learning

It is wiser for educators to present small amounts of new material incrementally rather than larger amounts at one time. Learners should be encouraged to read instructional materials to give them exposure to information over time so they have a more thorough understanding. This also provides an opportunity to ask questions of the educators.

Recency Influences Retention

The more recently learners have been exposed to information or have practiced a skill, the greater the possibility that they will recall it correctly. Retention is the ability to repeat information or grasp or hold on to information or a skill.

Primacy Affects Retention

People tend to learn the first few items best; this concept is referred to as primacy. Learners pay more attention to and devote more energy to items presented first. The human mind is capable of retaining a limited number (five to seven) of new bits of information at one time. When these new bits of information have been associated with other more solidly retained memories, learners are better able to grasp and retain other sets of facts.

Arousal Influences Attention

Arousal is affected by novelty. The human mind is attracted to change and glitches in patterns. Other sources of stimuli besides novelty include sensory intensity, emotional arousal, and other sources of tension. A certain amount of tension enhances learners' ability to focus. This tension is caused by fear, anger, anxiety, curiosity, and amusement. When tense, a client's neurochemistry changes. Chemicals are released that improve circulation, provide sugar to the brain and muscles, and enhance visual acuity. Clients vary in how much tension is ideal for them. This is illustrated in **Figure 3-5**. For example, too much tension interferes with learning, whereas a moderate level of tension is motivating (Cassady & Johnson, 2002; Stephenson, 2006). With too much tension, clients may become immobilized or restless and engage in behavior that further obstructs learning. Fear of punishment, such as job loss, usually impedes learning and interferes with the ability to apply learning to new situations.

Accurate and Prompt Feedback Enhances Learning

Learners need to know how well they are meeting learning objectives. Self-assessments are helpful; consider how frequently newspapers and magazines publish self-scoring tests and questionnaires. Clients want to know how their attitudes compare with others and their level of knowledge. Feedback is necessary for clients and educators to determine if learning occurred.

FIGURE 3-5

Arousal and Learning. **A moderate amount of tension enhances learning. Too little tension fails to engage learner's attention. Too much tension interferes with learning.**

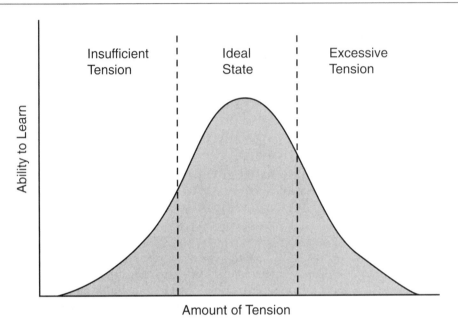

Prompt feedback reinforces desired behaviors and gives clients feelings of satisfaction when they are successful. Even when correction is necessary, feedback can reduce tension because learners know what is learned and what is still to be mastered.

Application of New Learning in a Variety of Contexts Broadens the Generalization of That Learning

Application of knowledge helps to broaden and generalize learning. An example is practicing crutch walking in a lab setting and then applying the skill in actual practice settings, such as walking up and down steps. Exposure to a particular concept, attitude, or skill in varying situations assists learners to retain new material and develop the ability to apply the material in a wider variety of situations.

The Learner's Biologic, Psychologic, Sociologic, and Cultural Realities Shape the Learner's Perception of the Learning Experience

Health affects energy level and ability to concentrate. Self-esteem and previous experiences with learning affect the willingness to risk, tolerance for temporary failure, and expectations of success. If clients are at a developmental level in which memorization and concrete processing are necessary, educators must respect that. Nurses as educators need to listen and be observant of the signs that learners are handling all they can.

Societal norms and learners' previous experiences with healthcare institutions affect the ability to learn. Clients' attitudes toward learning, their beliefs about personal responsibility for health, and the learning climate are all influenced by their culture.

SUMMARY

This chapter examined prominent theories of learning as they relate to the teaching and learning process of the nurse–client relationship in the Miller–Stoeckel Client Education Model. The theories are behaviorism (stimulus–response and operant conditioning), cognitivism (gestalt and information processing), and social cognitive theory. With each theory, application was made to how nurses as educators could apply that information in a clinical setting when working with clients as learners. Selecting which theory works best for clients and what is taught is your job as the educator. The chapter concluded with a discussion of principles of learning that are broadly applicable in a wide variety of health education situations.

EXERCISES

Exercise I: Integrating Learning Theories and Principles

Purpose: Apply learning theories and principles in preparation for client education.
Directions: Divide into groups and choose which assignment your group will prepare.

Group Assignment A

What learning theories and principles would you apply in each of the following situations? Act out one of the following scenes.

1. You are going to teach home safety and accident prevention to an elderly client after hip replacement surgery before she goes home.
2. As a nurse working in the gynecology clinic, you are to teach breast self-examination to a group of women in the waiting room.
3. As a public health nurse, you are to teach a group of young parents at a day care center about behavior modification using the propositions of behavioral theory. The objective is to translate the most important concepts into plain English and give practical examples.

Group Assignment B

You are a group of nurse entrepreneurs who have been granted an interview with a TV station program producer. Select two members to collaborate in playing the role of station program producer.

1. Your task is to talk the TV producer into buying your television program package. Prepare the following information:
   a. Identify the target audience. Who are the viewers? Are they in school? If so, which grade level? Are they at the work site? If so, which one? Why did you choose this audience?
   b. What population trends make your program feasible?
   c. Suggest how often your program should be shown. Daily? Monthly? What day? What hour? Provide your rationale.
   d. List the topics you would cover with your target audience.
   e. Identify the sponsors you would approach.
2. Place yourself in the role of the producer. Identify questions and concerns you have. Consider issues such as profit; market acceptability; risk; controversy; sensitivities of various cultural, ethnic, and age groups; and timeliness. Present these concerns to the nurse entrepreneurs.

Group Assignment C

Conduct the following activities on your regular television health program:

1. Your first guest is a self-styled fitness expert or nutritionist who is very popular but whose scientific base you question. Conduct the interview in a way that will promote critical thinking in your audience.
2. Create a commercial break in which you do the following:
   a. Market nurses as health educators, consultants, and care providers
   b. Advertise a health product or system with which you would like to be associated
3. Interview a nurse colleague about the changing trends in health care and what that means for the average citizen.

Exercise II: Compare and Contrast Learning Theories

Purpose: Examine behaviorism, cognitivism, and social cognitive theories.
Directions: Divide into small groups of four to five and discuss the theories of learning described in this chapter. Discuss the following questions:

1. How are the theories alike?
2. How are they different?
3. What is the difference between learning, teaching, and health education?
4. Do people think like computers?
5. How have computers influenced your way of thinking?

Exercise III: Reflecting on Self-Learning

Purpose: Reflect on how you learn.
Directions: Form dyads with someone in the class who you have not worked with before. Take a few minutes and reflect individually on how you learn; then share with your partner. Listen to how he or she learns. Compare the ways your learning is alike and different.

Exercise IV: Information Processing and Memory

Purpose: Contemplate on the information processing model.

Directions: Form small groups of three or four; then do the following:

1. For 5 to 10 minutes, think alone about how you memorize lists and new information.
2. Discuss your thoughts and memory aids with others in your group and compare how your memorization strategies are alike and different.
3. Did you learn new strategies that will help you in the future?

Exercise V: Role Modeling

Purpose: Reflect on role models and role modeling.

Direction: Reflect on the following for 5 to 10 minutes; then form small groups and discuss your responses:

1. Who are your present role models in your social life? Who are your present role models in your role as a student?
2. What have you observed them doing that has helped you?
3. What have you observed them doing that you wish to avoid?
4. In what ways are you a role model to others?

REFERENCES

Babcock, D. E., & Miller, M. A. (1994). *Client education: Theory and practice.* St. Louis, MO: Mosby.

Bandura, A. (1986). *Social foundations of thought and action: A social cognitive theory.* Englewood Cliffs, NJ: Prentice Hall.

Bandura, A. (2001). Social cognitive theory: An agentic perspective. *Annual Review of Psychology, 52,* 1–26.

Cassady, J. C., & Johnson, R. E. (2002). Cognitive test anxiety and academic performance. *Contemporary Educational Psychology, 27*(2), 270–295.

Edelman, C. L., Kudzma, E. C., & Mandle, C. L. (2014). *Health promotion throughout the life span* (8th ed.). St. Louis, MO: Elsevier Mosby.

Guthrie, E. R. (1935). *The psychology of learning.* New York, NY: Harper & Row.

Guthrie, E. R. (1952). *The psychology of learning* (rev. ed.). New York, NY: Harper & Row.

Knowles, M. S., Holton, E. F., III, & Swanson, R. A. (2005). *The adult learner* (6th ed.). Burlington, MA: Elsevier.

Merriam, S. B., Caffarella, R. S., & Baumgartner, L. M. (2007). *Learning in adulthood* (3rd ed.). San Francisco, CA: Jossey-Bass.

Olson, M. H., & Hergenhahn, B. R. (2013). *An introduction to theories of learning* (9th ed.). Upper Saddle River, NJ: Pearson Prentice Hall.

Ormrod, J. E. (2012). *Human learning* (5th ed.). Boston, MA: Pearson.

Piaget, J. (1972). Intellectual evolution from adolescence to adulthood. *Human Development, 15*(1), 1–12.

Rush, K. L., Kee, C. C., & Rice, M. (2005). Nurses as imperfect role models for health promotion. *Western Journal of Nursing Research, 27*(2), 166–187.

Santrock, J. W. (2014). *A topical approach to life-span development* (7th ed.). Boston, MA: McGraw-Hill.

Selder, F. (1989). Life transition theory: The resolution of uncertainty. *Nursing and Health Care, 10*(8), 437–451.

Slavin, R. E. (2012). *Educational psychology theory and practice* (10th ed.). Boston, MA: Pearson.

Spencer, C. (2007). Should nurses model healthy behaviour? *Kai Tiaki Nursing New Zealand, 13*(7), 14–15.

Squire, L. R., Knowlton, B., & Musen, G. (1993). The structure and organization of memory. *Annual Review of Psychology, 44,* 453–495.

Stephenson, P. I. (2006). Before the teaching begins: Managing patient anxiety prior to providing education. *Clinical Journal of Oncology Nursing, 10*(2), 241–245.

Webster's All-In-One Dictionary and Thesaurus (2nd ed.). (2013). Springfield, MA: Federal Street Press.

III

Assessment for Health Education

4

Learner and Setting Assessment

OBJECTIVES

Upon completion of this chapter, you will be able to do the following:

- Explain how your perceptions and those of the client affect teaching and learning.
- Identify three aspects of readiness to learn.
- Describe how the theories of learning relate to motivation to learn.
- Explain how you will apply Maslow's hierarchy of needs to a teaching and learning situation.
- Describe how the following levels of wellness affect teaching and learning: acute illness, convalescence, chronic illness, and full health.
- Describe how to assess a client's psychosocial vital signs.
- Describe how socioeconomic factors, cultural factors, and educational level affect health education.
- Describe ways to assess a client's background knowledge.
- Identify four types of client communication challenges that affect teaching and learning.
- Describe the ideal teaching and learning environment in terms of space; temperature; visual, auditory, and olfactory stimuli; equipment; resources; furniture arrangement; physical comfort; and time.
- Compare and contrast the effect of the following environmental settings on teaching and learning: hospital, long-term care or assisted living facility, private home, school, work site, and community.
- Apply the CCCC/AOL Quick Assessment Tool for Teaching Individuals and the Assessment Tool for Teaching Groups.

KEY TERMS

culture
developmental readiness
ethnicity
ethnocentrism
experiential readiness

hierarchy of needs
level of wellness
motivation
psychosocial vital signs
socioeconomic factors

teaching and learning
 environment
values

INTRODUCTION

In this chapter we examine factors to consider when assessing the client and the learning environment in preparation for health education. Thorough assessment is essential in the effectiveness of the nurse–client relationship in the Miller–Stoeckel Client Education Model. First we look at the client's readiness to learn. This includes the client's and educator's perceptions that affect learning. Then we focus on the client's motivation to learn, level of wellness, psychosocial vital signs (PVS), socioeconomic factors, cultural factors, and educational level. Generational differences are identified, and communication challenges are discussed. Learning is affected by the client's background knowledge, and methods to assess background knowledge are presented. Psychological and physical factors that affect the teaching and learning environment are described and clarified. The chapter concludes by describing assessment factors in different settings, such as the hospital, long-term care or assisted living facility, private home, school, work site, and community where teaching and learning occur.

ASSESSMENT OF LEARNERS

In preparing for health teaching, the nurse as educator must first assess factors that influence the learner's response to health education. Assessment is the first phase of the nursing process, an essential step before developing a teaching plan. The assessment of clients in a variety of settings should take into consideration multiple factors. **Figure 4-1** illustrates the factors that comprise the assessment and analysis stage of health education. Each factor is examined in more depth.

Perception

Assessment of the educator's and client's personal perceptions is critical when preparing for health teaching. Perception is the ability to receive stimuli through sight, hearing, taste, touch, and smell, and to give meaning to those sensations. Perceptions are the parts of the universe to which we attend. They result from our biologic, psychologic, sociologic, and cultural history. The following example illustrates how perceptions can affect client learning.

Christine was an 18-year-old homeless client seen at an urban clinic. Her chief complaint was dysuria and frequency of urination with a history of smoking marijuana and taking stimulants and depressants. She was diagnosed with a urinary tract infection and was prescribed antibiotics. The nurse instructed her on how to take the medication and emphasized the importance of taking it all. Christine had difficulty understanding why she could not stop taking the

FIGURE 4-1

Assessment and Analysis Factors in Preparation for Health Education

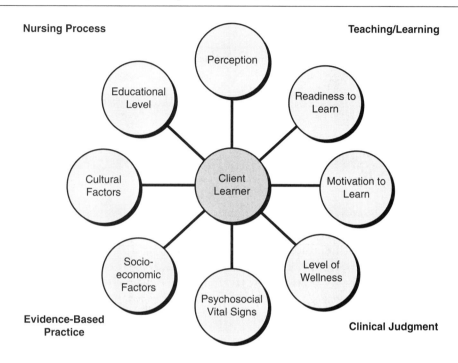

medication when her symptoms were relieved. She wanted to know what would happen if she failed to take the prescribed medication and verbalized that she might be harmed by taking it all. To Christine, the antibiotic represented a quick fix, and she could not see the need for medication when she felt better. Even though taking street drugs was a regular "safe" part of her life, she distrusted the healthcare system and did not see the need for taking all the medication. The nurse's knowledge influenced her perceptions of the need for the medication, whereas Christine based her perceptions on fear of the healthcare system and her experience of taking street drugs for a desired effect. It was important for the nurse to be aware of Christine's perceptions as she prepared a teaching plan.

As a healthcare professional, your perceptions are shaped by your personal history, nursing knowledge, and the amount of meaningful clinical and teaching experience you have accumulated. The ability to perceive a client's situation in preparation for teaching will grow as you expand your repertoire of life experiences and nursing skills. The development of empathy and the ability to put yourself in the shoes of another is achieved by purposefully gaining experiences that expand life perceptions. This may involve selecting service learning experiences that offer the chance to broaden your life experiences and deepen your understanding of the human condition.

Perceptions of clients not only shape the way you view them, but they also influence clients' self-perceptions. Clients and team members tend to perceive themselves in response to your reaction to them. What you know about their biological, psychosocial, and cultural

TABLE 4-1

Variables That Affect Listening Perception

Listening Is Enhanced	*Listening Is Diminished*
When a person is motivated to listen	When a person is not motivated to listen
When the listener is attentive	When the listener is inattentive or distracted
When the speaker is perceived as trustworthy	When a speaker is perceived as not trustworthy
When the speaker is perceived as knowledgeable	When the speaker is perceived as uninformed
When the message or speaker is important to the listener	When the message or speaker is not important to the listener
When the message fits the listener's beliefs	When the message conflicts with the listener's beliefs
When the message makes sense to the listener	When the message does not make sense to the listener

characteristics will greatly influence how you perceive them. Be alert to the fact that it is easier to hear messages that already fit your belief system and that come from people whom you like and respect. To illustrate this, consider how you might react differently to clients who are perceived as mentally challenged or smart, unmotivated or motivated, hopeless or hopeful, uncooperative or cooperative, and ignorant or informed. It is important to validate your perceptions before acting upon them.

Nurses' emotional states also affect their perceptual fields. When you are feeling confident and self-actualized, you are better able to be perceptive of client assessment data. When you are tired or rushed, you may become distracted, which can cause you to perceive information selectively. This may contribute to the nurse as educator failing to perceive important client data that are needed to develop the teaching plan. **Table 4-1** identifies variables that affect listening perception by the client and the nurse as educator.

Readiness to Learn

Readiness to learn is based on the client's or team member's willingness and ability to engage in a given learning activity. It includes an aroused interest or curiosity to learn, the learner's experiential background, and physiological or developmental maturation. Readiness to learn is most intense when the learner's life situation creates the desire or necessity to acquire new knowledge, attitudes, and skills. It is important to assess readiness to learn because it greatly impacts the learning situation.

The nurse as educator assesses clients' readiness to learn by listening to the concerns they express and the questions they ask. Clients often express their health concerns and ask questions while the nurse is administering medications, performing nursing procedures, or delivering nursing care. This is an unplanned opportunity to note the client's openness and readiness for informal health education. Team members also indicate their interest in learning while they are on the job and are engaged in client care activities.

To assess learner readiness, first ask learners what they want to know, or explain the learning needs that you have observed. Ask for background information and history of the issue. After

TABLE 4-2

Levels of Readiness for Health Education

Level 1

Client verbalizes no interest in health education and avoids the topic.

Client holds the healthcare team responsible for his or her health.

Client lacks physiologic or developmental abilities required for learning.

Level 2

Client verbalizes some interest in health education but is easily distracted and unable to stay on the topic.

Client is willing to follow some healthcare team directions.

Client has limited physiologic or development abilities.

Level 3

Client verbalizes more interest in health education and is able to stay on topic for brief periods of time.

Client seeks and follows healthcare team directions.

Client has the requisite physiologic or developmental skills.

Level 4

Client verbalizes great interest in health education and asks many questions.

Client follows healthcare team directions and assumes responsibility for his or her own health.

Client has full physiologic and developmental ability to learn.

completing an assessment of the learner's understanding, determine if you can build on what they already know. Inaccuracies or misunderstandings that could affect health status should be immediately and politely corrected. Ask whether they are interested in learning new material. Do they verbalize willingness to take the time to learn? Do they see themselves as playing a role in the learning process? Do they consider themselves instrumental in their own healing? What is their attitude about making life changes? Do they believe they will receive support to make changes from friends, family, and coworkers? Will their culture be a supportive or inhibiting factor in learning new behaviors? What is their perception of healthcare professionals? Readiness to learn can be assessed and classified according to learners' verbalizations. **Table 4-2** reviews the levels of readiness for health education. The guide can be readily adapted to individual client situations and addresses a client's cognitive skills, desire to learn, and psychomotor abilities.

Levels of readiness to learn are adaptable to fit a wide variety of teaching and learning situations. For example, Bonner and colleagues (2002) developed an educational intervention to improve asthma management; they used four levels to assess clients' readiness to manage asthma. Educational interventions are indicated at each level. The four readiness levels, based on family attitudes and behaviors about the diagnosis of asthma, are as follows:

- Level 1: Asthma symptom avoidance, no recognition of asthma as a chronic disease
- Level 2: Asthma acceptance, acknowledges asthma symptoms when they occur
- Level 3: Asthma compliance, uses preventive pharmacotherapy but considers fluctuations to be treatment failures
- Level 4: Asthma self-regulation, applies asthma actions plans when symptoms change

The authors reported successful educational interventions based on this readiness to learn model.

Motivation to Learn

Motivation is "an internal state that arouses, directs, and sustains human behavior" (Glynn, Aultman, & Owens, 2005, p. 150). It is important to assess an individual's motivation before providing health education. Glynn and colleagues (2005) identified four theoretical orientations to motivation: behavioral, humanistic, cognitive, and social. Behavioral, cognitive, and social orientations are components of learning theories. In behavioral theory, behavior that is reinforced tends to recur, whereas behavior that is ignored or punished tends to be suppressed. When certain behaviors are repeatedly reinforced, individuals are motivated to continue behaving in that manner. When these behaviors are health promoting, the nurse can continue to reinforce them. When these behaviors are not healthy, the nurse is challenged to teach the client new health-promoting behaviors.

In the cognitive view of learning, the individual's goals, plans, and expectations are important. Clients who are undergoing life changes and health problems are often in the process of reconstructing and reorganizing their perceptions of themselves and reality. The nurse's role is to assist clients to change their cognitive view to a more appropriate and healthful one. In the social cognitive orientation to motivation, individuals learn new behaviors by observing others as role models. To model new behaviors, clients must believe they are capable of performing the new behaviors successfully. In social cognitive theory, this is called the self-efficacy expectation.

Abraham Maslow, a prominent figure in the humanistic movement, proposed a theory of human motivation based on a **hierarchy of needs**. His theory has been widely adopted in nursing education (Maslow, 1954, 1987). His concept of self-actualization refers to human motivation to achieve personal growth and self-determination. Maslow's hierarchy has five levels of human needs that people tend to satisfy in sequence, beginning with the physiologic needs. See **Table 4-3** for an illustration of how these needs apply to health education.

In Maslow's hierarchy, the needs at each level must be at least partially met before needs are satisfied at the next higher level. Maslow distinguishes between deficiency needs and growth needs. Deficiency needs are things people lack and that need to be met by others or events in the environment. They are critical to physical and psychological well-being. They include the first four levels of the hierarchy: physiologic, safety and security, love and belonging, and self-esteem. After these needs have been satisfied, the individual is motivated to seek out new experiences that involve self-actualization, which Maslow called growth needs. Motivation to meet growth needs is intrinsic and comes from within the individual. Needs are rarely completely satisfied. Maslow believed people strive toward self-actualization, a condition that is made possible when the individual's deficiency needs have been satisfied (Ormrod, 2012; Slavin, 2012). Your role as an educator is to assess which needs are most important to the client so you can ascertain his or her motivation.

The last motivation model we discuss is the ARCS model. It is a useful, easily applicable model to assess motivation when a person is involved in a specific learning activity. Developed by Keller (1987, 2008), the model identifies four conditions that are essential for sustaining motivation in a learning situation. The acronym comes from the letter of each condition: attention, relevance, confidence, and satisfaction. Attention addresses arousing the client's curiosity and capacity to participate in learning. Relevance addresses whether or not the educational activity is meaningful to the client. Confidence addresses whether or not the client believes he or she is capable of learning the material. Satisfaction addresses the emotional response the client has toward the learning experience—whether positive or negative.

TABLE 4-3

Maslow's Hierarchy of Needs Applied to Health Education

Maslow's Hierarchy of Needs	Application to Health Education
Physiologic needs (oxygen, food, hydration, warmth, exercise, and sleep)	Clients who are tired, hungry, in pain, or critically ill have little motivation to focus on health education. Postpone teaching until a more appropriate time.
Safety and security needs	Clients who do not feel safe and secure are not open to health education. Inform them about routines and procedures.
Love and belonging needs	Clients who do not feel accepted by the healthcare team are not open to health education. Accept and welcome them to health education opportunities.
Self-esteem needs (feeling respected, valued, and appreciated)	Clients who do not feel respected, valued, or appreciated are not receptive to health education. Listen and appreciate their viewpoint and address their learning needs.
Self-actualization (achieving one's potential)	Clients who focus on lower-level needs will not achieve their full potential. Help them achieve their full potential by focusing on higher-level needs to improve their lives.

Level of Wellness

Clients' readiness for health education is related to their health status, and health education must be appropriate to their level of wellness. **Level of wellness** refers to the health status of an individual at any point in time. Health is a dynamic state and can be conceptualized on a bipolar continuum, with a high level of wellness at one end and acute and preventable illnesses at the opposite end. Individuals move freely along the continuum, depending on their current health status and their willingness to engage in health-promoting activities. The Stoeckel Wellness–Illness Functional Continuum could be used as a tool to assess a client's perception of wellness level.

The wellness level of acutely and chronically ill clients may change daily as they respond to medical and nursing care. These clients have the potential for achieving a higher level of wellness. It is important to remember that the highest level of wellness is specific to each client (Zuluaga, 2000). Nurses as educators need to be aware of how an individual client's level of wellness affects the teaching plan.

Acutely ill clients are concerned with physical survival. Clients are frequently in pain, confused, anxious, and fearful. They can receive medications that cloud their thinking. Medications can also interact with one another and cause problems. Clients at this level are not receptive to formal teaching. They benefit from information that will ease their fears and help them maintain orientation to their condition, surroundings, and time of day. Nursing interventions and teaching that make them more comfortable are welcome. In the case of very ill individuals, the family may be the client who is receptive to teaching.

Clients who are recovering are more receptive to health education than those who are acutely ill. These clients are found in subacute or home care shortly after the acute illness stage. Public health nurses encounter clients who are still recovering when they are sent home. These clients and their families need much support, supervision, and teaching. Families need instruction about how to give care and perform procedures that were previously done by skilled nurses and physicians. Recovering clients and their families are likely to be interested and motivated learners. They are usually motivated to learn whatever is necessary to resume normal life as soon as possible. In general it is believed that clients recover more quickly in their own homes, where they are surrounded by familiar support systems.

Chronically ill clients vary in their openness to receiving health education, depending on their acceptance of the reality of their illness. Some clients with long-term illnesses may have researched their disease and have an increased understanding of diagnosis and treatment. These clients want to be active participants in their care and expect a collaborative relationship with healthcare professionals. The nurse is a resource person and care manager.

When chronic illnesses wax and wane, clients may become weary and discouraged. It reduces physical and psychic energy. The nurse as educator's role in such situations is listener and collaborator for learning. Together the nurse and client experiment with adaptations designed to make the best of the client's abilities and energies. Clients are likely to be more motivated when their aggravating symptoms subside.

The nurse as educator also encounters clients who are physically well and interested in preventing illness and maintaining health. Today many clients realize that the way they conduct their lives is directly related to their health, longevity, and well-being. You will encounter potential clients among the visiting friends and relatives of clients who are in the hospital, at home, in freestanding surgical and medical clinics, and at workshops and classrooms. You will also encounter them in your neighborhood. **Figure 4-2** illustrates how a client's needs and learning ability change depending on the level of wellness related to the client's healthcare needs. When a client is acutely ill and has little energy, learning needs are very limited and concrete. During recovery clients are interested in what they can do to promote their own recovery and return to optimum health. Those with chronic illnesses are greatly affected by the reality and constraints of their illness. Those in good health are open to a wide range of health education (O'Brien, 2007).

Psychosocial Vital Signs

The nurse as educator works with clients who experience a variety of psychological and social stressors. Anxiety is a normal reaction to stressful situations (Connolly, Simpson, & Petty, 2006). It allows people to react quickly and thus prevents them from becoming hurt in dangerous situations or perceived threats. Causes of anxiety can be a result of biological and psychological factors that are intertwined in a complex manner. Tummala-Narra (2009) found that anxiety is felt both by learners and instructors. To enhance learning effectiveness, teachers are encouraged to identify anxiety-provoking situations and provide a supportive learning environment so learners can devote their complete working memory resources to the learning tasks. Anxiety consumes the resources of working memory, thus impeding a learner's ability to perform effectively. To assist the nurse as educator in nurturing the nurse–client relationship, an assessment tool will help to gauge the client's psychosocial state.

FIGURE 4-2

Levels of Wellness Related to Healthcare Needs. **A client's energy and readiness to learn increases as his or her level of wellness increases.**

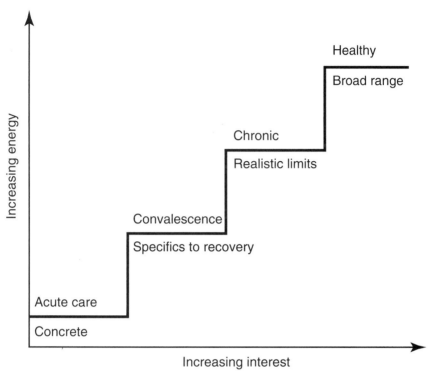

Source: Data from Maureen Sullivan RN, BS.

Psychosocial vital signs (PVS) is an assessment model that combines the measurement of a client's psychological experiences with the nurse's observations of anxiety and human responses as part of a holistic view of the client's health status (Spade & Mulhall, 2010). Each client completes a self-report of their perceptions on a 1–10 scale in four areas: client's perception of the situation, client's sense of support, client's coping ability, and client's anxiety level. Nurse observations include anxiety level measured as mild, moderate, severe, or panic. Nurse observations of human responses include cognitive, affective, spiritual, behavioral, and physical. This assessment tool engages clients through effective communication in a "collaborative patient centered relationship" (p. e150). You will find the PVS model in Appendix A.

Regardless of the number on the PVS scale, the nurse must observe a client's level of anxiety. Even if a client states that he or she is calm but behavior or thinking is at more than a mild level of anxiety, the client will have difficulty learning. A client with an anxiety level of severe or panic will be incapable of learning. These instances require the nurse to use therapeutic communication skills to facilitate clear thinking and delay health education to a more appropriate time.

Socioeconomic Factors

Nurses as educators need to consider **socioeconomic factors** when planning for health education because they have a significant impact on the health status of clients, especially minority groups. Socioeconomic factors include the client's living situation, financial status, health insurance or lack thereof, occupation or employment status, education, and the impact of these factors on the nature of the illness. Sufficient income affects the location and quality of housing, the level of education acquired, and occupational status. Clients' financial resources influence health status and health education. Middle- and high-income clients who are employed and have health insurance can purchase necessary services and supplies. A goal of Healthy People 2020 is to address health equity and disparities. Health equity is defined as the "attainment of the highest level of health for all people. Achieving health equity requires valuing everyone equally with focused and ongoing societal efforts to address avoidable inequalities, historical and contemporary injustices, and the elimination of health and healthcare disparities" (National Partnership for Action, 2011, para. 1). Health equity ensures that all people have access to health care regardless of their socioeconomic status, which is a goal of the Patient Protection and Affordable Care Act that passed in 2010 and was implemented in 2013.

Educational level has a profound impact on health status. The Centers for Disease Control and Prevention (CDC) reported a number of health differences between those with less than a high school education and those with a bachelor's degree or higher. Consider these examples:

- Obesity among boys and girls aged 2–19 years decreased as the educational level of the head of household increased. Obesity of boys decreased from 24% to 11%; obesity of girls decreased from 22% to 7%.
- Among 25-year-old women, the obesity range decreased from 39–43% to 25% for those with more education.
- The range of adults aged 50–75 years of age who reported a colorectal test or procedure increased from 45% to 67% among those with more education.

Similar findings related to the level of education were reported for life expectancy, depression, smoking, and other health problems (National Center for Health Statistics, 2011). Clients living alone need to be more independent in meeting their healthcare needs than clients living with supportive families and significant others. Clients living alone need realistic options that are suitable for their living situations. For example, a client living alone without neighbor or family support who needs a dressing change must be taught how to do so safely and independently. A client living with supportive family members may wish to have a family member learn how to do the dressing change. Homeless clients and those living in shelters present additional health education challenges (Bassuk, Volk, & Olivet, 2010). A difference in health perception is illustrated when nursing students serving in a homeless shelter were puzzled when they observed a 5-year-old child rolling an apple around on the floor. When the student spoke with the child's mother, she explained that her child had never seen an apple before and thought it was a toy. Regardless of the living situation, health education must be appropriate to the client's actual situation. **Box 4-1** provides basic information needed to offer financially appropriate health suggestions.

Nurses as educators need to be more sensitive, creative, and adaptable in meeting the health education needs of clients with limited financial resources. Nurses should be aware that decreasing the number of prescriptions, not taking prescribed medications, and skipping

BOX 4-1
Rapid Socioeconomic Assessment Tool

- What is your occupation?
- Is your monthly income sufficient to meet your expenses?
- Do you have health insurance?
- Do you have unmet financial needs related to health care?

doctor visits are common behaviors of clients with limited financial resources (Brown, 2008; Roberts-Grey, 2008). Part of your assessment is to verify whether clients are taking all their medications and teach them the importance of taking their medications as prescribed. A trusting nurse–client relationship will encourage the client to discuss his or her needs so the education can be appropriate.

In addition to socioeconomic factors affecting illness, clients' illnesses can impinge on their socioeconomic well-being. Individuals who are obese or suffering the effects of AIDS or hepatitis C may find that their diagnosis is a barrier to employment, social freedom, and other sources of socioeconomic support. Illnesses that family and friends perceive to be contagious can impinge on clients' socioeconomic well-being and lead to social isolation.

Cultural Factors

Culture is defined as "the totality of socially transmitted behavior, patterns, arts, beliefs, **values,** customs, lifeways, and all other products of human work and thought characteristic of a population of people that guides their world view and decision-making" (Purnell, 2013, p. 6). Cultural factors include beliefs, values, moral principles, habits, dress, language, rules for behavior, economics, politics, dietary practices, and health care (Burchum, 2002). Not only do cultural factors relate to race and **ethnicity,** but also to behaviors and beliefs characteristic of particular social, ethnic, disabled, age, and gender groups. Cultural factors are important to take into consideration when providing health education. The United States is increasingly multicultural and is often described as a melting pot (Racher & Annis, 2007).

The U.S. Census Bureau (2012) projects an older, more diverse nation by 2060. The number of those aged 65 years and older is expected to double from 43.1 million in 2012 to 92 million in 2060. The Hispanic population is projected to more than double, from 53.3 million in 2012 to 128.8 million in 2060; nearly one in three U.S. residents would be Hispanic. The black population is expected to increase from 41.2 million to 61.8 million over the same period; this represents an increase from 13.1% to 14.7% of the total population from 2012 to 2060. The Asian population is projected to more than double, from 15.9 million to 34.4 million over the same period; this represents an increase from 5.1% to 8.2% of the total population from 2012 to 2060.

Every region in the United States has a culturally diverse population. For nurses to be effective educators, it is important to assess cultural factors that will affect teaching and learning. Each person attributes his or her beliefs, values, and customs to cultural factors, and all nurses are affected by the culture of nursing and the healthcare delivery system. Within cultures there are many similarities and differences. Not all members of a single group hold the

---

BOX 4-2

Cultural Assessment for Health Education

- Do you identify with a particular ethnic or cultural group?
- Are you an immigrant or first- or second-generation citizen in this country?
- What do you believe is the cause of your health problem?
- What do you believe makes you healthy?
- What do you believe makes you sick?
- What remedies have you used to treat your health problems?
- What is your religious affiliation?
- Do you engage in any religious practices that you believe affect your health?
- Do you read and write in English, or do you prefer another language?
- What foods do you prefer, and what foods do you avoid?
- Do you have sufficient income (money) to meet your needs?
- Do you have family or friends who are available to support you if you need help?

---

same worldview or values (Burchum, 2002). Believing that your culture is superior to all others is called **ethnocentrism**. It is a barrier to critical thinking because it devalues the beliefs and values of people from other cultures and contributes to many social ills that are embodied in prejudice, discrimination, and racism (LaMar, 2013).

How nurses view health promotion, illness prevention, disease treatments, and care for the dying is determined by their culture (DeRosa & Kochurka, 2006). Nurses should strive to understand a client's cultural background and provide culturally congruent health education in cross-cultural situations. Culturally congruent health education is providing education that is meaningful and useful for individuals, families, groups, and communities, as well as for team members. It is identifying what is important to the client, the client's values, and how the client sees his or her present health situation (Cutilli, 2006).

As a busy educator, you will need to do an initial cultural assessment that covers the pertinent cultural factors related to teaching and learning. The questions in **Box 4-2** will guide you as you work with culturally diverse clients. The answers to these questions will give you direction in selecting teaching content, help you identify teaching strategies, and give you information to determine what instructional materials you will share with the client.

Educational Level

Approximately 30 million people older than 16 years in the United States cannot read better than the average third grader, 14% read at or below the fifth grade level, and 29% read at the eighth grade level, according to ProLiteracy Worldwide (2014). Health literacy is a concern in working with clients who need supplemental written material but are unable to read at a level sufficient to understand. Health literacy has profound implications for nurses as educators while they communicate with clients and provide health education reading materials.

The vocabulary that clients use is, to some extent, a measure of their health literacy and educational level. Those with large vocabularies are more apt to comprehend what you are saying.

Clients with less education are less likely to comprehend more abstract and technical language that you might inadvertently use. Concrete answers and examples are more likely to be meaningful to those with less education. A client's vocabulary impacts the type of health education materials that you provide, such as booklets and pamphlets (Seligman et al., 2007).

As you interact with clients, assess their knowledge about health and illness. Such an assessment provides clues that can guide health education activities. The client's level of education is often related to knowledge about health and illness. In general, the higher the level of education, the more likely the client is to engage in health-promoting behaviors such as exercise, proper diet, and smoking cessation (National Center for Health Statistics, 2011).

Clients who research health problems may have comprehensive knowledge of their illnesses. Nurses report this phenomenon more often in this era of increased availability of information on the Internet and the vast availability of materials and publications from libraries and healthcare providers. Clients are often articulate and well informed about the latest treatments for disease and are eager to collaborate with healthcare providers.

Because health literacy is so important in health education, we have included an easy-to-administer tool to assess health literacy, called the Newest Vital Sign (NVS), published by the American Academy of Physicians (Weiss et al., 2005). The tool takes approximately 3 minutes to administer and involves clients reading a nutrition label and then answering six questions. Four or more correctly answered questions indicate adequate literacy. The tool is also available in Spanish (**Figures 4-3 and 4-4**). **Box 4-3** summarizes the research that created the Newest Vital Sign tool.

Assessing health literacy is also a concern when teaching team members—not those who have years of formal educational preparation, but for team members in support roles such as nursing assistants. Team members may have limited knowledge of health and illness and often possess inaccurate information. They benefit from in-service activities that advance their understanding of their responsibilities. When preparing educational activities for team members, it is helpful to know what kind of theoretical and experiential preparation they have for their respective roles. This will help you plan educational activities that build on their current level of knowledge. If clients or team members are from a different culture or have limited English-speaking ability, this can affect their vocabulary and communication skills.

Health literacy and educational level are only approximations of what an individual client or team member can grasp. As educators, nurses must monitor the feedback from clients as they engage them in educational activities to determine their effectiveness. Also keep in mind that emotions may influence clients' ability to understand. For example, clients and their families have repeatedly stated to us that their anxiety level and other concerns interfered with their ability to comprehend material that would be quite understandable under normal circumstances.

ASSESSMENT OF GENERATIONAL DIFFERENCES

Nurses as educators must consider the age of the client as an important assessment factor when preparing health education offerings to adult learners. It is important to be aware of potential factors that can impede or promote learning. When building a teaching plan, it is helpful to consider fundamental generational differences beyond learners' control to choose effective teaching methods and strategies. **Table 4-4** examines the psychological and generational differences among the silent, baby boomer, generation X, and millennial generations. This is not intended to describe an individual, but rather to understand a cohort of learners.

FIGURE 4-3

Newest Vital Sign: Nutrition Information

Nutrition Facts	
Serving Size	1/2 cup
Servings per container	4
Amount per serving	
Calories 250	Fat Cal 120
	%DV
Total Fat 13g	20%
Sat Fat 9g	40%
Cholesterol 28mg	12%
Sodium 55mg	2%
Total Carbohydrate 30g	12%
Dietary Fiber 2g	
Sugars 23g	
Protein 4g	8%

* Percent Daily Values (DV) are based on a 2,000 calorie diet. Your daily values may be higher or lower depending on your calorie needs.

Ingredients: Cream, Skim Milk, Liquid Sugar, Water, Egg Yolks, Brown Sugar, Milkfat, Peanut Oil, Sugar, Butter, Salt, Carrageenan, Vanilla Extract.

Source: Reprinted with permission from "Quick Assessment of Literacy in Primary Care: The Newest Vital Sign," December, 2005, Annals of Family Medicine. Copyright 2005 American Academy of Family Physicians.

ASSESSMENT OF BACKGROUND KNOWLEDGE

It is important for the nurse as educator to check the client's background knowledge. Doing so is grounded in learning theories (Ausubel, Novak, & Hannesian, 1968; Dewey, 1938) and is supported by research on the learning process (Dochy, Segers & Buehl, 1999; Fisher & Frey, 2009; Tobias, 1994). The theory of constructivism supports this view of learning and proposes that new knowledge is constructed from old (Brooks & Brooks, 1993). It holds that as nurse educators, it is essential that we make connections among new information that is being presented and clients' prior experiences. Determining what clients already know allows you to do the following:

FIGURE 4-4

Newst Vital Sign Scoring Sheet

	ANSWER CORRECT?	
	YES	NO

READ TO SUBJECT: This information is on the back of a container of a pint of ice cream.

QUESTIONS

1. If you eat the entire container, how many calories will you eat?

    Answer ☐ 1,000 is the only correct answer   _____   _____

2. If you are allowed to eat 60 g of carbohydrates as a snack, how much ice cream could you have?

    Answer   Any of the following is correct: _____   _____
           ☐ 1 cup (or any amount up to 1 cup)
           ☐ Half the container

           Note: If patient answers "2 servings," ask "How much ice cream would that be if you were to measure it into a bowl?"

3. Your doctor advises you to reduce the amount of saturated fat in your diet. You usually have 42 g of saturated fat each day, which includes 1 serving of ice cream. If you stop eating ice cream, how many grams of saturated fat would you be consuming each day?

    Answer   33 is the only correct answer   _____   _____

4. If you usually eat 2,500 calories in a day, what percentage of your daily value of calories will you be eating if you eat one serving?

    Answer   10% is the only correct answer   _____   _____

Pretend that you are allergic to the following substances: Penicillin, peanuts, latex gloves, and bee stings.

5. Is it safe for you to eat this ice cream?

    Answer ☐ No   _____   _____

6. (Ask only if the patient responds "no" to question 5): Why not?

    Answer   Because it has peanut oil.   _____   _____

                            Total Correct   _____

TABLE 4-4

Generational Differences

Years	Silent 1925–1945	Boomer 1946–1964	Generation X 1965–1980	Millennial 1981–2000
Other names	Veterans Traditionalists	Consciousness generation Me generation	Lost generation Latchkey Slacker generation	Generation Y Echo boom Generation next

Family life	Earliest to marry
	  and have
	  children
	Divorce common
	Large number of
	  women entered
	  the workforce
		Religious and
		  spiritually
		  oriented
		Health conscious
		Defer childbirth
		  until later in life
		Attentive to
		  children;
		  helicopter
		  parents
			Adult oriented at
			  an early age
			Less parental
			  supervision
			  than earlier
			  generations
			Little peer
			  interaction in
			  childhood
			Balance work and
			  family
				Children
				  considered
				  special and
				  are eagerly
				  anticipated
				Families with fewer
				  children
				Balance work and
				  family

Work	Many entered
	  the helping
	  professions
	Hard work is good
	Respect authority
	Sacrifice
	Duty before fun
	Adhere to the rules
		Workaholics
		Career focused
		Work efficiently
		Personal
		  fulfillment
		Desire quality
		Will question
		  authority
			First to seek
			  balance
			   between work
			  and life
			Self-reliant
			Want structure
			  and direction
			Skeptical
			Challenge others
			Work is a difficult
			  challenge
				Financially
				  oriented
				More discretionary
				  income than any
				  previous group
				Multitasking
				Tolerant
				Goal oriented

Learning
preferences and
interactive style
	Like traditional
	  structure
	Will not contradict
	  instructor in
	  public
	Do not like being
	  singled out in
	  discussions
	Prefer to practice
	  alone
	May not ask
	  questions in
	  discussions
	May struggle with
	  technology
	Prefer learning
	  individually
		Enjoy working
		  creatively and
		  independently
		Sensitive to
		  criticism
		May have
		  significant
		  professional
		  experience
		Like interaction,
		  discussion, and
		  group work
		May dislike
		  authoritarian
		  teachers
		Prefer learning as
		  part of a team
			Self-reliant
			Like frequent
			  feedback
			May lack
			  interpersonal
			  skills
			Largest segment of
			  online learners
			Often impatient
			  but adaptable
			  and informal
			Technologically
			  capable
			Value autonomy
			Prefer an informal
			  learning
			  approach
				Team oriented, like
				  group work
				Multitask and
				  technological
				  experts
				Goal and
				  achievement
				  oriented
				Require more
				  structure and
				  mentoring
				Enjoy active
				  learning
				Prefer participative
				  learning

(continues)

| TABLE 4-4 |

Generational Differences (Continued)

Years	Silent 1925–1945	Boomer 1946–1964	Generation X 1965–1980	Millennial 1981–2000
Communication style	Formal Memo	In person	Direct Immediate	Email Voice mail
Teaching strategies	Emphasize important points in the teaching plan Use font large enough to see writing, and read handouts Fastest-growing group learning to use the Internet Encourage periodic movement while teaching	Give time to practice skills Use font large enough to see for older learners May not like role-playing exercises Enjoy most team projects Like being group leaders Like well-organized materials with headings	May resist group work outside of a formal class Give individual attention Prefer information in short lectures (15–20 minutes) Like working in small groups to review information Prefer graphics that are visually appealing and reflect the culture Want to have explanation for learning and skill acquisition	Present information and activities in steps Use up-to-date technology and resources Make learning relevant to real-life situations Encourage creativity and be creative in presentations Give supplemental reading and instructional materials

Sources: Modified from Baker College Effective Teaching and Learning Department (2004); Campbell and Brooks (2008).

- Target specific knowledge gaps (Angelo & Cross, 1993).
- Become aware of the diverse backgrounds of your clients.
- Create a bridge between clients' previous knowledge and new material.
- Check for misconceptions that may hinder learning new material (Ambrose et al., 2010).

For clients, understanding their starting point makes it easier for them to see what they have learned by the end of the teaching session. Awareness of their background knowledge can help them recall past learning and construct bridges between old and new knowledge (Angelo & Cross, 1993). The nurse educator determines from the assessment of background knowledge what clients already know in order to identify the specific knowledge and skills that are needed. From this information, pertinent learning objectives are developed. We think of background knowledge as falling into two categories: incidental and core. Incidental knowledge may be interesting but peripheral to the main concepts, and core knowledge is essential to understanding new concepts (Fisher & Frey, 2009). Both types of background knowledge help establish learning objectives.

There are different techniques to check background knowledge. Plan your assessment by asking the following questions:

BOX 4-3

Evidence-Based Research: Newest Vital Sign

Weiss et al. (2005). Quick assessment of literacy in primary care: The newest vital sign. *Annals of Family Medicine, 3*(6), 514–522.

Purpose: The purpose of this research was to develop a quick and accurate screening test, available in English and Spanish, for patients with limited literacy.

Method: To create the tool, candidate items for the new instrument and the Test of Functional Health Literacy in Adults (TOFHLA) were administered to 250 English-speaking and 250 Spanish-speaking primary care patients. Statistical tests were used to determine which of the candidate test items from the new instrument best correlated with results of the TOFHLA.

Results: The final instrument, the Newest Vital Sign (NVS), is a nutrition label that is accompanied by six questions and requires 3 minutes for administration. It is reliable in English and Spanish and correlates with the TOFHLA. The NVS is suitable for use as a quick screening for limited literacy in primary healthcare settings.

The NVS is available online at http://www.annfammed.org/content/3/6/514.full.

- What do you assume clients already know?
- What kinds of questions will help you confirm your assumptions?
- What are some common misconceptions related to the topic?
- How are you going to analyze and respond to the data your assessment provides?

You can choose from a variety of methods to assess clients' background knowledge and skills. Some methods are direct measures of clients' capabilities, such as written tests. Other methods use indirect measures, such as clients' self-reports of what they know. The method of assessment will depend on what is to be learned. Classroom Assessment Techniques (CATs) are a set of specific activities that educators use to quickly gauge learners' comprehension (Angelo & Cross, 1993). They are used to assess individual or group understanding of the material, and with minor modifications they apply to teaching in healthcare settings.

The following sections are a sample of different background learning assessment techniques using Bloom's taxonomy categories of knowledge, skills, and attitudes. These techniques may be used with individuals or groups. The three main areas of background knowledge assessment include assessing recall and understanding (knowledge); assessing skills in analysis, critical thinking, and performance (skills); and assessing awareness of attitudes and values (attitudes).

Assessing Recall and Understanding (Knowledge)

Assessing recall and understanding of knowledge can be done in several ways. A primary approach to determining prior knowledge is through the Background Knowledge Probe. This consists of short, simple questions that can be administered either verbally or written and are usually referred to as a pretest. This approach is helpful in determining the most effective starting point for learning and the appropriate level to begin instruction. Constructing a pretest serves several purposes, including: (1) current knowledge status, (2) guidance for future activities, (3) means of comparison for posttest results, and (4) determination of whether prerequisite knowledge is achieved.

To prepare a pretest, determine what key ideas and concepts you are trying to teach. Establish learning outcomes and objectives. Review the client's record or the group's course outline to help with this step. Brainstorm 10 to 15 questions that would effectively assess prior knowledge based on the learning outcomes and objectives you reestablished. A simple strategy to use in preparing questions is to reword the learning outcomes or objectives as questions. Be sure to select a variety of types of questions (multiple choice, true–false, fill in the blank, etc.). Varying the types of questions will peak the clients' interest in learning the material. Base your types of questions on your assessment and the information being taught.

Another approach to assessing prior knowledge is a technique called muddiest point. Here the individual or group is asked to share either verbally or in writing what questions confuse them about the proposed topic. For example, in an initial meeting the nurse educator says: You have heard about the different treatment options for acne. What questions would you still like answered regarding these treatment options?

A memory matrix could also be used to help determine how clients recall content and organize information. A matrix is created with rows, columns, and empty cells. This strategy assesses the ability of the learner to recall content and display skill in organizing information. This method can be presented on a white board or with cardboard figures and pictures on a desk or table. For example, a memory matrix for food characteristics would look like this (**Table 4-5**):

TABLE 4-5

Characteristic	Eating Healthy	Eating Unhealthy
Carbohydrates		
Proteins		
Fats		

Assessing Analysis, Critical Thinking, and Performance (Skills)

Assessing skill in analysis, critical thinking, and performance is done through a variety of approaches, depending on what aspect of skill is being assessed. In the problem recognition task, clients are presented with examples of common problems and are asked to identify the particular type of problem in each example. Clients read or are told the scenario; then they identify the problem. A sample problem is presented below. Identify and explain Mrs. Simpson's problem.

> Margaret Simpson is an 86-year-old woman who has lived alone in her own home for the past 20 years. Her son and daughter both live in different states but have frequent telephone contact and yearly visits. They are concerned about their mother and believe it is time for her to move into an assisted living facility where she will receive regular meals and routine assistance with activities of daily living. This is a sensitive topic, and the children are having a difficult time persuading their mother to see the benefits of moving.

FIGURE 4-5

Series of Events Chain

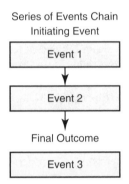

Series of Events Chain
Initiating Event

Event 1

↓

Event 2

↓

Final Outcome

Event 3

Assessing critical thinking skills can also be assessed by the series of events chain (see **Figure 4-5**). This method describes states of something in a linear procedure or the goals, actions, and outcomes of a behavior. Clients can be assessed either individually or as a group. Key questions for this activity could include the following: What is the object, procedure, or initiating event? What are the stages or steps? How do they lead to one another? What is the final outcome? From the answers, prior knowledge can be assessed regarding the order of events.

Assessing performance skills can be achieved in a number of ways, including client demonstrations, client products, and work samples. To demonstrate skills, clients are given scenarios and are asked to perform skills such as checking blood glucose levels. Abilities are assessed through direct observation. Skills can also be assessed through past performance and past documentation, such as medical records or nurses' notes.

Assessing Attitudes and Values (Attitudes)

Assessing clients' awareness of their attitudes and values can be accomplished using the opinion poll strategy. This approach provides anonymity for clients and allows the educator to understand their opinions. Examples of survey statements are as follows: (1) it is important to stop smoking, and (2) drinking five beers a day is a safe amount of alcohol.

Another strategy to determine values is through a self-confidence survey. This type of survey consists of a few simple questions aimed at getting a rough measure of the client's self-confidence in relation to a specific skill or ability. Examples of questions are as follows: How confident are you about breastfeeding your baby? Do you feel comfortable giving your baby medication for a high fever?

In addition to using tools to determine background knowledge, each healthcare team member has valuable information about clients and their learning needs and abilities. Collaborating with others who care for the client gives you a better picture and helps you design more effective teaching strategies. Determining learning needs, preferred learning style, and learning readiness are all requirements included in The Joint Commission standards for client and family education. The process of assessing needs begins when healthcare team members identify a need for a client to learn new skills or acquire more information. If a client asks a question (What exactly will this operation involve? How will I handle this when I go home?), he or she is already identifying the information need. If you, rather than the client, identify the need, your job will be not only to deliver the information in such a way that the client is able to understand it, but also to demonstrate to the client why the information is important.

In some instances there are differences between the client's and the nurse educator's view of the need to know. The educator may perceive the need for information when the client does not. For example, a nurse tries to give the client medication information during discharge teaching. The client's response is, "Oh, I don't need to know that. I trust my doctor. Whatever he ordered is fine. There is no reason why I should know all the details." In this example the best approach may be for the nurse to start with why the information is important and explain that the physician depends on the client knowing information before taking the medication.

Do not be tempted to overlook background knowledge when teaching new information. To do so is to build on an unstable foundation. Background knowledge has a profound influence on clients' abilities to comprehend what they are taught and believe. Its effect can be defined directly (such as knowledge of the topic) and indirectly (through clients' abilities to resolve problems). Determining background knowledge is a part of the learning needs assessment that influences the nurse as educator's approach to teaching clients.

COMMUNICATION CHALLENGES DURING ASSESSMENT

To assess clients accurately, you must be skilled at both verbal and nonverbal communication. It facilitates health education or hinders it. Words convey a variety of meanings and can be misinterpreted, especially by members of different cultural groups. Never assume that all clients from one ethnic group hold the same beliefs. Nurses can overcome these problems by asking clients how they interpreted the health message. Nonverbal communication (body cues, tone of voice, facial expression, and space between communicants) sends a message. Nurses who answer clients' or team members' questions but appear to be in a hurry will stifle communication (Horowitz, 2014).

Communication difficulties become challenges for nurses to overcome as they provide health education. The sources of these challenges come from clients and nurses (Pohl, 1981). This section addresses common communication problems affecting the teaching and learning process and suggests solutions.

Hearing Impairment

Approximately 17% of American adults (36 million) report some degree of hearing loss. Hearing loss increases with age. According to the National Institute on Deafness and Other Communication Disorders (2013), 18% of American adults aged 45–64 years, 30% of adults aged 65–74 years, and 47% of adults aged 75 years and older have hearing loss. The prevalence of hearing trouble is defined as a little trouble, a lot of trouble, or deaf. Clients with long-standing hearing deficits tell nurses what modes of communication work best for them. During the initial assessment, nurses can identify various ways that clients communicate. Clients or family members can provide this information, but family members should not be used as interpreters if confidentiality is a concern (Lieu, Sadler, Fullerton, & Stohlmann, 2007). To quickly assess a client's hearing, talk to the client in a normal tone of voice and note his or her reaction. If the client answers appropriately, you will know the client's hearing is sufficient for teaching and learning. Another assessment strategy is to cover your mouth and ask a question, again in a normal tone of voice. A client with a hearing impairment will not hear to answer you.

Check to see if the client wears a hearing aid. If so, make sure it is turned on and that the batteries are working. Creating other means of sound augmentation, such as cupping your hands around the client's ears or using the stethoscope in reverse, are other options.

When working with hearing-impaired clients, position yourself close on the same level as the client, and face the client so that person knows you are communicating with him or her. The client should be able to see your face and read your lips. Avoid standing in an area with a background glare because that interferes with the client's ability to read your lips. Remember to enunciate clearly and slowly. Clients who are proficient lip readers discern less than half of what you say and depend on the context and guesses to determine your meaning (Lieu et al., 2007).

Clients who rely on American Sign Language (ASL) require the assistance of a qualified sign language interpreter. This is considered a reasonable accommodation that healthcare institutions are required to offer under the Americans with Disabilities Act. Communication tools, such as flash cards, pencils and pads, and a laptop computer, are all helpful to clients who know how to write and have the strength to do so. If you are using writing, remember to choose simple words and phrases and write legibly (Lieu et al., 2007). The most important thing is to find a way to elicit responses that help you assess the client's hearing abilities and comprehension.

Vision Impairment

According to the CDC (2014), approximately 14 million people aged 12 years and older have a visual impairment, and 80% of those problems could be corrected to good vision with refractive lenses. The prevalence of visual impairment increases with age, particularly among those aged 40 years and older, based on 2010 census figures. The most common problems in this age group are cataracts, refractive errors, diabetic retinopathy, glaucoma, and age-related macular degeneration. The number of visually impaired people is expected to increase due to the increasing incidence of diabetes and other chronic diseases in the rapidly aging U.S. population (National Eye Institute, n.d.; Prevent Blindness America, 2012).

As clients live longer and visual impairment becomes more common, it is an important consideration for nurses providing health education. To quickly assess a client's vision, provide a magazine or newspaper and have the client read a paragraph out loud. As the client does so, note the distance between the paper and the client's face. Holding the paper more than 14 inches away may indicate presbyopia or hyperopia. This will give you a sense of the client's visual capabilities and how to adapt your teaching plan.

People who have been blind for some time develop other senses, particularly hearing, to compensate. Their acute hearing makes being shouted at a painful experience, and it does not aid their comprehension. Clients who are blind are unable to make use of body language or lip reading. If you are accustomed to expressing yourself with your hands and shaking your head, be aware that such clues are unavailable to blind clients. We recommend that you learn to use more verbal descriptions and psychomotor learning strategies that might not be necessary with a sighted client.

Blind people can often discern if a door is open or closed by the sound in a room. A door halfway ajar, however, can be deceiving and dangerous. We recommend that you close doors or open them all the way. It is also courteous to announce your presence and your purpose; for example, "My name is Fred Jones, and I'm your nurse for today. I'm going to teach you about . . . , then later we'll review. . . . Tell me what you are most interested in learning."

Speech Impairment

Speech problems impact clients who have a pathologic impairment in their ability to communicate. The type of impairment is related to the location and type of brain lesion. There are other forms of speech impairment related to a psychological etiology, but our reference here is to clients with brain pathology resulting in dysphasia, which is impairment of speech consisting of lack of coordination and failure to arrange words in the proper order. If a client has a form of dysphasia as an aftermath of stroke, consult with a psychologist and neurologist to determine the best way to deal with the speech impairment. One client may understand your words and not be able to answer. Another may not understand your words but can interpret your pantomime, drawings, flash cards, or objects. Shouting is not helpful in communicating with clients who are speech impaired.

Nurses as Educators' Contribution to Communication Challenges

The final communication problem we address is the one that nurses might inadvertently create. Mumbling, using technical jargon, or talking when you should be listening interferes with effective communication. Learn to recognize signs of poor client communication: confused facial expression, lack of attention, and questions that indicate a lack of understanding.

Suggestions to reduce this barrier include the art of active listening and observing. Listening includes not only hearing what the client is saying and the tone with which it is said, but also observing body language. It is developing a sensitivity to the spoken and unspoken meaning of the client's communication. Listening is an active, not a passive, process. Listening is an essential skill required of effective nurses in the educator role. Nurses may not agree with everything a client or team member says, but it is important to listen and respect the individual. Give complete attention to the learner and do not be preoccupied with your own thoughts. As educators, it is easy to think we should do the talking, but it is just as important to listen (Stuart, 2005).

As you listen, learn from the client's story and experience with the health problem. The problem may manifest in a manner that is not entirely consistent with the textbook description, which is called a variant of normal. Learn how the health problem is affecting the client's activities of daily living, and consider ways that you can help improve the client's adjustment and reaction. When you are a practicing nurse, you will be exposed to a broad range of human adaptations to health problems.

ASSESSMENT OF THE TEACHING AND LEARNING ENVIRONMENT

The **teaching and learning environment** is composed of the psychological environment and physical environment in which teaching and learning takes place. It is the nurse's responsibility to establish the psychological and physical environment to maximize learning.

Psychological Environment

As educators, nurses create the emotional tone for the learning environment. A positive, enthusiastic tone does much to make clients comfortable and helps to create a therapeutic environment. If the nurse is stressed, clients pick up on it and may assume that the stress is related to them. Conversely, if the nurse enjoys teaching and shows enthusiasm, that perception is conveyed as well.

Showing respect for learners and valuing their questions and input are all part of creating a positive teaching and learning environment. The nurse's attitude should be nonjudgmental. However, that does not mean the nurse agrees with or condones the client's beliefs and statements. Respect is accepting and valuing the client. The nurse has a responsibility to correct misinformation.

Physical Environment

As educators, nurses are responsible for assessing the physical environment and making it as conducive to learning as possible (Hall, 2013). The physical environment includes space; temperature; visual, auditory, and olfactory stimuli; equipment; resources; furniture arrangement; physical comfort; and sufficient time for learning.

Space is needed so you can display and get maximum use of your instructional materials. This is true whether you are speaking to an individual, a family, or a group in a living room or an auditorium. Examine the space for sight and sound barriers. Pillars will make it difficult for clients to see you. Poorly placed partitions may act as sound barriers that will prevent sound from getting through.

Temperatures that are too hot or too cold interfere with learning. Clients who are distracted by heat spend their time fanning themselves; if they are cold they clutch their arms instead of listening to you.

Visual stimuli are distracting and interfere with vision. Do not place yourself in front of a sunny window. The glare behind you turns you into a shadowy figure. Your audience will be squinting and wanting to look elsewhere. Try to pick a spot where you can control the appearance of the learning situation. If you cannot control all the stimuli, look for ways to control the area in which you intend to teach. In the hospital you may draw the curtain around the client's bed. One way to modify sound in a client's room is to hang a sign on the door that says, "Client teaching in progress. Please return in X minutes. Thank you."

If your client is a family, you may be able to cordon off a corner of the waiting room. In a dining area of an extended care facility, you may be able to use moveable screens to provide privacy. Auditory stimuli may or may not be under your control. Choose a quiet place and turn off your cell phone. Olfactory stimuli are distracting and can be deflected by a fan. You could try cutting a lemon or putting a drop of cinnamon oil on a nearby heated surface, such as a light fixture, or use a room deodorizer.

The availability of equipment and teaching resources influence your options. Find out what equipment, expertise, and resources are available in the hospital or community to enhance teaching. Observe where the electrical outlets are if you will need them, and arrange the room to allow access to the outlets.

Arrange furniture in a way that is conducive to learning. Be sure to take into account the learning objectives and teaching strategies. Do you plan to have the clients interact with one another? Do you wish a relative to see everything you are doing for the client? Do you plan to make a presentation to a group or have a guest lecturer? Nurses should be involved in designing the spaces where teaching occurs.

Physical comfort is an important variable in enhancing the teaching and learning environment. Teach clients after the morning routine when they are comfortable and relaxed. You will find that your clients learn better when they are sufficiently medicated to not be distracted by pain but not too sleepy to pay attention. Lighting and temperature also affect comfort. You will want the lighting to be bright enough to allow lip readers to see your face but not so strong that it creates glare.

Time is a factor to consider. Be sure you have sufficient time to teach. If time is limited, be selective about what you teach, focusing on only the most important topics. Do not make your teaching session too long. A mistake we have seen busy nurses make is trying to include too much information too quickly in the available time.

TEACHING AND LEARNING SETTINGS

The teaching and learning settings that we consider here include the hospital, long-term care or assisted living facility, private home, school, work site, and community. Each has unique characteristics that affect the way health education is delivered.

Hospital

The value of health education is supported by hospitals. Although the quantity and quality are frequently affected by policies and administrative support, the importance of health education in acute care settings is reflected in role expectations and job descriptions. The mission and philosophy of hospitals reflect the importance of client education. Hospital administrators are now required to meet The Joint Commission standards by providing necessary support and resources for patient teaching. Every hospital has an education department that focuses on client and staff education. They are responsible for discharge planning and case management for clients and competency training for staff. Hospitalized clients have teaching needs that revolve around acute illness and discharge planning. Some hospitals also offer classes for the community related to health promotion.

Long-Term Care and Assisted Living Facility

Long-term care facilities include nursing homes, assisted-living homes, and other facilities in which care is provided for clients over a prolonged period of time. Long-term care includes a wide range of services that are provided over an extended period of time to clients who need help to perform normal activities of daily living because of a variety of health problems. Services within long-term care include rehabilitative therapies, skilled nursing care, palliative care, and social services, as well as supervision and a wide range of supportive personal care provided by family caregivers or home care agencies. Most long-term care and assisted living facilities also have education departments.

The goals of long-term care include training to help clients adjust to or overcome limitations. Like hospitals, health education in long-term care and assisted living facilities can occur individually or in groups. Effective educational programs can prevent minor illnesses or injuries from progressing to the point of needing professional intervention. Increased client awareness through education can also result in earlier detection of problems and timelier outpatient intervention, thus decreasing hospitalizations. Clients with chronic illnesses who have been empowered through health education programs generally have better coping skills and are usually less reliant on healthcare providers.

Assisted living facilities for the rapidly aging population are becoming more popular. They provide apartment-type living for those who need only selected services, which are individualized to the client. For example, some clients may take one or all meals a day in a central dining room. Others may need assistance only with bathing or dressing. General housekeeping laundry service is also available. If additional services are needed, such as checking on selected clients more frequently, that can be arranged.

Private Home

Many health problems are being treated at home as chronic illnesses increase in an aging population. Home care is a formal, government-regulated program of care that provides a range of services offered by different agencies and are delivered by a variety of healthcare professionals. Among clients aged 65 years and older, cancer was more common among men, and essential hypertension was more common among women. In this group women were more likely to be aged 85 years and older, and men were more likely to receive home care as postacute care (CDC, 2012). Common chronic diseases that are prevalent in this age group include heart disease, cancer, chronic lower respiratory diseases, and stroke. Also increasing in frequency is Alzheimer's disease and diabetes mellitus (CDC, 2010). This shows the importance of addressing health education in private homes.

Home visits for elderly clients have been found to have direct benefits when measured in terms of morbidity and admission to long-term institutional care. Clients are discharged from acute care settings with increasingly complex treatment and learning needs. Families are expected to learn skills and information that, only a decade ago, were reserved for healthcare personnel. Home care visits are also made by community health nurses to women with newborns to teach them proper baby care. The nurse also observes and assesses progress in child growth and development.

Clients often find it easier to learn in familiar surroundings. Remember that in the client's home you are a guest and are not in charge, as you are when the client is in a healthcare institution. During home care nursing it will be easier for you to be realistic in your teaching because you can see the reality of the client's environment. Family dynamics that may enhance or impede recovery will be more evident in the home, which means you will likely be more realistic in teaching the family and the client.

School

School is an ideal site for health education because it is a focal point for reducing health risk behaviors and improving the heath status of youth. Based on the potential to reach a large number of youth, schools are logical sites for interventions that help them develop skills, change health behaviors, and empower them to take responsibility for their own health. Some of the most effective health education efforts for youth incorporate peer support. Although most schools require health education, teachers are often not comfortable with sensitive subjects and need the contributions of school nurses in addressing certain topics.

If you are teaching a class, you will want to find out more information about the group of students. Ask about the culture of the classroom. What ages are the children? Are they accustomed to discipline and to giving polite attention? Are they able to sit and listen? What are their learning style preferences? What health education tools are already available? This is important information for the teaching plan.

Schools are often good settings for teaching and learning with multiple audiovisual aids. Teaching disease prevention and providing anticipatory guidance are excellent topics. Nurses are informed role models to address today's concerns about how to avoid communicable diseases and substance abuse, and teach behaviors that promote healthful living. Learn the age of the group you will speak to and address age-appropriate topics. Ideally health education begins in grade schools.

Work Site

Work site settings are beneficial to managers, employees, and the community. Nurses in work site settings are effective providers of health education. These educational programs provide an opportunity to support health while reducing healthcare costs, increasing worker productivity, and decreasing absenteeism. Interventions in the workplace may target behavioral change, the development of policies to facilitate a healthier and safer workplace, and environmental support to maintain behavioral changes.

Concerns that nurses in work site settings can address include consultation about cost-effective insurance plans, infection and accident control, and health promotion and maintenance programs. These nurses can also conduct physical assessments, teach prevention to employees, provide screening services, produce health newsletters, and inform employers about major health hazards in the setting. The political system at the work site greatly affects the ability of the nurse as an educator to be effective. Self-help groups for alcoholism, smoking cessation, stress management, prevention of accidents, and safety precautions are all worthy topics for consideration.

Community

Health education in the community focuses on health problems identified as a priority by the public health department or other community agency responsible for community health planning. The focus of nurses as educators in public health is to provide direct care through a process of evaluation and assessment of the needs of individuals in the context of their population group. Regardless of the environment within the community where nurses work, the health education process can be used to establish partnerships with clients so nurses can provide education and counseling to promote self-management. Nurses as educators work with other care providers to plan, develop, and support systems and programs in the community that emphasize health promotion, disease prevention, and access to care.

Community assessment focuses on populations rather than individuals. Those individuals who make up a population share one or more personal or environmental characteristics. A population can be categorized as a population at risk or a population of interest (Keller, Strohschein, & Briske, 2008). A population at risk shares an identified risk factor or risk exposure that threatens its health. For example, all individuals who smoke are at risk for developing respiratory and cardiovascular health problems.

A population of interest may be basically healthy but could improve its health and prevent illness from developing. Examples include making home visits to new mothers to encourage breastfeeding or working with adolescents to prevent sexually transmitted diseases by offering programs in public schools. Other populations of interest may be needs-based, such as mothers and infants or cancer survivors; age-based groups, such as adolescents, older adults (65 years and older); gender-based groups, such as men or women; and ethnic groups, such as African American, Hispanic American, Asian American, and American Indian.

ASSESSMENT TOOLS FOR TEACHING INDIVIDUALS AND GROUPS

Box 4-4 is an assessment tool for nurses who find themselves in a teachable moment with clients. It is for those unplanned opportunities that arise in the course of nursing practice when the nurse needs a tool for guidance. It is a quick teaching assessment guide that is useful in a variety of settings in which the teaching is informal and spontaneous. For example, the guide can be useful for nurses at the bedside, in a client's home, at a clinic, at a school, at a work site, and in a doctor's office. Practicing nurses are busy; it is not always possible to conduct a thorough assessment as outlined in this chapter. The tool addresses client Concerns and Client knowledge, then moves on to Create a teaching plan and Carry out a teaching plan. Each area requires the nurse to Ask, Observe, and Listen (CCCC/AOL Quick Assessment Tool for Teaching Individuals). The purpose of this tool is to guide nurses as educators in quickly assessing and teaching a client when health education is indicated.

Table 4-6 is an assessment tool, called the Assessment Tool for Teaching Groups, for nurses who are planning health education for a group of people. Interested groups may be found in hospitals, long-term care facilities, schools, work sites, and community settings. We recommend that nurses review teaching priorities, goals, objectives, and content with a representative at the facility before the presentation. Careful assessment of the educational needs and communication with a representative at the facility will help bring about a successful educational offering.

BOX 4-4

CCCC/AOL Quick Assessment Tool for Teaching Individuals

Assess Client Concerns
Ask: What are your concerns?
Observe: Nonverbal behavior
Listen: Spoken and unspoken words

Assess Client Knowledge
Ask: What do you understand about the condition?
Observe: Nonverbal behavior
Listen: Determine accuracy of knowledge and teaching needs

Create Teaching Plan
Ask self: What type and amount of information is needed?
Observe: Context of client situation
Listen: Reflect on appropriateness of teaching plan

Carry Out Teaching Plan
Ask: What is your understanding of what I have explained?
Observe: Nonverbal cues to understanding or not understanding; return demonstration
Listen: Client feedback, evaluate teaching effectiveness, determine additional educational needs

TABLE 4-6	

Assessment Tool for Teaching Groups

Assessment Steps	Action Steps
1. Identify the educational need.	1. Assess group members' perceptions and knowledge base through surveys and focus groups. 2. Examine and clarify educational needs.
2. Identify group characteristics.	1. Determine the group size. 2. Determine the group's educational level. 3. Determine the group's pertinent cultural aspects. 4. Determine the group's other pertinent characteristics.
3. Identify current evidence-based practice research.	1. Review the literature for evidence-based research on the topic. 2. Evaluate the current evidence-based practice research that is applicable to the educational need.
4. Identify goals, objectives, and content.	1. Formulate goals and objectives based on educational need. 2. Prepare a content outline.
5. Determine facility support.	1. Does the facility agree with the educational need? 2. Does the facility support the content you are proposing in the educational offering? 3. Will the facility provide space and resources for the educational offering? 4. Are facilities and resources available to hold the class? 5. Does the facility have a plan to ensure that group members can participate in the educational offering?

An example of using this tool is a situation in which a nurse gives a presentation on preventing back injuries to a group of registered nurses. With the facility's support the nurse surveys the registered nurses to determine their perceptions and knowledge of the topic. The nurse reviews the literature for evidence-based research related to the topic and develops a teaching plan that includes learning objectives, content, and teaching strategies.

The next step in the assessment process is to determine the facility's support and approval of the educational offering. The nurse seeks facility support throughout the assessment process. This tool can be used for nurses planning educational programs in clinics, community centers, schools, work site settings, and for civic groups. Health education is appropriate in any place where there is an educational need. The tool applies to groups of students, clients, employees, and healthcare team members in a multitude of settings.

SUMMARY

This chapter covered a multitude of factors that nurses as educators must take into consideration when planning for health education, be it with individuals, families, groups or communities, or health team members. The assessment of clients and their teaching and learning needs are greatly influenced by your perception of their ability to learn. We provide tools to assess readiness to learn, motivation to learn, level of wellness related to healthcare needs, PVS, socioeconomic factors, cultural factors, and health literacy. Clients who are members of different generations require special recognition about how their lived experiences affect teaching and learning. In addition, how to assess a client's background knowledge and how it impacts learning was discussed.

Communication is an essential component in client assessment. Clients with hearing, vision, and speech impairments require special adaptations. Nurses also might inadvertently create communication problems. Nurses as educators are expected to create a positive teaching and learning psychological and physical environment. Teaching and learning occurs in a variety of settings, each of which has unique characteristics that impact learning. Settings discussed included the hospital, long-term care facility, private home, school, work site, and community. The CCCC/AOL Quick Assessment Tool for Teaching Individuals and the Assessment Tool for Teaching Groups provides guidance to the nurse as educator in planning health education.

EXERCISES

Exercise I: Perception in Assessment

Purpose: Examine how your interpretations of what you see and hear affect your interactions with clients.
Directions:

1. Share one example in which the client's perception of his or her health status was significantly different from yours.
2. Describe a situation in which it was easy to relate to a client. What factors in you and the client made it easy to relate?
3. Describe a situation in which it was difficult to relate to a client. What factors in you and the client made it difficult relate?
4. How did this affect your assessment of the client's learning needs?

Exercise II: Assessing Readiness to Learn

Purpose: Apply the knowledge of readiness to learn to clients.
Directions:

1. In a small group, differentiate among **experiential readiness**, emotional readiness, and physiologic and **developmental readiness**.
2. Give an example of each type of readiness.
3. How will you apply this knowledge to teaching a client about diabetes care?

Exercise III: Assessing Levels of Wellness

Purpose: Examine how a client's level of wellness affects his or her readiness to learn.

Directions:

1. Working alone, assess your own level of wellness using the Stoeckel Wellness–Illness Functional Continuum. Plot the continuum for each factor to determine strengths and weaknesses. Give yourself a score between 0 and 10.
2. Give an example of teaching content that would be appropriate for each of the needs you have identified.

Exercise IV: Critical Thinking and Health Education

Purpose: Apply critical thinking to health education in a variety of situations.
Directions: Form small groups of three to four members and assign each group one of the following examples. After a discussion period, return to the whole class and share the solutions generated by each group.

1. You are concerned about clients being discharged early from the surgical unit before they have dealt with any of the stages of emotional adjustment to trauma, and you have grave doubts about the effectiveness of the teaching you are expected to do. Identify a real situation and work on creative ways to assess clients and achieve reasonable educational goals.
2. You are working with an unemployed, homeless client who lives on the streets and needs daily insulin injections. He is mildly retarded but seems motivated to help himself. Provide creative, workable solutions for this client.
3. You are a home care nurse visiting a client with slowly advancing dementia who lives alone and has no family and few neighbors. She insists on living in her home. You find very little food in her cupboards and spoiled food in the refrigerator. What creative solutions can you find to help this client?

Exercise V: Teaching and Learning Settings

Purpose: Assess the impact of teaching and learning settings on health education.
Directions: You are preparing to teach clients the importance of eating a healthy diet to include the food categories and daily nutritional requirements needed to maintain health. Discuss how your teaching approach will change in the following settings:

1. Hospital, convalescent, and nursing home
2. Client's private home
3. High school
4. Work site setting
5. Community setting

Exercise VI: Apply the Quick CCCC/AOL Assessment Tool for Teaching Individuals and the Assessment Tool for Teaching Groups

Purpose: Apply the assessment tools for teaching individuals and groups.
Directions: Divide the class into at least two groups. Assign one group to discuss how they will apply the CCCC/AOL Quick Assessment Tool for Teaching Individuals. Assign the other group

to discuss how they will apply the Assessment Tool for Teaching Groups. Allow approximately 15 minutes. Reconvene the class and let each group report on their discussion.

REFERENCES

Ambrose, S. A., Bridges, M. W., DiPietro, M., Lovette, M. C., Norman, M. K., & Mayer, R. E. (2010). *How learning works: Seven research-based principles for smart teaching.* San Francisco, CA: Jossey-Bass.

Angelo, T. A., & Cross, K. P. (1993). *Classroom assessment techniques: A handbook for college teachers* (2nd ed.). San Francisco, CA: Jossey-Bass.

Ausubel, D., Novak, J., & Hannesian, H. (1968). *Educational psychology: A cognitive view* (2nd ed.). New York, NY: Holt Rinehart & Winston.

Baker College Effective Teaching and Learning Department. (2004). Teaching across generations. Retrieved from http://www.mcc.edu/pdf/pdo/teaching_across_gen.pdf

Bassuk, E. L., Volk, K. T., & Olivet, J. (2010). A framework for developing supports and services for families experiencing homelessness. *The Open Health Services and Policy Journal, 3,* 34–40.

Bonner, S., Zimmerman, B. J., Evans, D., Irigoyen, M., Resnick, D., & Mellins, R. B. (2002). An individualized intervention to improve asthma management among urban Latino and African-American families. *Journal of Asthma, 39*(2), 167–179.

Brooks, J. G., & Brooks, M. G. (1993). *In search of understanding: The case for constructivist classrooms.* Alexandria, VA: Association for Supervision and Curriculum Development.

Brown, S. B. (2008). A dangerous bind for American workers. *Hospitals and Health Networks, 82*(11), 54.

Burchum, J. L. R. (2002). Cultural competence: An evolutionary perspective. *Nursing Forum, 37*(4), 5–15.

Campbell, J., & Brooks, C. (2008). Tools for effective teaching. Retrieved from https://cache.trustedpartner .com/docs/library/000223/Transforming%20Behaviors%20Conference%20Materials/Effective%20 Teaching%20Stategies_J%20Campbell_C%20Brooks_11_21_08.pdf

Centers for Disease Control and Prevention. (2010). Deaths and mortality. Retrieved from http://www .cdc.gov/nchs/fastats/deaths.htm

Centers for Disease Control and Prevention. (2012). National home and hospice care survey. Retrieved from http://www.cdc.gov/nchs/nhhcs.htm

Centers for Disease Control and Prevention. (2014). Vision health initiative (VHI). Retrieved from http:// www.cdc.gov/visionhealth/

Connolly, S., Simpson, D., & Petty, C. (2006). *Anxiety disorders.* New York, NY: Chelsea House.

Cutilli, C. C. (2006). Do your patients understand? *Orthopaedic Nursing, 25*(3), 218–224.

DeRosa, N., & Kochurka, K. (2006). Implement culturally competent healthcare in your workplace. *Nursing Management, 37*(10), 18–26.

Dewey, J. (1938). *Experience and education.* New York, NY: Collier Books.

Dochy, F., Segers, M., & Buehl, M. (1999). The relation between assessment practices and outcomes of studies: The case of research on prior knowledge. *Review of Educational Research, 69*(2), 145–186.

Fisher, D., & Frey, N. (2009). *Background knowledge: The missing piece of the comprehension puzzle.* Portsmouth, NH: Heinemann.

Glynn, S. M., Aultman, L. P., & Owens, A. M. (2005). Motivation to learn in general education programs. *The Journal of General Education, 54*(2), 150–170.

Hall, A. M. (2013). Client education. In P. A. Potter, A. G. Perry, P. A. Stockert, & A. M. Hall (Eds.), *Fundamentals of nursing* (8th ed., pp. 328–347). St. Louis, MO: Mosby Elsevier.

Horowitz, J. A. (2014). The therapeutic relationship. In C. L. Edelman, E. C. Kudzma, & C. L. Mandle (Eds.), *Health promotion throughout the life span* (8th ed., pp. 81–102). St. Louis, MO: Mosby Elsevier.

Keller, J. M. (1987). Development and use of the ARCS model of instructional design. *Journal of Instructional Development*, *10*(3), 2–10.

Keller, J. M. (2008). First principles of motivation to learn and e-learning. *Distance Education*, *29*(2), 175–185.

Keller, L. O., Strohschein, S., & Briske, L. (2008). Population-based public health nursing practice: The intervention wheel. In M. Stanhope & J. Lancaster (Eds.), *Public health nursing: Population-centered health care in the community* (7th ed., pp. 187–214). St. Louis, MO: Mosby Elsevier.

LaMar, J. (2013). Culture and ethnicity. In P. A. Potter, A. Perry, P. A. Stockert, & A. M. Hall, *Fundamentals of nursing* (8th ed., pp. 101–115). St. Louis, MO: Mosby Elsevier.

Lieu, C. C., Sadler, G. R., Fullerton, J. T., & Stohlmann, P. D. (2007). Communication strategies for nurses interacting with patients who are deaf. *Dermatology Nursing*, *19*(6), 541–551.

Maslow, A. H. (1954). *Motivation and personality*. New York, NY: Harper & Row.

Maslow, A. H. (1987). *Motivation and personality* (3rd ed.). New York, NY: Harper & Row.

National Center for Health Statistics. (2011). Health, United States, 2011: With special feature on socioeconomic status and health. Retrieved from http://www.cdc.gov/nchs/data/hus/hus11.pdf

National Eye Institute. (n.d.). Prevalence of adult vision impairment and age-related eye diseases in America. Retrieved from http://www.nei.nih.gov/eyedata/adultvision_usa.asp

National Institute on Deafness and Other Communication Disorders. (2013). Health information. Retrieved from http://www.nidcd.nih.gov/Pages/default.aspx

National Partnership for Action. (2011). Health equity and disparities. Retrieved from http://www.minorityhealth.hhs.gov/npa/templates/browse.aspx?lvl=1&lvlid=34

O'Brien, P. G. (2007). Patient and family teaching. In S. L. Lewis, M. M. Heitkemper, S. R. Dirksen, P. G. O'Brien, & L. Bucher (Eds.), *Medical-surgical nursing* (7th ed., pp. 53–65). St. Louis, MO: Mosby Elsevier.

Ormrod, J. E. (2012). *Human learning* (6th ed.). Boston, MA: Pearson.

Pohl, M. L. (1981). *The teaching function of the nursing practitioner*. Dubuque, IA: Wm. C. Brown.

Prevent Blindness America. (2012). Vision problems in the U.S. Retrieved from http://www.visionproblemsus.org/introduction.html

ProLiteracy (2014). The Crisis, Adult Literacy Facts. Retrieved from http://www.proliteracy.org/the-crisis/adult-literacy-facts

Purnell, L. D. (2013). *Transcultural health care: A culturally competent approach*. Philadelphia, PA: F. A. Davis.

Racher, F. E., & Annis, R. C. (2007). Respecting culture and honoring diversity in community practice. *Research and Theory for Nursing Practice: An International Journal*, *21*(4), 255–270.

Roberts-Grey, G. (2008). Got coverage? *Essence*, *39*(7), 160–164.

Seligman, H. K., Wallace, A. S., DeWalt, D. A., Schillinger, D., Arnold, C. L., Shilliday, B. B., . . . Davis, T. C. (2007). Facilitating behavior change with low-literacy patient education materials. *American Journal of Health Behavior*, *31*(Suppl. 1), S69–S78.

Slavin, R. E. (2012). *Educational psychology theory and practice* (10th ed.). Boston, MA: Pearson.

Spade, C. M., & Mulhall, M. (2010). Teaching psychosocial vital signs across the undergraduate nursing curriculum. *Clinical Simulation in Nursing*, *6*(4), e143–e151. doi 10.1016/j.ecns.2009.10.002

Stuart, G. W. (2005). Therapeutic nurse–patient relationship. In G. W. Stuart & M. T. Laraia (Eds.), *Principles and practices of psychiatric nursing* (8th ed., pp. 15–49). St. Louis, MO: Mosby Elsevier.

Tobias, S. (1994). Interest, prior knowledge, and learning. *Review of Educational Research*, *64*(1), 37–54.

Tummala-Narra, P. (2009). Teaching on diversity: The mutual influence of students and instructors. *Psychoanalytic Psychology*, *26*(3), 322–334.

U.S. Census Bureau. (2012). U.S. Census Bureau projections show a slower growing, older, more diverse nation a half century from now. Retrieved from http://www.census.gov/newsroom/releases/archives/population/cb12-243.html

Weiss, B. D., Mays, M. Z., Martz, W., Castro, K. M., DeWalt, D. A., Pignome, M. P. M. J., & Hale, F. A. (2005). Quick assessment of literacy in primary care: The newest vital sign. *Annals of Family Medicine, 3*(6), 514–522.

Zuluaga, B. H. (2000). Implementation of the Zuluaga-Raysmith (Z-R) Model for assessment of perceived basic human needs in home health clients and caregivers. *Public Health Nursing, 17*(5), 317–324.

5

The Child Learner

Upon completion of this chapter, you will be able to do the following:

- Describe the biologic changes, psychosocial stages, and developmental tasks that are characteristic of newborns through adolescents.
- List health education topics for newborn through adolescent clients related to biologic changes, psychosocial stages, and developmental tasks.
- Define pedagogy and apply it to teaching newborns through adolescents.
- Describe five steps that nurses as educators take to streamline the process of providing efficient yet personalized health care teaching to children in a variety of settings.
- Identify health education topics when working with clients who have special needs.
- List ways that nurses as educators work with families, are involved in the community, and work with health team members.

KEY TERMS

autonomy versus shame
   and doubt
centering
developmental task
formal operations
identity versus role
   confusion
industry versus inferiority

irreversibility
medical play
operant conditioning
parallel play
pedagogy
preoperational stage
psychosocial stages
reflex

reinforcer
schema
sensorimotor stage
separation anxiety
transductive reasoning
trust versus mistrust

INTRODUCTION

Understanding the development of children, including biologic characteristics, psychosocial stages, and developmental tasks, is fundamental to effective client education. A **developmental task** is a set of skills and competencies that are peculiar to each developmental stage and that children must accomplish or master to deal effectively with their environment (Wong, Hockenberry-Eaton, Wilson, Winkelstein, & Schwartz, 2008). Young clients react differently depending on their developmental stage. Differences in development not only affect clients' reactions to their condition, but also their responses to and motivation for carrying out treatment recommendations. As the educator, you need to take into account the client's developmental stage based on an understanding of the health issues faced at that stage. Another important aspect of effectively teaching children is to know how children learn at different stages. This chapter describes child development in five major stages: infants (0–1 years), toddlers (1–3 years), preschoolers (3–4 years), school-age children (5–12 years), and adolescents (13–19 years). It looks at the concept of pedagogy and children's styles of learning at various stages. Your role as the educator is examined in working with pediatric clients who have special needs, within families, groups, communities, and health team members.

BIOLOGIC CHARACTERISTICS, PSYCHOSOCIAL STAGES, AND DEVELOPMENTAL TASKS

Children grow, develop, and learn throughout their lives, from birth through adulthood. Development of the child learner refers to change or growth that occurs in a child during the life span from birth to adolescence. A developmental task represents our culture's definition of normal development at different points in the life span. A child's development is measured through biologic characteristics, psychosocial stages, and developmental milestones or tasks. Although there are universally accepted assumptions about human development, no two children are alike. Children differ in physical, cognitive, social, and emotional growth patterns. They also differ in their genetic background and the ways they interact with and respond to their environment. **Psychosocial stages** emphasize the development of healthy personality traits (Erikson, 1963). Developmental changes normally occur in an orderly sequence, in predictable patterns that are age related; however, there are differences in the rate or timing of the changes from one child to another. It is important to have an understanding of the sequence of development so you can respond to the learning needs of young clients and their parents. It is also important to be aware that regression in development may occur with stress and illness.

Infants (Birth to 1 Year)

Biologic Characteristics

Infants at birth have reflexes as their sole physical ability. A **reflex** is an automatic body response to a stimulus that is involuntary; that is, the infant has no control over the response. Many reflexes disappear within a few weeks or months after birth. The presence of reflexes at birth is an indication of normal brain and nerve development. If reflexes are not present or if the reflexes continue past the time they should disappear, this is

TABLE 5-1

Common Infant Reflexes

Reflex	Response
Blinking	In response to a puff of air, the infant closes both eyes. The reflex disappears as the neurologic system matures within the first year.
Babinski	In response to stroking the side of the foot, the infant twists the foot inward and fans out the toes. The reflex disappears at about 1 year.
Grasping	In response to an object pressed against the palm, the infant attempts to grasp the object. The reflex disappears at 5 to 6 months.
Moro	In response to surprise movement or loud noise, the infant startles with the legs and head extending while the arms jerk up and out with the palms up and thumbs flexed. The reflex disappears at 3 to 6 months.
Rooting	In response to stroking the cheek, the infant turns the head toward the touch and attempts to suck. The reflex disappears at about 4 months.
Stepping	In response to holding the infant so the feet barely touch a surface, the infant makes stepping movements. The reflex disappears at about 10 to 15 months.
Sucking	In response to inserting a finger or nipple into the mouth, the infant begins sucking. Voluntary movement occurs at around 2 months.
Glabellar	In response to tapping the forehead, the infant blinks. The reflex disappears as the neurologic system matures within the first year.
Plantar	In response to touching the ball of the foot, the infant curls the toes under. The reflex disappears at 9 to 12 months.
Tonic neck	In response to turning the head to one side, the reflex causes a relaxed baby to straighten the arm on that side and bend the other arm in the fencing position. The reflex disappears at 4 to 9 months.

Source: Adapted from Wong et al. (2008).

considered an abnormal finding, and the infant should be seen by a healthcare provider for further evaluation (Wong et al., 2008). **Table 5-1** reviews the major infant reflexes and when they normally disappear.

There are a number of growth landmarks and physical changes that occur as infants grow in the first year. The weight gain of infants is particularly important. A newborn generally weighs between 6 and 9 pounds. A baby's size is influenced by a variety of factors, including the parents' size, gender, birth order, mother's health and nutrition, lifestyle choices during pregnancy, and medical problems. Babies often lose a few ounces in the first week after birth, but they regain the weight by the second week. By the end of the first month, newborns will generally have gained about 15 ounces. Between the ages of 1 and 3 months, a newborn generally gains about 6 ounces per week. Between the ages of 4 and 7 months, the weight gain is about 1.5 to 2 pounds per months. This rate typically slows a bit around 6 months of age to between 1.25 pounds per month. By 8 months the baby usually weighs around 2.5 times the birth weight. Between the ages of 8 and 12 months, weight gain is steady but at a slower pace. By the first birthday, an infant should weigh around three times the birth weight.

Psychosocial Stages

Erikson's theory of psychosocial development (1963) focuses on how children socialize and how this affects their sense of self. According to the theory, successful completion of each stage results in a healthy personality and successful interactions with others. Failure to successfully complete a stage can result in a reduced ability to progress; however, stages can be resolved successfully at a later time. Of the nine stages identified by Erikson, five relate to children (**Table 5-2**). The task

TABLE 5-2

Erikson's Stages of Psychosocial Development

Stage	*Description*
Trust versus mistrust Age birth to 1 year	■ Learns to trust others based on caregiver response. ■ If trust develops, gains confidence and trust; is able to feel secure when threatened. ■ Unsuccessful completion results in inability to trust and fear of the world.
Autonomy versus shame and doubt Age 1 to 3 years	■ Asserts independence, walks away from mother, and makes choices. ■ If encouraged, becomes confident and secure in own abilities. ■ If criticized, overly controlled, or not given the opportunity to assert self, may feel inadequate, become overly dependent, lack self-esteem, and feel shame or doubt.
Initiative versus guilt Age 3 to 6 years	■ Asserts self more frequently. ■ Plans activities, makes up games, and initiates activities with others. ■ Develops a sense of initiative, feels secure in ability to lead others and make decisions. ■ If discouraged through criticism or control, develops a sense of guilt; will remain a follower and lack self-initiative.
Industry versus inferiority Age 6 to puberty	■ Develops pride in accomplishments. ■ Initiates and completes projects, feels good about achievements. ■ Teachers play an increased role in development. ■ If encouraged and reinforced, feels industrious and confident about achieving goals. ■ If discouraged, feels inferior, doubts abilities, and may not reach potential.
Identity versus role confusion Puberty to adolescence	■ Transition from childhood to adulthood. ■ More independent, looks to the future: career, relationships, family, housing, and so forth. ■ Explores possibilities and forms own identity based on outcomes of explorations. ■ Can be hindered, resulting in a sense of confusion about self and role in the world. ("I don't know what I want to be when I grow up.")

Source: Adapted from Erikson (1963).

in infancy is the development of **trust versus mistrust**. From the time of birth to 1 year, infants begin to learn to trust others based on the consistency of the responses of their caregivers. If trust develops successfully, the child gains confidence and security in the surrounding world and is able to feel secure in future relationships. Unsuccessful completion of this stage can result in an inability to trust, fear, anger, and a sense of insecurity about the world. It may result in anxiety and a feeling of mistrust in the surrounding world.

The most important social task for the infant is the development of attachment to the primary caretaker, most often the child's mother. This forms the basis for attachment, which is the cornerstone of emotional development. **Separation anxiety** is another attachment behavior of infants characterized by the infant showing distress by crying when a familiar caregiver leaves (Wong et al., 2008). The first signs of separation anxiety appear at about 6 months of age and are clearly evident by 9 months of age. Separation anxiety is the strongest by 15 months of age and then begins to gradually weaken.

Developmental Tasks

Infant developmental tasks for this age group include the areas of motor development and cognitive development. Motor development follows cephalocaudal and proximodistal patterns, so that motor skills become refined first from the center and upper body and later from the extremities and lower body (Wong et al., 2008). Physical development is orderly and occurs in predictable sequence. The motor sequence of new movements for infants involves the following approximate sequence:

- Lack of head and trunk control: First few months after birth
- Lifts chin while lying flat: 1 month
- Raises chest while lying flat: 2 months
- Grasps rattle: 4th month
- Sits with support: 4th month
- Rolls over: 5th month
- Sits upright in a high chair: 4th to 6th month
- Sits without assistance: 8th month
- Crawling: 9th month
- Stands with help: 10th month
- Walks with help: 12th month
- Stands alone: 14th month
- Walks alone without support or help: 15th month
- Walks up stairs with help and runs clumsily: 18th month

The ages for each motor skill milestone are averages; the rates of physical and motor developments differ among infants depending on a variety of factors, including heredity, the amount of activity the infant participates in, and the amount of attention the infant receives (**Figure 5-1**).

Cognitive development refers to intellectual or mental development. It includes the activities of thinking, perception, memory, problem solving, language, and speech. Jean Piaget's theory of cognitive development in the 1920s challenged the then-prevalent thinking that children think like adults. Piaget's theory (1952) is based on the idea that a developing infant builds cognitive structures, or schemes, to understand and respond to physical experiences within

FIGURE 5-1

Infants Develop at Different Rates

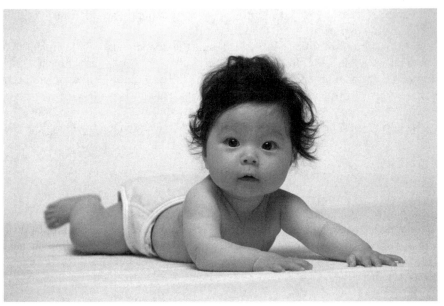

© Photodisc

the environment. Piaget posits that an infant's cognitive structure increases in complexity with development, moving from displaying reflexes, such as sucking and grasping, to highly complex mental activities, such as speech. Piaget's four stages of cognitive development are included in **Table 5-3**. The infant is in the **sensorimotor stage**, in which infants begin to understand the information entering their senses and are able to interact with the world. During this stage, the infant learns to manipulate objects, although he or she will fail to understand the permanency of these objects if they are not within the infant's current sensory perception. Object permanence develops toward the end of the first year.

The most intensive period of speech and language development occurs during the first 3 years of life when the brain is developing and maturing. These skills appear to develop best when the infant is exposed to sounds, sights, and the speech and language of others. The beginning signs of communication occur during the first few days of life when an infant learns that crying will bring food, comfort, and companionship. The newborn also begins to recognize important environmental sounds, such as the mother's voice. As they grow, infants sort out the speech sounds or phonemes that compose the words of their language. Most infants recognize the basic sounds of their native language (National Institute on Deafness and Other Communication Disorders [NIDCD], 2014). **Table 5-4** reviews the developmental milestones of speech development of the infant.

TABLE 5-3		

Piaget's Stages of Cognitive Development

Stage	Age	Characteristics of Stage
Sensorimotor	0–2	The child: ■ Learns by doing: looking, touching, and viewing ■ Learns through physical interaction with the environment ■ Builds a set of concepts about reality and how it works ■ Has a primitive understanding of cause-and-effect relationships ■ Develops object permanence at about 9 months
Preoperational	2–7	The child: ■ Is not able to conceptualize abstractly and needs concrete physical situations ■ Uses language and symbols, including letters and numbers ■ Is egocentric ■ Conservation marks the end of the preoperational stage and the beginning of concrete operations
Concrete operations	7–11	The child: ■ Starts to conceptualize, creating logical structures that explain physical experiences ■ Demonstrates conservation, reversibility, serial ordering, and a mature understanding of cause-and-effect relationships ■ Begins abstract problem solving and continues with concrete thinking
Formal operations	12+	The child: ■ Begins to develop an abstract view of the world ■ Is able to apply reversibility and conservation to both real and imagined situations ■ Demonstrates abstract thinking, including logic, deductive reasoning, comparison, and classification ■ Has an increased understanding of the world and the idea of cause and effect; can develop theories about the world

Source: Adapted from Piaget (1963).

Toddlers (1 to 3 Years)

Biologic Characteristics

During the toddler period, weight gain slows to about 4 to 6 pounds per year as the activity level increases. The physical appearance of the toddler includes a protuberant abdomen, accentuated lumbar lordosis (inward curvature of the spine), and a characteristic gait in which feet are placed wide apart and the child appears to walk flat footed. The birth weight quadruples by the age of 2.5 years. A steady growth in height of 2 to 4 inches per year is expected. During this time the child perfects the gross and fine motor skills that emerged during the first year by developing balance, coordination, stability, and an improved ability to manipulate objects. Emotional and physical readiness for toilet training begins at around 18 months.

TABLE 5-4

Language Development: First Year

Age	Infant Response
Birth to 5 months	■ Reacts toward sounds ■ Turns head toward sounds ■ Cries, coos, laughs ■ Makes noise when talked to ■ Looks at faces ■ Turns head toward sounds
6 to 11 months	■ Understands "no" ■ Says "da-da" and "ma-ma" ■ Tries to communicate by making gestures ■ Tries to imitate sounds

Source: Adapted from National Institute on Deafness and Other Communication Disorders (2009).

Psychosocial Stages

Toddlers are in Erikson's stage of **autonomy versus shame and doubt**. From the ages of birth to 1 year, children begin to learn how to trust others based on the consistency of the responses of their caregivers. Toddlers strive to develop a sense of autonomy within the boundaries of a trusting parental relationship. If trust develops successfully, the child gains confidence and security in the surrounding world. The child is then better able to develop affectionate and trusting relationships with family members and with adults outside the family. Unsuccessful completion of this stage can result in an inability to trust, and therefore a sense of fear about the world.

Developmental Tasks

Toddlers are in Piaget's **preoperational stage** of cognitive development. A hallmark of this stage is egocentrism, or the tendency of children to recognize their environment only in terms of their own point of view. Toddlers think that parents and others share their thoughts. The toddler applies new knowledge of language and begins to use symbols to represent objects, such as pretending a broom is a horse. They may experiment with objects in their minds, first predicting what will happen if they do something to an object, then transforming their plans into action. To some degree mental prediction and planning replace overt trial and error as growing toddlers experiment and attempt to solve problems. The toddler is now better able to think about things and events that are not present. Language development is proceeding rapidly in the toddler, but the ability to understand language is greater than the ability to express it, which creates frustration. **Table 5-5** reviews the milestones for language development at this stage.

Preschool (3 to 4 Years)

Biologic Characteristics

The preschooler has a steady growth rate of approximately 4 pounds of weight and 2 inches of height per year. The body lengthens and the protuberant abdomen disappears. In terms of

TABLE 5-5

Language Development: Toddler Years

Age	Toddler Response
12 to 17 months	■ Attends to a book or a toy for a few minutes ■ Follows simple directions ■ Answers simple questions nonverbally ■ Points to objects, pictures, or family members ■ Says two to three words to label a person or object (pronunciation may not be clear) ■ Tries to imitate simple words
18 to 23 months	■ Enjoys being read to ■ Follows simple commands without gestures ■ Points to simple body parts ■ Understands simple verbs ■ Makes animal sounds ■ Starts to combine words such as *more milk*
2 to 3 years	■ Knows about 50 words at 24 months ■ Knows some spatial concepts such as *in* and *on* ■ Knows pronouns such as *you*, *me*, and *her* ■ Knows descriptive words such as *big* and *happy* ■ Says about 40 words at 24 months ■ Speech is becoming more accurate but may still leave off ending sounds; strangers may not be able to understand much of what is said ■ Answers simple questions ■ Begins to use more pronouns such as *you* and *I* ■ Speaks in two- to three-word phrases ■ Uses question inflection to ask for something (e.g., *my ball?*) ■ Begins to use plurals such as *shoes* or *socks* and regular past-tense verbs such as *jumped*

Source: Adapted from National Institute on Deafness and Other Communication Disorders (2009).

physical abilities, a 3-year-old can kick a ball, jump in place, build a tower of nine cubes, copy a circle, put on most clothing and shoes, and eat without assistance. By the age of 4 years, the child can climb a ladder, throw a ball overhand, hold a pencil, cut and paste, wash and dry hands, brush teeth, and ride a bike with training wheels. Most basic gross motor abilities have emerged. Existing skills are practiced and perfected, and the child develops mastery in applying motor skills to increasingly challenging and complex situations.

Psychosocial Stages

The preschooler moves through two of Erikson's stages of psychosocial development: the stage of autonomy versus shame and doubt, and the stage of initiative versus guilt. After developing basic trust, the child goes on to begin to plan activities, make up games, and initiate activities with others. If given this opportunity, the preschooler develops a sense of initiative and feels secure in the ability to lead others and make decisions. If this tendency is not encouraged, either through criticism or control, the child develops a sense of guilt. The child may feel like an annoyance to others and therefore remain a follower lacking in self-initiative.

At 2 years and older the preschooler develops rudimentary relationships with other children, which are usually characterized by **parallel play;** that is, play in the presence of rather than in interaction with other children. As the child progresses, social relationships increase outside the family, and interactive and cooperative play skills with peers are expanded. The preschooler also begins to imitate and practice social roles. Concepts of right and wrong are learned as the child begins to understand the nature of rules, which causes the child to experience guilt when doing wrong.

Developmental Tasks

Preschoolers are in Piaget's preoperational cognitive stage. A concrete thought process is evident in this stage by what Piaget calls **transductive reasoning,** which describes how the preschooler cannot think from the general to the particular or from the particular to the general. Piaget also describes the concept of **centering** as lacking in the preschooler's thinking. The child cannot consider more than one factor at a time when solving a problem or connect a reversible operation to the original act. This is called **irreversibility**. Piaget describes preschool-age children as preoperational because they do not yet use logic. They understand the world through magical thinking and have difficulty distinguishing between wishes and what really happens. They believe that thoughts and strong feelings can make things happen.

A major accomplishment in the preschool stage is the perfection of language skills and the use of language to communicate with others. During the preschool years language progression depends on aptitude, the opportunity for using language, the quality and quantity of language used at home, and the child's range of experiences using language to communicate. It is also at this stage that grammar and syntax are refined, and the vocabulary increases rapidly (**Table 5-6**).

School Age (5 to 12 Years)

Biologic Characteristics

The school age child gains an average of 6 pounds and grows approximately 2 inches per year. Growth is marked by spurts and times of little growth as dictated by genetics. During these years boys and girls are of similar size, but school-age children tend to be concerned about their rate of growth and what their height and weight will be. The child practices, refines, and masters complex gross and fine motor skills. Examples of gross motor skills for school-age children include balancing on one foot, tandem walking, hopping on one foot, pedaling a bicycle, and bathing self. Fine motor skills for this age group include drawing a person with three to six parts, cutting with a knife, tying a bow, drawing a diamond, and having good eye–hand coordination. This is also a time when the school-age child begins to lose baby teeth and the permanent teeth emerge.

TABLE 5-6	

Language Development: Preschool Years

Age	Preschooler Response
3 to 4 years	▪ Groups objects, such as food and clothes, together ▪ Identifies colors ▪ Uses most speech sounds but may distort some of the more difficult sounds, such as *l, r, s, sh, ch, y, v, z,* and *th*; these sounds may not be fully mastered until age 7 or 8 years ▪ Uses consonants in the beginning, middle, and end of words; some of the more difficult consonants may be distorted, but attempts to say them ▪ Strangers are able to understand much of what is said ▪ Able to describe the use of objects such as *fork, car,* and so forth ▪ Has fun with language; enjoys poems and recognizes language absurdities such as *Is that an elephant on your head?* ▪ Expresses ideas and feelings, rather than just talking about the surrounding world ▪ Uses verbs that end in -ing such as *walking, talking* ▪ Answers simple questions such as *What do you do when you are hungry?* ▪ Repeats sentences

Source: Adapted from National Institute on Deafness and Other Communication Disorders (2009).

Psychosocial Stages

School-age children are in Erikson's stage of **industry versus inferiority**. In this stage children begin to develop a sense of pride in their accomplishments. They initiate projects, see them through to completion, and feel good about what they have achieved. During this time teachers play an increased role in the child's development. If children are encouraged and reinforced for their initiative, they begin to feel industrious and confident in their ability to achieve goals. If this initiative is not encouraged, if it is restricted by parents or teachers, the child will begin to feel inferior, doubting his or her abilities, and may not reach full potential. Relationships with people outside the family become more important to the school-age child. They develop friendships and participate in peer group activities. The child imitates, learns, and adopts age-appropriate social roles, including those that are gender specific. The child develops an understanding of rules that can be relied on to dictate proper social behavior and govern social relationships and activities. The child develops a sense of self as an individual with awareness of likes and dislikes and with special areas of skill. Introspection is possible at this age.

Developmental Tasks

School-age children are in Piaget's stage of concrete operations. During this stage accommodation (ability to modify schema to fit the world) increases. The child develops an ability to think abstractly and make rational judgments about concrete or observable phenomena that in the past the child needed to physically manipulate in order to understand. Some specific skills that

FIGURE 5-2

The School Age Child Learns to Solve Problems

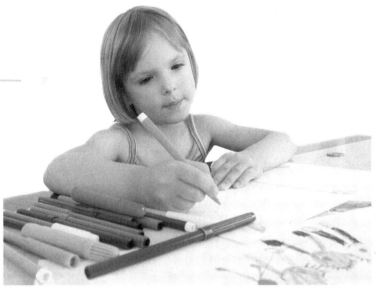

© Pavel Siamionau/Dreamstime.com

develop at this time are the ability to classify items and put them in a series, recognize logical relationships among elements in a serial order, and understand that the quantity, length, or number of items is unrelated to the arrangement or appearance of the object or items (conservation). The school-age child can take into account multiple aspects of a problem to solve it. He or she understands that numbers or objects can be changed and then returned to their original state (reversibility). The child moves toward more cooperative interactions and develops the ability to understand other people's perspectives (**Figure 5-2**).

School-age children generally enter this developmental stage with the ability to understand and speak a language. School focuses on learning to read and write. Success in school depends on three things: the child having the visual ability to read, the auditory ability to perceive language spoken to him or her, and the fine motor skills for handwriting.

Adolescent (13 to 19 Years)

Biologic Characteristics

Adolescence is a time of accelerated physical growth in weight and height; 15–20% of adult height and 50% of adult weight is achieved. This is also the time of onset of puberty, or sexual maturity, which signals the ability to reproduce. Females usually begin puberty 2 years earlier than males and experience their growth spurt earlier. Physiologic changes in puberty include development of secondary sex characteristics. In females the first sign of puberty is often breast development. Other signs are the growth of hair in the pubic area and armpits. Menarche, the onset of menses in girls, usually happens later in puberty, at around 13 years of age. In males puberty usually begins with the testicles and penis getting larger. Then hair grows in the pubic area and armpits. Muscles grow, the voice deepens, nocturnal emissions begin, and facial hair develops as puberty continues. Even though the physical changes are usually sequential in nature and are mediated through the hormonal regulatory system, there are individual variations for onset and duration of puberty. Some adolescents may begin puberty earlier than normal, a condition called precocious puberty. Others may have delayed puberty, meaning the process begins later than normal.

Psychosocial Stages

The adolescent is in Erikson's stage of **identity versus role confusion**. This is a period of transition from childhood to adulthood. Adolescents want more independence and begin to look to the future in terms of career and future relationships. Social relationships center on their peer group, with decreased time spent with family. Group values often guide their individual behavior, and acceptance by peers becomes a critical part of self-esteem. Adolescents explore possibilities and begin to form their own identities based on the outcome of their explorations. Identity is defined as a coherent conception of the self, made up of committed goals, values, and beliefs. This sense of who they are can be hindered, which can result in a sense of confusion about themselves and their role in the world. Toward the end of this stage, identity becomes more individualized, and the adolescent develops a more stable sense of self that is separate from either family or peer group.

Developmental Tasks

Piaget's stage of **formal operations** describes the adolescent's cognitive development. This stage brings cognition to its final form. Adolescents no longer require concrete objects to make rational judgments. Abstract, theoretical, philosophical, and scientific reasoning become possible. At this time they also develop an understanding of long-term cause and effect. Adolescents question, reinterpret, and revise their previous knowledge base. At this point they are capable of hypothetical and deductive reasoning. There are many possible options for teaching adolescents because they can consider options from different perspectives. It is common for them to challenge current thinking and have a sense of idealism about the world as they move toward a formal thinking process.

Language development is largely complete by adolescence. Language at this stage exhibits evidence of reflective and abstract thought, with increasingly complex grammatical construction of speech and writing. Adolescents have the ability to define and discuss abstractions such as health, love, and peace. They are also aware that words can have multiple meanings. The use of slang is common. This is considered to be an opportune time developmentally to learn other languages.

IMPLICATIONS FOR HEALTH EDUCATION

It is critical to understand child development to provide effective health education to children, their parents, and their caregivers. Knowledge of child development enables you to prepare teaching plans based on realistic child expectations, and it increases the chances of adherence and success in promoting, retaining, and restoring health. As an educator your knowledge and understanding of cognitive and perceptual behavior serves as a guide in counseling. Use this knowledge to influence behavior by listening to parental concerns, respecting values, and modeling behaviors that support the overall health of the child. As the child grows and is able to independently communicate, use understanding of growth and development to interact with the child in ways that acknowledge his or her verbal and physical abilities and encourage self-reliance.

Use age-specific strategies to prepare teaching plans. Infants expand their gross and fine motor skills by being encouraged to reach and grasp and move toward objects. An example of this is placing toys safely in the crib that are black and white or brightly colored to attract attention and stimulate movement. Younger children, toddlers through preschool, have language skills that require concrete examples to help them understand information. A younger child will respond well to being told, "We always wash our hands before meals." An older child will want more explanation, to which the nurse can respond by discussing that this prevents germs that can make you sick. As the child's gross and fine motor skills develop, it is helpful to supplement explanation with objects that the child can manipulate. When teaching about how to take blood pressure, having the child hold and examine the blood pressure cuff lets him or her gain familiarity with the equipment and gives a sense of mastery and trust. The preschool child enjoys pretend play, which is when the child remembers past experiences and replays them (Graca, Fowler, & Rosenstock, 2009). By pretending, the child is able to share fears and concerns and can gain a sense of mastery over the environment. Use this time to clear up misconceptions that are common in this age group because of magical thinking. Older children enjoy activities that involve peers and that are repetitive and entertaining. Games, including those on the computer, are fun and create a sense of mastery. **Table 5-7** summarizes psychosocial, cognitive, language, and teaching implications.

Promote and Retain Health

The focus of promoting health is on prevention of illness, whereas the focus of retaining health is on maintaining the present health status, assuming it is satisfactory. **Table 5-8** lists suggested topics to promote and retain health that are appropriate for children at various stages of development. These suggestions are not all inclusive and need to be adapted to the circumstances of the individual client.

Restore Health

Restoration of health for children refers to working with children who have an acute or chronic illness or disability. The purpose of health education at this time is to help clients understand the nature of their health problem, the treatment regimen, and the limitations imposed by the health problem, disability, or injury. This may involve not only working with the client, but also with family members. **Table 5-9** explains the approach used by nurses as educators when teaching different age groups. The developmental stage is taken into account, and both the parent and the child are viewed as clients.

TABLE 5-7

Teaching Implications for Various Developmental Stages

Age	Psychosocial (Erikson)	Cognitive (Piaget)	Language	Teaching Implications
Infancy	■ Trust versus mistrust ■ 5–6 weeks: Responsive smile to families' faces and voices ■ Emotionally symbiotic with main caretaker ■ Individual temperament emerges in earliest weeks of life ■ Needs balance of rest, exercise, nutrition, love, strokes ■ Cuddliness varies	■ Sensorimotor: Basic reflex habits (i.e., sucking nipple within 2 weeks) ■ Higher levels later: 2–3 months ■ Looks for sounds ■ At 8–9 months develops object permanence ■ Thinks in pictures	■ Prelanguage sounds ■ Inner language: Recognizes objects ■ Audioreceptive: Recognizes spoken words	■ Teach parents and caregivers ■ Calibrate for their anxiety when child is very ill ■ Anticipatory guidance about growth and development, safety, and stimulation (talk and touch)
Early childhood 2 to 3 years	■ Autonomy versus shame and doubt ■ *No!* ■ Frustrated by personal and external limits ■ Egocentric ■ Needs to explore safely and to succeed	■ Sensorimotor: Still thinks in pictures ■ Starts development of object formation, representation, extension	■ Single three-word sentences: Nouns, verbs and adjectives (*ball, carry, soft*) ■ At age 3, understands time (*yesterday*)	■ Needs safe play space, love, security ■ Find out routines, special words, comfort toy ■ Give positive, simple command ■ Read or make up relevant picture books ■ Most teaching through parent
3 to 6 years	■ Initiative versus guilt ■ Fears: Unknown, separation, strangers, disapproval, pain, punishment, own aggression ■ Roles: Male, female	■ Sensorimotor: ■ Expanding imagination and concepts	■ Rapid growth ■ By 5 years has usual speech patterns	■ Encourage play to assess child and to teach ■ Give simple explanations (*You will smell icky perfume*) ■ See, hear, feel: Make tape and picture books, objects ■ Use timing: Tell child soon enough to allow processing but not to get panicky; allow only one stall ■ Positive commands (*You hold Band-Aid*)

(continues)

TABLE 5-7

Teaching Implications for Various Developmental Stages (Continued)

Age	Psychosocial (Erikson)	Cognitive (Piaget)	Language	Teaching Implications
Late childhood 6 to 12 years	■ Industry versus inferiority ■ Makes things ■ Peer influence is important ■ Developing parents and ego states	■ Concrete operations ■ Inductive reasoning ■ Memory ■ Conscience teachable in many cultures	■ Good command of language; can use it to tell stories, ask questions, argue, tease	■ Assess child's reading ability ■ Likes mechanical explanations ■ Help child gain content by participating in self-care and procedures ■ Can pay attention to teaching ■ Can do own hygiene, choose good food, recognize signs of illness
Adolescence	■ Identity versus role confusion ■ New and more mature relationships ■ Sexual identity ■ Changing body ■ Becoming emotionally independent from parents ■ Preparing for adult responsibilities, career, love ■ Workable value system ■ Social responsibilities ■ Mood swings and ambivalence ■ Fears loss of face	■ Formal operations ■ "One's thinking takes wings" (Piaget)	■ Depends on IQ, culture, socioeconomic group ■ Slang	■ Ask for meaning of slang ■ Use peers to teach and persuade ■ Protect face privacy ■ Expect mood swings ■ Be honest and straightforward ■ Try to read between the lines of what a teenager is trying to say or does not say

Source: Adapted from Babcok, D. E., & Miller, M. A. (1994). Client education: Theory and practice. St. Louis: Mosby.

TABLE 5-8

Suggested Topics to Promote and Retain Health

Nursing Assessment	Health Education Topics
Infant	■ Promotion of infant–parent bonding ■ Infant nutrition: Breastfeeding, formula feeding, introduction of solid food and weaning ■ Developmental milestones ■ Elimination patterns ■ Activity and exercise through stimulation and play ■ Sleep needs ■ Injury prevention ■ Sensory stimulation to promote cognitive and social development ■ Vaccinations
Toddler	■ Nutritional needs and preferences ■ Toilet training ■ Appropriate toys and activities ■ Rituals and security objects ■ Need for autonomy, temper tantrums ■ Parental frustration ■ Safety issues, injury prevention ■ Vaccinations
Preschooler	■ Nutritional needs and preferences ■ Dental care ■ Appropriate play activities and exercise ■ Choosing TV shows ■ Managing bedtime concerns ■ Imaginary friends and magical thinking ■ Vision and hearing screenings ■ Gender identification ■ Injury prevention ■ Health screenings
School age	■ Understanding of health ■ Balanced nutrition, prevention of obesity ■ Nocturnal enuresis, encopresis, and shy bladder ■ Sports activities, TV, video, and computer games ■ Developing socialization skills ■ Sleep walking, sleep talking, night fears ■ Health screenings ■ Attention-deficit hyperactivity disorder (ADHD) ■ Questions about sex ■ Coping strategies ■ Accident prevention
Adolescent	■ Physical changes: Puberty ■ Common health issues: Acne, scoliosis ■ Diet and exercise: Prevention of obesity and eating disorders

(continues)

TABLE 5-8

Suggested Topics to Promote and Retain Health (Continued)

Nursing Assessment	Health Education Topics
	■ Sexual behavior, contraception
	■ Sexually transmitted diseases
	■ Body image issues
	■ Substance abuse: Alcohol and drugs
	■ Injury and violence prevention
	■ Health screening
	■ Vaccinations

ORIENTATION TO LEARNING

Learning in Children

Most theorists believe that learning is something that occurs as the result of certain experiences that precede changes in behavior (Olsen & Hergenhahn, 2013). The experiences that precede learning are interactions with the environment. Athey (2007) and Piaget (1963) agree that children's interactions with their environment lead to mental actions through which they construct ideas or **schema** about what they are encountering. As they come across objects, situations, people, and ideas, they adjust and structure their knowledge to try to make sense of their experiences. Using this cognitive learning process, they build a framework for thinking and learning. Children's direct experiences and interactions with things and people around them are central to their learning (David, Goouch, Powell, & Abbott, 2003).

B. F. Skinner posits that learning is a change in overt behavior that occurs in response to events or stimuli that occur in the environment (1968). Reinforcement is the key element in Skinner's theory of classical conditioning. A **reinforcer** is anything that strengthens the desired response. It could be a smile, verbal praise, a good grade, or a feeling of increased accomplishment. Skinner also identifies negative reinforcers, which result in the increased frequency of a response when it is withdrawn (different from adverse stimuli or punishment, which results in reduced responses). Babies generally respond well to **operant conditioning**, which is a process of gradually shaping the infant's behavior. An example of this is an infant who learns that smiling elicits positive parental attention, which in turn causes the infant to smile at his or her parents more (Skinner, 1968). Babies generally respond well to operant conditioning. Cognitive and behavioral theories are applied to teaching in **Table 5-10**.

Learning Styles in Children

Learning occurs as children respond to environmental, social, emotional, and physical stimuli when trying to understand new information. Learning styles are the way individuals process information. Learning styles refer to three perceptual pathways or modalities of learning: visual (sight), kinesthetic (body, sensation, motion), and auditory (sound). The visual modality occurs when information is received best through visual stimulation (reading, pictures, movies, etc.).

TABLE 5-9

Teaching Approach with Different Age Groups

Age Group	Clients–Parents	Nursing Approach
Infant (0–1)	Child	▪ Observe the infant's physical condition: Weight and appearance ▪ Observe child–caregiver interaction: Look for bonding behaviors

	Parent	▪ Establish rapport
		▪ Use good listening skills to identify parent's concerns
		▪ Address parental anxiety and stress with calm demeanor
		▪ Assess parental educational level, literacy level, cultural influences
		▪ Encourage enjoyment of infants
		▪ Discuss balance of work and home life
		▪ Share knowledge of:
		  ● Community resources
		  ● Developmental milestone
		  ● Importance of play for development
		  ● Preventive teaching
		  ● Infant safety
		  ● Nutrition
		  ● Health screenings and vaccinations schedule

Toddler (1–2)	Child	▪ Assess the quality of the parent–child relationship ▪ Observe the physical status and growth of the child ▪ Talk to and interact with the child on his or her level to initiate a relationship

	Parent	▪ Establish rapport
		▪ Listen to parental concerns and encourage questions
		▪ Determine parental knowledge, literacy level, cultural influences
		▪ Be sensitive to signs of frustration with child's behavior
		▪ Provide appropriate teaching tools and resources
		▪ Share knowledge of:
		  ● Community resources
		  ● Developmental milestones
		  ● Importance of play for development
		  ● Safety
		  ● Techniques of discipline and limit setting
		  ● Toilet training

Preschooler (3–4)	Child	▪ Talk to and interact with the child on his or her level to establish a relationship ▪ Observe the child at play; listen to vocalizations and observe imaginary play ▪ Observe the physical status and growth of the child ▪ Teach children about procedures to be performed ▪ Keep explanations simple ▪ Allow children to express their fears

(continues)

TABLE 5-9

Teaching Approach with Different Age Groups (Continued)

Age Group	Clients–Parents	Nursing Approach

	Parent	▪ Establish rapport
		▪ Listen to parental concerns and encourage questions
		▪ Determine parental knowledge, literacy level, cultural influences
		▪ Teach parents ways to respond to their child's questions
		▪ Provide appropriate teaching tools and resources
		▪ Share knowledge of:
		  ● Normal developmental milestones
		  ● Child's sexual curiosity
		  ● Imaginary play and magical thinking
		  ● Safety

School age (5–12)	Child	▪ Observe the physical status and growth of the child ▪ Develop rapport with the child by introducing yourself and asking about his or her interests and friends ▪ Ask the child about his or her health and encourage questions ▪ Explain procedures or teaching in clear, logical ways ▪ Include child in the patient education process ▪ Use appropriate tools and resources

	Parent	▪ Establish rapport
		▪ Listen to parental concerns and encourage questions
		▪ Determine parental knowledge and literacy level
		▪ Help parents to foster child independence and praise accomplishments
		▪ Give parents tools for teaching
		▪ Share knowledge of:
		  ● Normal developmental milestones
		  ● School adjustment
		  ● Enuresis, encopresis
		  ● Sleepwalking, sleep talking
		  ● Learning disabilities
		  ● Obesity, nutritional teaching
		  ● Dental health
		  ● Safety, accidents, drowning, bicycles
		  ● Drugs, alcohol, smoking, sexual activity
		  ● Health screening: Vision, hearing
		  ● Use of TV, computer, cell phones, and video games

Adolescent (13–19)	Child	▪ Focus on establishing rapport based on openness and trust ▪ Ask about bodily changes and sexual adjustment ▪ Ask about family support and facilitate the family relationship ▪ Ask about peer group and social, cultural influences ▪ Ask about health concerns and answer questions ▪ Advocate for the adolescent client

(continues)

TABLE 5-9		

Teaching Approach with Different Age Groups (Continued)

Age Group	Clients–Parents	Nursing Approach
		▪ Be mindful of modesty and privacy issues
		▪ Use empathetic understanding; no lecturing
		▪ Provide appropriate teaching tools and resources
		▪ Share knowledge about:
		● Physical change in puberty
		● Sexual issues and contraception
		● Body image and eating disorders
		● Health issues and safety
		● Body piercing and tattooing
		● Scoliosis, acne
	Parent	▪ Establish rapport
		▪ Listen to parental concerns and encourage questions
		▪ Determine parental knowledge, literacy level, cultural influences
		▪ Assist parents in understanding adolescent behavior
		▪ Encourage limit setting and fostering of adolescent independence
		▪ Help parents redefine their role in this transition phase

Source: Adapted from Falvo, D. R. (2004). Effective patient education: A guide to increased compliance. Sudbury, MA: Jones and Bartlett.

Approximately 40% of secondary students are visual learners. The kinesthetic modality occurs when information is received best via touch and hands-on activities (computer-assisted instruction, models, field trips, etc.). Approximately 50% of secondary students are kinesthetic learners. The auditory modality occurs when information is best obtained by hearing (being read to aloud, listening to songs, puppet shows, reciting songs or poems, etc.). Approximately 10% of secondary students are auditory learners (Carbo, Dunn, & Dunn, 1986). There is no right or wrong learning style. Most children show a preference for one style, as do nurses and parents. It is not unusual for the nurse and parents to prefer learning styles different from that of the child. To work effectively with children, it is important for you to understand your own, the child's, and possibly the parents' preferred learning styles. This understanding helps to produce more efficient, productive learning opportunities for children. Including activities that use other styles can be helpful in expanding children's areas of interest and ability to learn.

The Role of Play in Learning

Jones and Reynolds state that "young children learn the most important things, not by being told but by constructing knowledge for themselves in interaction with the physical world and with other children—and the way they do this is by playing" (1992, p. 1). In play, children expand their understanding of themselves and others, their knowledge of the physical world, and their ability to communicate with peers and adults. Children experience play through all

TABLE 5-10

Application of Cognitive and Behavior Learning Theories for Children

Learning Theory	Principles	Teaching Application
Cognitive theories of learning	Jean Piaget's cognitive development theory	■ Children will provide different explanations of reality at different stages of cognitive development. ■ Cognitive development is facilitated by providing activities or situations that engage learners and require adaptation. ■ Learning materials and activities should involve the appropriate level of motor or mental operations for a child of a given age; avoid asking children to perform tasks that are beyond their current cognitive capabilities. ■ Use teaching methods that actively involve children and present challenges.
Behavioral theory of learning	B. F. Skinner's operant conditioning theory	■ Behavior that is positively reinforced will reoccur; intermittent reinforcement is particularly effective. ■ Information should be presented in small amounts so responses can be reinforced (shaping). ■ Reinforcements will generalize across similar stimuli (stimulus generalization), producing secondary conditioning.

Source: Adapted from Kearsley (1994 to 2004).

the developmental stages. Infants and toddlers engage in activities that stimulate their senses and develop motor skills. Preschoolers play with other children, develop and refine motor skills, and use basic academic skills such as counting, reading, and writing. School-age children play formal and informal games with their peers, such as hopscotch, jump rope, and board, card, and computer games. Through these activities they enhance their coordination and physical abilities, refine their social skills, and build concepts such as cooperation and competition. In adolescence play is more organized and structured as the need for orderly thinking is expressed through games with rules and in organized sports.

Play is so important that its significance in children's lives is recognized by the United Nations as a specific right (United Nations, 1989). The Association for Childhood Education International (ACEI) issued a position paper outlining the following beliefs about the importance of play in children's development (Isenberg & Quisenberry, 2002):

■ Play is a dynamic, active, and constructive behavior and is an essential and integral part of all children's healthy growth, development, and learning across all ages, domains, and cultures.

■ Play enhances learning and development for children of all ages, cultures, and domains.

- The forms and functions of children's play must be considered in the context of our knowledge about age-related play behaviors. Knowledge about how children play at different ages should guide the practice of all adults who work with children.
- Play is a powerful, natural behavior contributing to children's learning and development, and no program of adult instruction can substitute for children's own observations, activities, and direct knowledge.

The nurse as educator uses this knowledge of the importance of play to support child learning. Graca and colleagues (2009) describe **medical play** as developmentally appropriate activities that provide insight into how the child is coping with health events and can be used as a tool in successful teaching. Medical play allows opportunities to deal with both the physical and emotional stressors of health care and act as a mechanism to increase understanding. An example of using medical play is rehearsing activities before surgery. The child can manipulate equipment, such as an oxygen mask, and rehearse what it is like to have the mask in place. The nurse as educator uses knowledge of developmental milestones to choose play strategies that fit the child's need (**Figure 5-3**).

Practices That Encourage Child Learning

As an educator you assume a big part in creating the climate and conditions that best promote children's learning. Involvement in learning is built on the confidence and trust that come from good relationships. First, build rapport with the child. It is important to promote self-esteem,

FIGURE 5-3

Children Explore the World Through Play

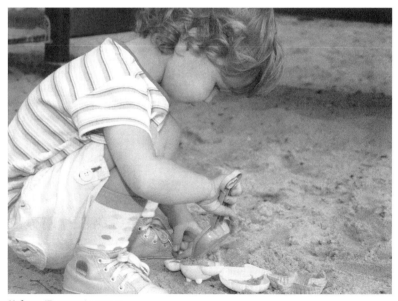

© Artyom Yefimov/Dreamstime.com

confidence, and trust to create an environment conducive to learning. It is also important to involve children both physically and mentally in the learning process (David et al., 2003). Children should be encouraged to explore their world through movement using all their senses to find out what they can do, what things are like, and what things mean. It is through this exploration that they achieve understanding and form ideas from sensory experiences. Learning strategies should include these types of activities.

Provide support to cultivate, sustain, and extend children's explorations and recognize their accomplishments. You should also be aware that part of the active learning process is to allow children to make decisions and have control and independence as part of the learning process. Allowing children to decide what and how they do things increases their engagement in the learning process (David et al., 2003). This does not mean that children are left on their own to decide what and how they will learn, but it does means the nurse can create situations for them to make decisions and then support them as they engage in learning activities. Making decisions helps children become managers of their own learning.

Another important aspect of active learning is to personalize the learning process. This means to build on what the child is familiar with, knows, and can do. Getting to know the child and his or her parents helps you understand how to stimulate and sustain the child's involvement and effort in learning (David et al., 2003). The pace and character of children's learning differs from one child to another because they have different interests, skills, and knowledge built on their experiences. This means that children learn the same thing in different ways, or learn the same thing at different times in their development. The range and character of learning activities should be planned to address these kinds of differences in a way that enables all children to find something that is relevant and that will engage and sustain their interest. Some children need additional support to become fully involved in learning activities.

It is important for you to consider how learning activities are presented. The context in which children experience things has a considerable effect on their willingness to become involved and their ability to connect with the ideas that are presented (David et al., 2003). Children want to understand the situation or circumstances in which they learn, so explanations should be simple and clear. When they find things that they already know about and can latch on to, they have a base from which to explore new things. A final important factor that you should consider is the importance of maintaining good working relationships with parents. Strong parental relationships provide essential information about the child's learning at home and help to provide insight into the things with which each child is familiar.

PEDAGOGY

Pedagogy is derived from the Greek word *paid*, meaning *child*, plus *agogos*, meaning *leading*, and is defined as the art and science of teaching children (Hiemstra & Sisco, 1990). In the pedagogic model, the teacher has full responsibility for facilitating learning, including what will be learned, when it will be learned, and whether the material has been learned. Pedagogy is also sometimes referred to as the correct use of teaching strategies and is described as being a didactic and traditional approach to teaching children. As the educator you will use pedagogic principles when teaching young clients. One-to-one teaching with the child facilitates individual learning needs, provides for child and family interaction with the nurse, and protects confidentiality.

Group teaching may be appropriate when the child can benefit from learning with others. Discussions and demonstrations often work well in groups.

Implications for Health Education

Health education occurs in a variety of situations, including clinics, hospitals, schools, colleges or universities, and community settings. Some situations offer the opportunity for advance planning, developing learning objectives, and arranging multiple teaching sessions. More often there is no time for a formal teaching approach in the practice area. Woodring emphasizes that "economic realities require nurses to use both their time with patients and their teaching opportunities more efficiently" (2000, p. 505). Nurses are often placed in the position of needing to maximize time to teach the child and family. There is also an expectation that the child and family have learned the information that is presented and that the learning will be evidenced by positive health outcomes (Woodring, 2000).

Step 1

There are six steps that nurses as educators can take to streamline the process of providing efficient yet personalized health teaching in a variety of settings. At the core of the teaching process remains the nurse–client relationship as described in the Miller-Stoeckel Client Education Model. The first step in building a trusting nurse–client relationship is to clarify the perceptions of the client and family about the health issue by asking questions. Questions regarding client perceptions are drawn from the health belief model (see Table 1-3). For example: What is the need for care? What do you know about the problem? What is the seriousness of the condition? What impact is it having on your life? What are your goals for effective treatment? What are potential barriers to treatment? Careful attention to the answers and observations of the client as he or she responds helps establish the need for health education and begins the process of building trust. It is important to be attentive to the client's cultural background as the nurse analyzes client responses.

Step 2

A second step is consideration of the assessment factors that influence learning. It is important to assess the child's physical, psychosocial, and language development. It is also helpful to determine family support for treatment. Tools are available to assess the learning styles and literacy levels of both the child and parent (Davis, Nur, & Ruru, 1994; James & Galbraith, 1984). Assessment factors will weigh heavily when planning learning activities later. It is possible that how the child and family members learn may be discerned simply by observing their responses to activities that occur within the usual care situation, but assessment tools provide an efficient and quick way to gather this information.

Step 3

As an educator you will draw on assessment data to establish mutual learning objectives that form the basis of the teaching plan as part of step 3. The learning objectives should be reviewed briefly with the child and family to answer questions and determine if all learning needs are identified.

You select teaching content appropriate to achieving the learning objectives and highlight the must-know information by separating information into small sections as part of the teaching plan. It is important to consider current evidence-based practices as part of the plan.

Step 4

Selection of teaching strategies and instructional materials to carry out the teaching plan is an important fourth step. Use assessment data to choose strategies and materials that accommodate learners' needs and abilities. It is important to take into account clients' cognitive stage, physical abilities, and language skills when planning activities. Reading capability and comprehension of the child and parent will help determine what instructional materials are appropriate. Learning materials should be age specific, interesting, and reflect the needs of the child. Remember that the cultural context of materials should be carefully considered as well. Brochures, pocket-sized flip charts, pamphlets, videos, and comic books depicting children of the client's race and ethnicity are suggestions for educational materials (Ebbinghaus & Bahrainwala, 2003). Samples of educational materials from pharmaceutical companies can be useful when return demonstrations are used.

Step 5

The fifth step is the implementation of the teaching plan. Select a conducive learning environment to meet the learning objectives of the teaching plan. Explanations should be simple and concrete with instructional materials that enhance understanding of the content. Speak slowly and clearly without extraneous noise interference. It is particularly important that you create an atmosphere that captures the child's interest. This may entail being adaptable and willing to offer the child options during the course of the teaching session. Pay close attention to body language that indicates distraction or lack of interest. It is particularly concerning if the child or parent does not ask questions. This is a clue that changes are needed in the teaching approach (Woodring, 2000). It is important for you to focus on the ultimate goal of the teaching session, child learning, not on maintaining a stubborn insistence on following the teaching plan. A good way to determine how the teaching session went is to ask the young client or parent to summarize what has been learned at the conclusion of the session so you can correct any misconceptions related to essential content. Questions such as, Tell me in your own words how you plan to . . . are helpful to evaluate understanding.

Step 6

Summative evaluation is the final step of the process. It not only evaluates content knowledge, but also allows the client to give the nurse feedback about what he or she liked or disliked about the whole teaching and learning experience. Client evaluation may include return demonstration, short quizzes, or checklists. Evaluation of the learning experience includes asking the child and family about factors such as the setting, teaching strategies, instructional materials, pace of learning activities, and the nurse–client interactions. Ideally you will see the child and family over time to assess long-term learning and provide reinforcement of essential content. This may involve scheduling follow-up teaching sessions, creating action plans for school use, and initiating a visiting nurse referral to provide ongoing education and support. **Figure 5-4** summarizes the steps of the health education process with children.

Stoeckel Health Education Process for Children

Step 1	Step 2	Step 3	Step 4	Step 5	Step 6
Nurse/Client Relationship	Assessing Learning Factors	Teaching Plan	Selection of Teaching Strategies & Instructional Materials	Implement Plan	Client Feedback

| Build trust

Get health perceptions

Cultural influences | Physical

Psychosocial

Language

Learning styles | Develop learning objectives

Develop content | Age-appropriate materials

Consider development stage

Assess reading capability and comprehension | Appropriate Learning Environment

Simple clear explanation

Formative Evaluation | Summative evaluation

Determine client likes and dislikes

Review of the teaching plan |

WORKING WITH CLIENTS WITH SPECIAL NEEDS

Nurses as educators may be asked to modify their approach to pediatric clients and their families to accommodate clients with special needs. Special needs clients include those with autism; cognitive limitations; learning disabilities; visual, hearing, or physical limitations; and emotional disturbances or behavior disorders. Nurse educators and parents need to consider how children with special needs respond to any form of stress brought on by illness or hospitalization. Children with disabilities generally have specific triggers, such as words, images, or sounds, that signal danger or disruption to their feelings of safety or security. These are specific to each child but come from past experiences associated with traumas or seeing fear in adults. These cues can serve as warning signals that adults can read (National Association of School Psychologists, 2002). Examples of cues include certain facial expressions, changes in speech patterns, sweating, or becoming quiet and withdrawn. When adults observe these cues, they should provide assurance, support, and attention as quickly as possible. If cues are missed, children may escalate their behavior and lose control. If this happens adults should remove the child to a safe place and allow him or her to calm down. Nurse educators and parents should work together to share information about triggers and cues.

Appropriate resources should be used that provide individual consideration for the child's developmental and emotional maturity. Acts of healing, such as making drawings or writing letters, may be important for children recovering from or facing illness. There are general guidelines that can be followed in preparation for teaching. They include preparing children for difficult vocabulary and concepts ahead of time. During the teaching session the nurse may give explanations in small distinct steps, provide written and oral instructions that are age appropriate, and have the child repeat directions. The nurse will have greater results by being concise with verbal information. This approach is demonstrated by wording requests in a concise way, such as

"Lisa please sit" instead of "Lisa would you please sit in the chair" (Bulloch, 2013). If a child has difficulty reading, the nurse can read or have a parent read. If a child has difficulty writing, oral responses can be accepted, or the child can dictate his or her thoughts to the nurse or parent.

All children benefit from concrete information presented at the proper level of understanding and maturity. The nurse educator and parents must consider how children with special needs respond to teaching and anticipate their reactions. Strategies that have been effective with special needs clients in the past are the best strategies to implement, but understand that the steps might need to be more concrete and immediate. The nurse as educator should consider triggers and cues and anticipate rather than react to them. The nurse educator should expect some regression and deal with inappropriate behaviors calmly and consistently. Children need to know that despite changes and disruptions, they have a constant caring support system.

WORKING WITH FAMILIES

Families have considerable influence on children's health practices and the success of health education. As an educator you must consider the family as part of the unit of care when addressing the health education needs of children. Preparing teaching plans for child clients without considering the family may result in less than adequate adherence to the treatment recommendations.

A family is a "group of individuals with a continuing legal, genetic, and/or emotional relationship. Society relies on the family group to provide for the economic and protective needs of individuals, especially children and the elderly" (American Academy of Family Physicians, 2003). Society's definition of family is rapidly expanding and has come to include single parents, biracial couples, blended families, unrelated individuals living cooperatively, and homosexual couples, among others.

It is important to determine who the immediate members of the family are, what roles they play within the structure of the family, their expectations about health care, and the nature of the relationships among family members. Not all families function the same way, so the nurse should assess this information by talking with clients and observing family interactions. Child health issues disrupt family functioning. The extent of disruption is dependent on the seriousness of the illness, the family's level of functioning before the illness, socioeconomic considerations, and the extent to which the illness disrupts family functioning.

When you are aware of how the family operates, you can work to address their health education needs. The most effective client education is that which is compatible with the family's frame of reference and with which the client or family feels most comfortable. The nurse should assess the family's response to health teaching because the group's reaction can have a significant influence on the child's and parents' motivation to continue and cooperate with recommended treatment.

WORKING WITH GROUPS AND COMMUNITIES

Nurses serve many different roles within the community. Public health nurses and school nurses assist children and families to take action to improve their health status. Often this takes the form of teaching parents and children about healthy lifestyle choices. Public health nurses assist people in incorporating improved health behavior in their everyday lives. Ensuring children's health is critical not only for reducing child morbidity and mortality, but also for increasing the likelihood of a healthier adult life. The primary goal of child health education in the community is to prevent major causes of disease, illness, and death during childhood. Health prevention teaching covers the topics of accidental injuries, infections, learning problems, and behavioral problems. The nurse may also work within school settings to develop action plans to support learning objectives.

Public health nurses educate clients concerning issues such as environmental risks, problems related to low family income, and psychological stress. Early detection and treatment of disease and disability require screening, counseling, and interventions for high-risk populations. For children from birth to age 10 years, screening includes measurement of height and weight, blood pressure, hearing, and vision. Counseling, or anticipatory guidance, relates to injury prevention, diet and exercise, substance use, and dental health. The nurse explains the importance of immunizations for children, which include diphtheria, tetanus, pertussis (DTaP); oral poliovirus; measles, mumps, rubella (MMR); H. influenza type B; hepatitis B; and varicella. For children older than age 10 years, additional screening recommendations include Pap smear and chlamydia screening for sexually active females and assessment of problem drinking for adolescents. Counseling with this age group covers sexual behaviors, smoking, drinking, and other drug use. Immunizations for this age group include tetanus–diphtheria booster for those aged 11 to 16 years. Hepatitis B and varicella vaccines should be given to those who did not receive them at earlier ages. High-risk populations include those who engage in high-risk sexual behavior or drug use and those with certain medical conditions.

Often the nurse will inform families about services available to them. The nurse needs to be knowledgeable about community programs, which include programs such as health services for low-income families, supplemental nutritional programs, child care services, safe houses for domestic violence, pediatric vaccine programs, and health education classes. One such nutrition program is the Women, Infants, and Children (WIC) program. WIC provides federal grants to states for supplemental foods, healthcare referrals, and nutrition education for low-income pregnant, breastfeeding, and nonbreastfeeding postpartum women. It also provides help for infants and children up to age 5 years who are found to be at nutritional risk. Another government service is Medicaid, which provides medical assistance for low-income families, mainly woman and children. State Children's Health Insurance Program (SCHIP) is insurance that is available for children who are not covered under Medicaid. A child must be younger than 19 years and be a member of a family whose income is 200% below the poverty level. It is important for you to become familiar with services that can support health education and evaluate funding requirements for which the family might be eligible.

WORKING WITH HEALTH TEAM MEMBERS

The nurse as educator works with multidisciplinary health team members in many settings. Each member of the team brings skills that contribute to the overall health of the child. Ideally the team collaborates to develop individualized and comprehensive treatment plans that serve as the foundation for health education. Team members should include the child, family, primary care physician, specialty physicians if necessary, the nurse (nurse practitioner, home care nurse), and other healthcare professionals, depending on the need. Other team members could include a social worker, patient care coordinator, pharmacist, dietitian, respiratory therapist, occupational therapist, physical therapist, speech pathologist, radiologist, psychiatrist or

Evidence-Based Nursing Practice

> Boweman, K. G., & Ruchala, P. L. (2006). A comparison of the postpartum learning needs of adolescent mothers and their mothers. *Journal of Obstetric, Gynecologic, & Neonatal Nursing* Nursing, 35(2), 250–256.
>
> **Purpose:** This study described postpartum learning needs of adolescent mothers and their mothers, and it compared the differences between the learning needs of the two groups.
>
> **Method:** A descriptive cross-sectional survey design was used to assess the postpartum learning needs of a convenience sample of 100 women (50 mother–daughter pairs) in three Midwestern hospitals over 1 year.
>
> **Results:** There were three group differences: emotional changes, resumption of sexual activity, and birth control. The results indicate that nurses may need to use different teaching strategies for adolescent mothers about resumption of sexual activity; however, teaching strategies for other topics may be the same.

psychologist, school teacher, and school nurse. It is important to view the child and family as an equal partner in the process of developing teaching plans. This type of client education is a family-centered and community-based approach (**Box 5-1**).

SUMMARY

This chapter reviewed the biologic characteristics, psychosocial stages, and developmental tasks of infants, toddlers, preschool children, school-age children, and adolescent children. Implications for health education were given for each age group. Orientation to learning in children involves how children learn, learning styles in children, and the role of play in learning. Specific teaching practices are used to promote child learning. Pedagogic concepts assist you as the educator in preparing teaching plans. Working with clients with special needs, families, groups, communities, and health team members brings together the importance of a multidisciplinary, holistic community-based approach to health education for children.

EXERCISES

Exercise I: Deepen Sensitivity to Child Clients and Their Families

Purpose: Practice application of child learning theory.
Directions: Visit a preschool and gather a group of 6 to 10 preschoolers to complete the following tasks:

1. You are teaching a health education class to a group of preschoolers. Compose a health promotion song with gestures, using the tune of a popular nursery song or popular song; for example, "Safety the Snowman" (to the tune of "Frosty the Snowman").
2. Use props you have on hand to enhance the meaning of the song (e.g., bicycle helmets, street signs, etc.).

3. Share the songs with members of the class.
4. Discuss how you think the children learned the information.

Exercise II: Pretend Play

Purpose: Practice applying theory, discussed in this chapter, with children.
Directions: Role-play a baby doll clinic. Involve a nurse, children, and their dolls in a preschool setting to complete the following tasks:

1. Have the "mothers" come and see the nurse by walking into the pretend clinic or making an appointment on the pretend phone.
2. Have the nurse notice concern for the doll's health and ask what the mother wants (doll checkup or illness).
3. Have the nurse perform an examination, treatment, or give advice.
4. Ask a health or safety question about the doll.
5. Use real equipment or pretend you are using equipment.
6. With your peers, discuss what you learned by doing this exercise.

Exercise III: Helping Children with Chronic Illness

Purpose: Use your knowledge of child development and learning strategies.
Directions: For small groups to complete the following tasks:

1. Describe an adolescent with a long-term chronic illness. Include information such as age, developmental needs, amount of regression, and how the illness interferes with normal developmental tasks.
2. Design substitute experiences that would enhance the child's chances for meeting appropriate developmental needs.

Exercise IV: Group Teaching with Children

Purpose: Apply child learning theory to working in groups.
Directions: Role-play the following teaching and learning scenario with school-age children:

1. You are working with a group of fifth or sixth graders discussing a topic of your choice.
2. Choose topics such as peer pressure, drugs, sex, abuse, eating disorders, or bullying.
3. Lead the children in role-playing and discussing a difficult situation.
4. Offer suggestions to address the problems that the children present; for example, how to develop refusal skills to drugs or how to seek help for bullying.
5. With your peers, discuss what you have learned by doing this exercise.

REFERENCES

American Academy of Family Physicians. (2003). Definition of family. Retrieved from http://www.aafp.org/online/en/home/policy/policies/f/familydefinitionof.html

Athey, C. (2007). *Extending thought in young children: A parent teacher partnership* (2nd ed.). London, England: Paul Chapman Educational.

Babcock, D. E., & Miller, M. A. (1994). *Client education: Theory and practice*. St. Louis, MO: Mosby.

Boweman, K. G., & Ruchala, P. L. (2006). A comparison of the postpartum learning needs of adolescent mothers and their mothers. *Journal of Obstetric, Gynecologic, & Neonatal Nursing, 35*(2), 250–256.

Bulloch, K. (2013). How to adapt your teaching strategies to student needs. Retrieved from http://www.ldonline.org/article/370

Carbo, M., Dunn, R., & Dunn, K. (1986). *Teaching students to read through their individual learning styles.* Englewood Cliffs, NJ: Prentice Hall.

David, T., Goouch, D., Powell, S., & Abbott, L. (2003). Birth to three matters: A review of the literature compiled to inform the framework to support children in their earliest years. Research Report 444. London, England: DfES.

Davis, E. C., Nur, H., & Ruru, S. A. (1994). Helping teachers and students understand learning styles. *English Teaching Forum, 32*(3), 12–15.

Ebbinghaus, S., & Bahrainwala, A. H. (2003). Asthma management by an inpatient asthma care team. *Pediatric Nursing, 29*(3), 177–183.

Erikson, E. (1963). *Childhood and society* (2nd ed.). New York, NY: W. W. Norton.

Falvo, D. R. (2004). *Effective patient education: A guide to increased compliance.* Sudbury, MA: Jones and Bartlett.

Graca, S., Fowler, K., & Rosenstock A. (2009). Play—an educational tool in health care. In A. Lowenstein, L. Foord-May, & J. D. Romano (Eds.), *Teaching strategies for health education and health promotion: Working with patients, families and communities.* Sudbury, MA: Jones and Bartlett.

Hiemstra, R., & Sisco, B. (1990). *Individualizing instruction.* San Francisco, CA: Jossey-Bass.

Isenberg, J., & Quisenberry, N. (2002). Play: Essential for all children. (A position paper of the Association for Childhood Education). Association for Childhood Education International, *79*(1), 33–39.

James, W., & Galbraith, M. (1984). Perceptual learning styles: Implications and techniques for the practitioner. *Lifelong Learning, 8*(4), 23.

Jones, E., & Reynolds, G. (1992). *The play's the thing: Teachers' roles in children's play.* New York, NY: Teachers College Press.

Kearsley, G. (2004). Explorations in learning and instruction: The theory into practice database. Retrieved from http://tip.psychology.org/index.html

National Association of School Psychologists. (2002). Coping with crisis-helping children with special needs: Tips for school personnel and parents. Retrieved from http://www.nasponline.org/resources/crisis_safety/specpop_general.aspx

National Institute on Deafness and Other Communication Disorders. (2014). Speech and language developmental milestones. Retrieved from http://www.nidcd.nih.gov/staticresources/health/voice/NIDCD-Speech-Language-Dev-Milestones.pdf

Olsen, M. H., & Hergenhahn, B. R. (2013). *An introduction to theories of learning* (9th ed.). Boston, MA: Pearson Prentice Hall.

Piaget, J. (1952). *The origins of intelligence in children.* New York, NY: International Universities Press.

Piaget, J. (1963). *The psychology of intelligence.* New York, NY: Routledge.

Skinner, B. F. (1968). *The technology of teaching.* New York, NY: Appleton-Century-Crofts.

United Nations. (1989). Convention on the rights of the child, G.A. res. 44/25, annex, 44 U.N. GAOR Supp. (No. 49) at 167, U.N. Doc. A/44/49 (1989). Entered into force Sept. 2, 1990. Retrieved from http://www1.umn.edu/humanrts/instree/k2crc.htm

Wong, D. L., Hockenberry-Eaton, M., Wilson, D., Winkelstein, M. L., & Schwartz, P. (2008). *Wong's essentials of pediatric nursing* (6th ed.). St. Louis, MO: Mosby Elsevier.

Woodring, B. C. (2000). If you have taught—have the child and family learned? *Pediatric Nursing, 26*(5), 505–509.

6

The Adult Learner

OBJECTIVES

Upon completion of this chapter, you will be able to do the following:

- Describe the biologic changes, psychosocial stages, and developmental tasks that are characteristic of early and middle adulthood.
- List health education topics for clients in early and middle adulthood related to biologic changes, psychosocial stages, and developmental tasks.
- Distinguish among goal-, activity-, and learning-oriented learners and state which category best fits your motivation.
- Distinguish between pedagogy and andragogy.
- Describe how adult and child learners are alike and different in two of the assumptions of andragogy.
- Apply andragogic theory to teaching adult learners.
- Identify teaching and learning implications of working with individuals, families, groups and communities, and health team members.

KEY TERMS

activity-oriented learner
andragogy
developmental task

extrinsic motivation
goal-oriented learner
intrinsic motivation

learning-oriented learner
pedagogy
psychosocial stage

INTRODUCTION

This chapter discusses learning in adulthood and divides this period into early and middle adulthood. Learning and development are lifelong processes with identifiable features, including biologic characteristics, psychosocial stages, and developmental tasks. Learning and development are multidimensional and unique for each client, with implications for those who are seeking to promote, retain, and restore health.

Nurses work with clients of all ages who have different learning needs at different stages of development. This information is important because it affects what you teach and how you teach it. The first section of this chapter examines biologic characteristics, psychosocial stages, and developmental tasks, and their implications for nurses as educators. **Andragogy,** a theory of adult learning, and its underlying assumptions are examined. We describe how andragogy differs from **pedagogy,** the theory of how children learn.

BIOLOGIC CHARACTERISTICS, PSYCHOSOCIAL STAGES, AND DEVELOPMENTAL TASKS

Adulthood is divided into two periods: early and middle. This division is made because the biologic characteristics, psychosocial stages, and **developmental tasks** that accompany these periods are distinct. **Figure 6-1** illustrates the overlapping influence of these factors.

FIGURE 6-1

Factors Influencing Development Across the Life Span

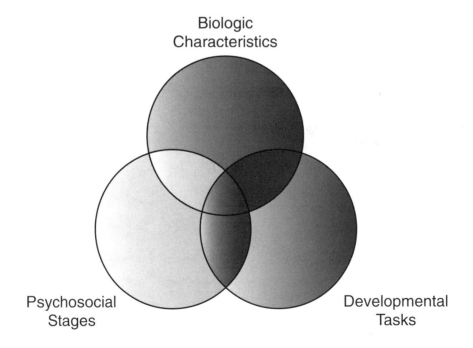

Early Adulthood (Early 20s through 30s)

Biologic Characteristics

Clients complete their physical growth and experience peak functioning of the musculoskeletal system in their 20s. Laboratory findings are generally within normal limits. The health status of men and women is generally uneventful unless severe illness or injury occurs. Women have additional health concerns during pregnancy and lactation. The occurrence of chronic disease is unusual but can occur in this period (Ruchala, 2013; Santrock, 2014).

Psychosocial Stages

Erikson's **psychosocial stages** for previous life stages are applicable to early and middle adulthood (1963). During puberty the psychosocial stage is identity versus role confusion, from which a sense of identity develops. As young adults continue to mature, they move into Erikson's next stage, intimacy versus isolation, which is characterized by an increasing ability to love and care about others. They seek meaningful friendships and intimacy with others (Balakas, 2013). It is also during this stage that young adults clarify their values, understand themselves and others better, and develop a philosophy of life (Knowles, 1990). It is the longest of Erikson's psychosocial stages, covering the ages of 40 to 65 years.

Developmental Tasks

Becoming economically independent, establishing a career, and developing job-related skills are important tasks during this time. Making new friends and selecting a mate or significant other, starting a family, and rearing children are common tasks. Learning to get along with others at work, one's mate, and friends are other tasks. Dealing with ethnic and gender factors, changing role expectations in the United States, and the need for two-career families are stressors that influence these tasks (Santrock, 2014).

Middle Adulthood (40s to Late 60s)

Biologic Characteristics

Clients in this stage begin to experience gradual physical changes, the rate of which can vary widely among individuals. Changes are influenced by genetic and lifestyle factors. Clients tend to gain weight, the skin begins to wrinkle and loosen, the hair turns gray, muscle mass and strength decline, and blood pressure and cholesterol levels may increase. Vision and hearing acuity decreases, women experience menopause, and men experience climacteric, which is similar to menopause. Cognitive functioning remains intact unless it is affected by illness or injury (Ruchala, 2013; Santrock, 2014).

Psychosocial Stages

Erikson's (1963) stage for this period is generativity versus self-absorption and stagnation, with a focus on helping the younger generation develop and lead useful lives. Generativity refers to the concern mature adults have for guiding the next generation. It includes being productive and creative. If they have children, parents may help them choose a suitable career. Cultural interests increase, as does social involvement and leadership responsibilities in organizations and the community (Knowles, 1990; Santrock, 2014).

Developmental Tasks

Clients are learning advanced job skills, often supervising others. Some are dealing with unemployment. If so, clients may be looking for new careers or educational opportunities to acquire new skills. Cultural interests increase, as does social involvement with others. As children leave home, spouses must readjust their marital relationship. If divorce occurs, further lifestyle adjustments are needed. Stay-at-home mothers may return to the job market. These clients may have living parents who require time and financial attention. Because adults in this stage are still involved with raising their children and caring for aging parents, they are called the sandwich generation (Knowles, 1990; Santrock, 2014).

IMPLICATIONS FOR HEALTH EDUCATION

How does this information help you become more sensitive and effective in your role as an educator? We now look at how this information helps you promote, retain, and restore the health of your clients.

Promote and Retain Health

The focus of promoting health is on prevention, whereas the focus of retaining health is on maintaining one's present health status, assuming it is satisfactory. With this in mind, **Table 6-1** lists suggested topics to promote and retain health that are appropriate for adult learners (Ruchala, 2013). These suggestions are not all inclusive and will need to be adapted to the circumstances of the individual client.

Restore Health

Restoration of health for individuals in adulthood refers to addressing the needs of those who are experiencing an acute or chronic illness or disability. The purpose of health education at this time is designed to help clients understand the nature of their health problem, the treatment regimen, and the limitations imposed by the health problem, disability, or injury. This may involve not only working with clients, but also with family members. **Table 6-2** suggests suitable topics related to the restoration of health (Ruchala, 2013). These suggestions are not all inclusive and need to be adapted to the circumstances of the individual client.

ORIENTATION TO LEARNING

Houle (1961, 1980) found that adults continue learning for a variety of reasons. He identified three categories that describe adults' general orientation to learning: goal-oriented learners, activity-oriented learners, and learning-oriented learners.

TABLE 6-1

Suggested Topics to Promote and Retain Health

Nursing Assessment	Health Education Topics
General health habits	▪ Eating nutritious diet with dietary changes to control weight ▪ Practicing regular oral hygiene and dental care ▪ Obtaining adequate sleep ▪ Knowing benefits of an exercise program ▪ Managing physical stress ▪ Coping with mental stress, such as depression ▪ Minimizing risks of disease for which there is a family history, such as diabetes mellitus and cardiovascular disease
General living conditions	▪ Avoiding exposure to hazardous cleaning supplies ▪ Maintaining home safety for elderly and children (slip-resistant rugs, night-lights, nonskid adhesive textured strips in tub and shower, handrails on steps, grab bars in bathrooms, electrical outlets, etc.) ▪ Maintaining cleanliness in the home ▪ Managing family stress or abuse
Medications	▪ Using prescription medications properly ▪ Minimizing use of caffeine, tobacco, alcohol ▪ The dangers of illicit drugs and avoiding them ▪ Promoting medication safety with children in the home
Sexual habits	▪ Preventing sexually transmitted diseases (STDs) ▪ Knowing mode of STD transmission ▪ Knowing partner's sexual history and practices ▪ Practicing safe sexual practices ▪ Recognizing STD symptoms
Pregnancy and children	▪ Knowing about family planning ▪ Addressing pregnancy and lactation issues ▪ Knowing child growth and developmental stages ▪ Obtaining immunizations ▪ Parenting skills
Work site and employment	▪ Maintaining safe occupational environment ▪ Avoiding exposure to hazardous substances ▪ Minimizing economic stress ▪ Minimizing job stress
Disease prevention	▪ Getting routine health screening, blood pressure checks ▪ Knowing serum cholesterol levels ▪ Performing monthly skin checks ▪ Obtaining monthly breast exam and annual mammogram ▪ Performing monthly male genitalia exam ▪ Obtaining annual flu shot ▪ Getting regular physical and screening exams

TABLE 6-2

Suggested Topics to Restore Health

Nursing Assessment	*Health Education Topics*
Acute illness	■ Knowing nature and cause of the health problem or disability ■ Common conditions: Upper respiratory infections, urinary tract infections, minor surgery, substance abuse ■ Understanding diagnostic tests ■ Supporting and explaining treatment regimen ■ Knowing hospital and clinic environment and routines ■ Preventing spread of communicable illnesses ■ Dealing with lifestyle changes ■ Supporting continued physician supervision
Chronic illness	■ Knowing nature and cause of the health problem or disability ■ Possible conditions: Multiple sclerosis, rheumatoid arthritis, hypertension, diabetes mellitus, AIDS, cancer, substance abuse ■ Understanding diagnostic tests ■ Using physical, occupational, speech therapies ■ Managing exacerbations and remissions ■ Preventing complications ■ Adapting to lifestyle changes ■ Making environmental adaptations ■ Using self-help devices ■ Supporting and explaining treatment regimen ■ Supporting continued provider supervision
Disability	■ Knowing strengths and limitations due to disability ■ Managing activities of daily living ■ Building on abilities
Accidents	■ Adapting to nature of injury and impact on function ■ Managing activities of daily living ■ Building on abilities ■ Addressing rehabilitation issues ■ Preventing accidents and injuries ■ Providing safe home environment (slip-resistant rugs, night-lights, nonskid adhesive textured strips in tub and shower, handrails on steps, grab bars in bathrooms, etc.)

Goal-Oriented Learners

Goal-oriented learners use their educational endeavors to accomplish clear and identifiable objectives. They often wait until their middle 20s to make a start on their education, and sometimes they wait much longer. Their educational activities tend to occur in episodes, each beginning with the realization of a need or an interest to expand their skills and knowledge. Houle (1961, 1980) found that learning was a recurring pattern in their lives. These learners were not restricted to an academic setting or to any one institution or topic. They sought courses of instruction or other forms of learning when they became aware of a need. Exploration on the Internet, attending night courses, and enrolling in workshops were ways to add to their level of expertise.

Activity-Oriented Learners

Activity-oriented learners select activities that are likely to meet their need for human contact. They are course takers and group joiners. The course content or purpose of the organization is secondary to their social needs. These learners often begin their educational activities when their need to reach out to others becomes pressing. For example, divorce adjustment groups attract people who are attempting to fill specific needs. A young mother joins a La Leche group to fulfill her need for socialization and for support and information to breastfeed successfully. A divorced man takes a class in astronomy to talk to other people and ease his loneliness.

When setting up health education programs for adult learners, it is helpful to assess their interests via a survey. Although many adults indicate specific interests, a substantial number just want something to do and seek out classes for social reasons. You should become aware of community support groups and consider this category of learning activities whenever social isolation and loneliness are encountered. Newspapers periodically print lists of self-help and special interest groups. You should include such lists in your resource files and maintain connections in the community.

Learning-Oriented Learners

Learning-oriented individuals seek knowledge for its own sake. Often they have been engrossed in learning all their lives and are avid readers. These individuals see themselves as lifelong learners and investigate everything of interest. They join groups, classes, and organizations they anticipate will be educational. An example of this is a learner who joins a book discussion group at the local library. When these learners travel, they prepare for trips by engaging in activities that make the trips more informative. They read about their destination in books, periodicals, or on the Internet, or they might take a language course.

Figure 6-2 summarizes Houle's (1961, 1980) three orientations to learning. Most people fit into each of the categories at different times in their lives. People find that they emphasize one category more often than others. Houle concluded that most adults engage in continuing education every year, which they plan themselves. He also noted that people do not have to fit into only one category. His generalizations were meant to clarify motivations rather than to confine people to categories.

ANDRAGOGY

Malcolm Knowles, known as the Father of Andragogy in the United States, posited that adults learn differently than children. To explain this process he developed a theory of adult learning, comprised of core adult learning principles that apply to all adult learning situations, called andragogy. His theory is about the art and science of how adults learn. Knowles's theory has its

FIGURE 6-2

Primary Orientations to Learning. Individuals learn for different reasons; three primary orientations
are goal, activity, and learning.

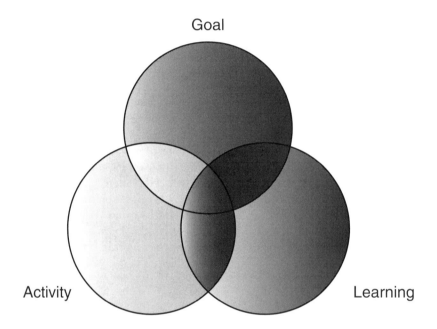

roots in the work of Abraham Maslow and Carl Rogers, who were concerned with self-actual-ization of the individual and a pragmatic philosophy that values knowledge gained from expe-rience rather than formal authority (Knowles, Holton, & Swanson, 2011).

Knowles contrasted how children learn (pedagogy) in the formal education system with how adults learn (andragogy). The forces that impinge on educating young children have more to do with achieving than with learning. He cited passing tests, scoring high on the Scholastic Aptitude Test, and getting into college or graduate school as the goals of much formal educa-tion (Knowles, 1990). He noted that many assumptions that underlie the teaching methods used for adults were derived from pedagogy and are inappropriate for adults. He observed that adults learn best in informal, comfortable, flexible, and nonthreatening settings, and he consequently popularized a different set of assumptions, also called core principles, that apply to all adult learning situations. The six core principles of andragogy are (1) the learner's need to know, (2) the learner's self-concept, (3) the role of the learner's prior experiences, (4) readiness to learn, (5) orientation to learning, and (6) motivation to learn.

These principles should be viewed in a general sense and applied only as they fit the learn-ers with whom you are working. They are also applied along with consideration of several variables, such as the context of the learning situation. For example, are you working with an individual or a group? Are you face to face with the learner or communicating online? A sec-ond variable to take into consideration is the differences in the nature of the subject matter.

For example, are you teaching knowledge content, performance skills, or attitudes and values? For each type of subject matter, you will select appropriate teaching strategies. A third variable to take into consideration is individual learner differences. For example, what are the abilities, learning styles, and preferences among your learners? How does each prefer to learn? These variables and core principles or assumptions (Knowles et al., 2011) are discussed in the following sections, and healthcare examples are provided.

The Need to Know

Adults want to understand why they should learn something new before they are willing to learn it. In this case you will need to be persuasive in explaining why your teaching is important. Others may recognize a gap in their current knowledge and realize they need more education in specific areas. Adult learners may also want to participate in setting the goals for learning. Adults who initiate new learning projects on their own spend considerable time and effort weighing the cost–benefit ratio before they expend large amounts of time and energy on new projects.

Application to Health Education

In your introductory remarks with adult clients in any individual or group teaching and learning situation, explain the importance of the instructional content and identify the benefits of learning it. Persuade them about the importance of learning the material by making it attractive and interesting. If you are working with a group, each individual has joined it for a different reason, so another approach would be to ask the clients what motivates them to be present and have them share their thoughts with the group. Some clients may want help developing learning objectives to address their self-identified knowledge gaps. As an educator, this gives you some sense of what motivates each individual and why they are present. Do this by asking questions such as the following:

- What do you hope to get from this lesson?
- What do you expect from our time together?
- What is the best outcome you hope for?
- Why have you come out on this beautiful (or awful) day?

Another approach is to set up situations in which clients discover for themselves the likely benefits of their efforts. For example, a first-time mother may have a multitude of questions about the care of her baby. As you work with the mother, ask her questions such as the following:

- What are your plans for caring for your baby at home?
- Have you thought about the equipment you will need at home to care for your baby?
- Will you have any help at home in caring for your baby?
- What are your concerns about the care of your baby?
- Is there anything that worries you about the care of your baby?

The Learners' Self-Concept

As individuals grow into adulthood, they increasingly see themselves as responsible beings in charge of their own lives and capable of making their own decisions. Having achieved maturity, adults wish to be respected and treated as being capable of self-direction. Any attempt to treat them as uninformed children in need of direction in the teaching and learning situation is considered demeaning. It is important to avoid talking down to clients.

Application to Health Education

This need for self-direction often presents a problem for you and clients because the situation may necessitate some client dependency. In the hospital you have information about the acutely ill client's physiologic status, and you will be in a better position to decide what information is helpful for them to know. During certain stages of illness the client may relinquish some control and trust your judgment and expert care. You can gently guide them in appropriate learning at this time.

Some clients who become dependent may respond with fear, bitterness, and sarcasm to relinquishing their independence. For example, an older man was rude to the nurses who cared for him while he was suffering from incontinence. He was accustomed to being the boss, and his strong self-concept was being challenged by the reality of his new dependency. The nurses were matter-of-fact and unperturbed while changing his soiled linen. As the nurses worked, they taught him that his incontinence was temporary and control would return with time and healing. They understood this response and treated him with respect and courtesy even though he was angry and rude.

Health problems may evoke feelings of unmet dependency needs in the client and complementary issues in you, such as the need to control. An example is a nurse who experiences a dependency problem when dealing with burn clients. The nurse thinks, "If only they would do what I say, they will learn that they will feel and look better in the long run. They do not understand that not moving will affect burn healing. It is up to me to teach them about the consequences of immobility before it is too late. They need to listen to me." This nurse wanted the clients to trust her advice and depend on her. In addition, the nurse is adamant about the nurse's role and her expected behavior of clients. In this case the nurse as educator needs to reflect on her need to control and take a more empathetic approach to the clients.

The Role of the Learners' Prior Experiences

As people mature they accumulate an expanding reservoir of experiences, both in quantity and quality. Based on these experiences, adults are able to handle more complex issues and make more thoughtful decisions that take into consideration a number of variables. Experience is something that happens to children, but for adults experience is what defines them. A way to check out this assumption is to ask people of various ages, "Tell me about yourself." You will hear differences in the way children and adults answer. **Figure 6-3** shows adults in an active learning role.

Application to Health Education

Adults bring a wide range of health experiences that nurses as educators can draw on as a group discusses common issues. Nurses guide the discussion by being a facilitator of learning and provide new information as appropriate. This is in contrast to lecturing to the group with little or no time for discussion. Some members of a group may have more experience with a

FIGURE 6-3

Experience Defines Older Adults

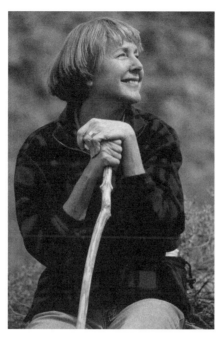

Source: © Steve Mason/PhotoDisc

particular issue than the nurse, and that person can become a resource for the group. For example, a small group of diabetic clients met weekly to discuss their experiences in dealing with this disease. The nurse shared information about the physicians' medical regimen. Several clients in the group who had grappled with diabetes for more than 10 years explained the difficulties of balancing insulin intake, exercise, and nutritional requirements. By encouraging clients to share their experiences, the nurse tapped into a rich reservoir of experience to take advantage of the expertise of group members.

Adult clients learn better when strategies are employed that respect a broad base of knowledge and experience and that make use of it in the teaching and learning situation. Strategies such as discussion, laboratory, simulation, field experience, team projects, and other action-learning approaches are more conducive to the way adults learn and have strong experiential and integrating components. A good place to start is to ask adults what experiences they have had on the topic and then listen to how they interpret that experience and what it meant to them. For example, in teaching team members about a new urinary catheterization procedure, the nurse asked what their past experience has been. Have they done a similar procedure before? Were they familiar with the new equipment? What was their reaction to the new procedure? The nurse listened carefully to what was said and prepared the teaching plan accordingly.

Sometimes having extensive experience is a hindrance to learning, according to Knowles (1990). Habits, biases, and presuppositions become a hindrance when the person is not open to looking at health issues in new and different ways. The nurse's role in these situations is to help clients examine troublesome and unresolved health issues and guide them in looking for alternative ways of doing things. Nurses can encourage clients to examine health habits that are not working for them and find creative ways to make changes.

In summary, it is important to recognize adult learners' experiences and contributions. If their experiences are ignored or devalued, they will likely reject efforts to learn in new ways. We believe this phenomenon is behind the resentment that some adults express when they return to school after years of earning a living and are not respected for what they have accomplished.

Readiness to Learn

It is assumed that children are ready to learn according to their biologic development and academic progress. Developmental readiness is also necessary for adult learning. The needs of adults, however, are related less to their biologic maturation and more to the developing roles in life that they have chosen or have had thrust upon them. A nurse's first pregnancy is an example. "I was a good student and did well in my OB/GYN experiences and state board examinations. Some years later, when I was pregnant, I went to childbirth education classes and was amazed at what I did not know. I listened with keen attention and made many associations that had not occurred to me when I was learning how to attend to women in labor and delivery. My increased interest was caused by a change in role. Now I was the one who was entering the role of pregnant woman and expectant parent."

Readiness to learn in the adult is associated with the ability to meet the developmental tasks associated with each stage in life. Adults face real-life situations and want to learn whatever will help them cope with their present circumstances and evolving social roles. Developing job skills and a professional identity, earning a living, meeting community responsibilities, establishing successful relationships, raising a family, and aging gracefully are some examples of these tasks.

Application to Health Education

Adults often seek out knowledge and skills based on a current health need at a particular time in their lives. Perhaps clients encounter a problem or situation and recognize that they do not have the knowledge or experience to handle it. Many adults are self-directed and find the information they need in the local library or in a class offering at a local college or community learning center. For example, a class titled "How to Remember" was offered in a setting that attracted retired citizens who had the time, energy, and resources to attend. The enrollment was high because the topic was on memory. Older people experience difficulty in remembering and find it a blow to their self-concept when they are forgetful. This workshop offered attendees an opportunity to address an important need.

Knowles (1990) noted that it is not always necessary to wait for readiness to learn to develop. You can foster readiness through experiences you create when you expose clients to successful role models. For example, encourage clients to participate in community-sponsored health fairs designed to prevent illness and detect early evidence of disease. When clients attend health education classes, they learn how to live more healthfully and how to prevent illness. By anticipating the future, clients can prepare themselves emotionally and intellectually if problems develop.

Orientation to Learning

Adults want to learn when it helps them perform a task or deal more effectively with current problems. This approach to learning is in contrast with learning that occurs in the formal educational system, in which the teacher decides what is to be learned and how the subject matter is to be organized. Adults want learning that helps them in the here and now, not learning that will be useful sometime in the future.

Andragogy assumes that adults learn better when life- or task-centered problems are the organizing factor. Adults are reluctant to expend their resources (time, money, and energy) to learn information, skills, and attitudes that they do not see as directly relevant to their current lives or problems they anticipate having. When you take a continuing education program or enroll in a degree-advancing program, you want to know how you can use it when you go to work tomorrow.

Application to Health Education

Adult clients expect nurses as educators to be knowledgeable and experientially familiar with the health issues they face. Clients expect health professionals to be in touch with real-life challenges in current society. They look for nurses who show empathy for their situation and respond to them in a professional manner. For example, one popular diabetic nurse was introduced to a group as "one of those nurses who works with diabetic clients in the clinic and has diabetes herself." Adults find information easier to grasp when it is presented in a practical life context. When clients ask for an example, they want you to present a real-life example to which they can relate. Another valuable approach is to set up a simulation or interactive exercise and offer clients the opportunity to role-play appropriate behavior in a safe setting.

Organization of content is important to learning and good teaching. Your challenge is to develop an effective teaching plan. A good place to begin is the development of learning objectives to meet the client's needs. This should be a collaborative effort between you and the client. After the objectives are developed, the teaching plan is organized. A good principle is to teach from the simple to the complex. Clients appreciate content that is presented from the simple to the complex and within a context to which they can relate. Other principles are to use a logical train of thought and to promote association. There are times when presenting the concept and then following it with more specific applications is the most effective way of teaching. There are other times when experiencing a number of events and then looking for their relationship to one another is more meaningful. The point is worth repeating. After the learning objectives are in place, organization of content is important. The most effective type of organization will vary with the objectives, the client, you, and the situation.

Motivation to Learn

According to Knowles (1990), the most effective motivators for adults are internal pressures and personal reasons; some examples are the desire for increased job satisfaction, self-esteem, quality of life, and so forth. Adults also respond to external motivators; for example, they may strive for a better job, a promotion, or a higher salary. Santrock (2014) calls these **intrinsic** and **extrinsic motivators.** Intrinsic motivators are like Knowles's internal pressures and are characteristic of an individual who does something for its own sake; for example, an adult may study literature because it is enjoyable. Extrinsic motivators are like Knowles's external motivators, which occur when an individual does something to obtain a reward or avoid a punishment, as noted.

Adults seek out learning experiences for a variety of reasons. Merriam, Caffarella, and Baumgartner (2007), quoting Boshier (1991), identify seven factors that motivate adults to continue learning: (1) improvement of verbal and written skills, (2) social interaction with others, (3) remediation of past deficiencies, (4) improvement of career or job status, (5) improvement of family relationships, (6) social stimulation, and (7) following interests and seeking new knowledge. These are broad-based and powerful motivators for adults seeking continued learning.

Carl Rogers (1961) and Abraham Maslow (1987) demonstrated that adults are motivated toward self-improvement and continued growth. In Maslow's terminology, adults strive for self-actualization. However, barriers such as negative self-concept, inability to access resources, time constraints, and programs that violate adult learning principles all interfere with the growth process. Our own experiences as clinicians and teachers working with clients of different ages and abilities leads us to believe that these principles have broad application. See **Figure 6-4**.

FIGURE 6-4

Adult Learners Are Motivated for Intrinsic and External Reasons

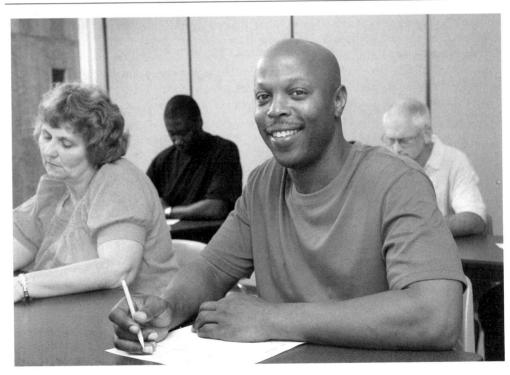

Source: © Lisa F. Young/ShutterStock, Inc.

Application to Health Education

During times of illness and stress, clients are more motivated to make changes and modifications to improve their health status. Often health-altering events cause clients to seek help for themselves or their family members. The nurse as educator asks, What is the nature of the client's problem, and what kind of adaptations will he or she have to make? How life-altering are these adaptations? Are they lifestyle changes, or do they involve a lengthy rehabilitation regimen? Is the client temporarily or permanently disabled? Depending on the seriousness of the health problem, clients undergo several stages of adjustment, and most become motivated to improve their health status.

Nurses also see clients who are undergoing stressful life situations that compound health problems they are experiencing. For example, consider clients who are going through role changes and life transitions, such as changing careers and requiring new skills, transitioning from childless couple to parents, and moving from being employed to unemployed. A life transition is the process that individuals undergo when their roles change dramatically, as in the death of a significant other, birth, marriage, divorce, moving from a stable environment, and making a radical work change. A life transition may force clients to make a paradigm shift in their thinking. As an educator you can capture these moments when clients are amenable and motivated to hear your suggestions and encouragement. These times are what educators call teachable moments. It is a time when you have clients' full attention.

Table 6-3 compares the different assumptions of pedagogy and andragogy as they affect the approach to learning. This information is important because it influences how you approach clients of different ages. It is the theoretical knowledge that undergirds your teaching plan and your approach to health education. Although the table makes a distinction between pedagogy and andragogy, the principles of andragogy have been reported to be effective in teaching younger clients (Knowles, Holton, & Swanson, 2005; O'Shea, 2003).

TABLE 6-3

A Comparison of Assumptions of Pedagogic and Andragogic Approaches to Learning

Assumptions About Learning	Pedagogy	Andragogy
Need to know	Teacher driven; accepted by learner	Learner driven
Self-concept	Accepts direction from teacher	Self-directed
Role of experience	Happens to the learner	Integrally involved with self-concept; must be acknowledged
Readiness to learn	Biologic and academic development	Evolving social and life roles
Orientation to learning	Subject centered; selected by the teacher	Life centered; task and problem centered
Motivation	External approval by the teacher	Internal drives and life goals

Source: Modified from Knowles (1990); Knowles et al. (2005).

EXPERIENTIAL LEARNING

Learning in adulthood is also viewed from experiential learning theory, an approach that combines experience, perception, cognition, and behavioral learning theories. Personal experiences serve as sources of learning and contribute to adult development. Although experiential learning theory is applicable to individuals in all life stages from childhood to old age, we believe it is especially suitable for working with adult clients who have accumulated a wealth of life experiences.

Kolb developed a model for experiential learning (1984). From adults' concrete experiences, they formulate observations and reflect on those experiences. This leads to the formation of abstract concepts and generalizations, theories about effectiveness and ineffectiveness. Following this, adults test the implications of new concepts in new situations. Through personal experiences they continuously modify their thoughts, concepts, and ideas of the world and their environment. In this model it is not necessarily the outcome that is important; the focus is on the process of learning.

Implications for Health Education

Teaching strategies that combine theory and practice with practical application are most effective for adults. Because learning is grounded in experience, not all experiences have resulted in accurate knowledge. Nurses as educators can implant new ideas and information to revise inaccurate perceptions. It is often helpful to begin teaching by asking learners what they know about the topic. If they express inaccurate beliefs and information, discuss them with the client. Nurses are responsible for modifying these beliefs by presenting accurate information, but they may encounter client resistance to new information. Clients must then decide if they will integrate, substitute, or reject this new information.

WORKING WITH FAMILIES

Illness affects not only the client, but also the client's family and significant others. When clients need assistance from others, nurses must be sensitive to their wishes about the degree to which they want family and significant others participating in their health education. Some clients value their privacy, whereas other clients want family and significant others involved. If clients require procedures and follow-up care that they are unable to do themselves, they may request that others be involved. In all cases it is important to avoid embarrassing clients by sharing unnecessary information with family or significant others. If clients want family and significant others involved, then reveal only information that is essential for communicating the health message.

WORKING WITH GROUPS AND COMMUNITIES

Many social groups, civic organizations, educational institutions, and industries are interested in health education and are looking for guest speakers. If you have a specialty area, consider making yourself available to these groups. It will build your confidence, and you will realize ways to contribute to your community. For example, nursing students were invited to present a program on healthful living to members of a local church. Each took a topic and kept their remarks pertinent and brief, and they supplemented the information with colorful audiovisual aids. They talked about the benefits of good nutrition, adequate sleep, daily exercise, and mental stimulation through a variety of activities. The audience listened and had questions following the students' presentation. Other nursing students met with female members of another church and taught them about early detection of breast cancer. They taught breast self-examination through a video presentation followed by demonstration of the technique on breast models. Both were successful events—many of the women scheduled mammograms at a nearby hospital.

When presenting health education to a group in the community, be sure to make it lively and interesting by using a variety of teaching strategies and instructional materials. Announce your presentation in advance by publishing it in a local newsletter or community newspaper to attract an audience. Doing so provides time for the audience to work it into their daily schedule. Also, give your presentation an interesting and catchy title, something that creates interest. Perhaps the place where you will make your presentation will help to advertise it. When making the presentation, use teaching strategies that encourage active participation, such as providing time for discussion. Also plan time for questions and clarification to ensure your message is understood. Active participation stimulates interest. Your presentation will be remembered longer if those attending actively participate.

WORKING WITH HEALTH TEAM MEMBERS

Some of today's care providers have little formal healthcare training, such as nursing assistants, who usually receive about 6 weeks of training. Consequently, some health education may be directed to team members with whom you work. In planning health education for team members, you must know the provisions of the nurse practice act in your state to know the scope of practice for each team member, such as the nursing assistant, licensed practical nurse, and registered nurse. You must also know the general policies and practice guidelines of your employer. Acute care institutions have in-service education departments that handle continuing education for employees, but long-term care facilities may or may not.

If it is your responsibility to provide health education to team members, you should first assess their learning needs through either a formal or informal survey. You can also determine learning needs by observing team members as you work with them. While developing learning objectives, keep in mind the three learning domains—cognitive, affective, and psychomotor— and consider in which domain team members need health education. For example, does a team member lack knowledge about the client's health problem and rationale for treatment (cognitive domain)? Is a team member biased in his or her attitude toward caring for certain patients (affective domain)? Does a team member need to refresh his or her skills in performing nursing care procedures (psychomotor domain)? After you have determined the learning domain in which health education is needed, write the learning objectives. Your next step is to determine how the content should be taught and whether or not it can be done informally on the job or formally away from the patient care unit. After this decision is made, select teaching strategies and instructional materials to meet the team members' needs. Following your teaching, you need to assess the effectiveness of your teaching. **Box 6-1** describes how evidence-based nursing practice feedback can improve client education.

BOX 6-1

Evidence-Based Nursing Practice

Dolansky, M. A., Moore, S. M., & Viscovsky, C. (2006). Older adults' views of cardiac rehabilitation programs. *Journal of Gerontological Nursing, 32*(2), 37–44.

Purpose: This study examined older adults' expectations and experiences with cardiac rehabilitation programs.

Method: A descriptive design was used with a convenience sample of 40 older adults from a large urban teaching hospital who had experienced an acute cardiac event to identify their views of cardiac rehabilitation programs using focus groups and individual interviews.

Results: The participants did not have an accurate understanding of what to expect in cardiac rehabilitation programs; however, their experiences with these programs were generally positive. The participants suggested that cardiac rehabilitation programs could be improved by including more socialization opportunities, offering varied forms of exercise, enhancing teaching about stress management, and adapting teaching strategies. A major finding was the report of adverse events during exercise that were experienced by individuals who did not go to a cardiac rehabilitation program.

SUMMARY

As adults deal with changes in their business, personal, and professional lives, they realize that learning is, indeed, a lifelong process. Learning in adulthood is influenced by needs related to biologic characteristics, psychosocial stages, and developmental tasks. Adults continue their learning for a variety of reasons, some to meet goals, others for social reasons, and still others for the love of learning. Health-related topics to promote, retain, and restore health are numerous and should be individualized for specific client situations.

The assumptions of andragogy were explored and contrasted to pedagogy. Adults engage in learning activities because they have a need to know, perhaps knowledge related to employment or personal issues. Adults want to be respected as competent and capable of self-direction, and they want to be valued for their life experiences. Other assumptions of andragogy include readiness to learn, orientation to learning, and motivation to learn. Health education opportunities occur with individuals, families, and groups or communities, as well as with health team members.

EXERCISES

Exercise I: Contrasting Pedagogy and Andragogy

Purpose: Test Knowles's ideas about adult learning.
Directions:

1. Identify children at different ages and say, "Tell me about yourself." Note the answer. If a child asks you, "What do you mean?" answer, "Oh, anything you want to tell me."
2. Repeat the preceding assignment with adults.

3. Note the differences and similarities between the responses of the children and the adults.
4. Discuss your findings with your colleagues.

Exercise II: Orientation to Learning

Purpose: Develop awareness of your own orientation to learning according to Houle.
Directions: Work in small groups to complete the following tasks:

1. Categorize your orientation to learning according to Houle's findings.
2. Discuss the implications this has for you as a learner and in your role as an educator.
3. Distinguish between andragogy and pedagogy.
4. Discuss how this information is useful with clients.
5. Discuss your reflections with your peers.

Exercise III: Reflection Questions

Purpose: Become aware of how your orientation to learning affects your motivation, learning strategies, and topics of interest.
Directions:

1. What is your motivation for studying health education in nursing?
2. What strategies help you learn?
3. What aspects of nursing interest you the most?
4. What do you hope to gain from your formal education?

Exercise IV: Teaching Team Members

Purpose: Apply adult learning theory to teaching team members.
Directions: Role-play the following teaching and learning situations:

1. A newly certified nurse assistant is assigned to care for a client with a hip replacement. On the first postoperative day, the client requests a bedpan and the nurse assistant asks you what she should do. How would you respond?
2. You observe a dietary aide responding to a client's request for more salt on her dinner tray. The client has congestive heart failure and salt is prohibited. You meet the dietary aide as she is about to enter the client's room to deliver the additional salt. How would you handle this situation?
3. You are supervising a new registered nurse graduate who is administering heparin for the first time to a client with a clotting disorder. She asks you to help her properly administer the subcutaneous injection.
4. Your colleague needs to change a complex dressing on a hospitalized client, which is a new procedure to her. You are familiar with the procedure and she asks you for help.

REFERENCES

Balakas, K. (2013). Developmental theories. In P. A. Potter, A. G. Perry, P. A. Stockert, & A. M. Hall (Eds.), *Fundamentals of nursing* (8th ed., pp. 130–138). St. Louis, MO: Mosby-Elsevier.

Boshier, R. (1991). Psychometric properties of the alternative form of the education participation scale. *Adult Education Quarterly, 41*(3), 150–167.

Dolansky, M. A., Moore, S. M., & Viscovsky, C. (2006). Older adults' views of cardiac rehabilitation programs. *Journal of Gerontological Nursing, 32*(2), 37–44.

Erikson, E. (1963). *Childhood and society* (2nd ed.). New York, NY: W. W. Norton.

Houle, C. O. (1961). *The inquiring mind.* Madison: University of Wisconsin Press.

Houle, C. O. (1980). *Continuing learning in the professions.* San Francisco, CA: Jossey-Bass.

Knowles, M. S. (1990). *The adult learner: A neglected species* (4th ed.). Houston, TX: Gulf.

Knowles, M. S., Holton, E. F., III, & Swanson, R. A. (2005). *The adult learner* (6th ed.). Burlington, MA: Elsevier.

Knowles, M. S., Holton, E. F., III, & Swanson, R. A. (2011). *The adult learner* (7th ed.). Burlington, MA: Butterworth-Heinemann, Elsevier.

Kolb, D. A. (1984). *Experiential learning.* Englewood Cliffs, NJ: Prentice Hall.

Maslow, A. H. (1987). *Motivation and personality* (3rd ed.). New York, NY: Harper & Row.

Merriam, S. B., Caffarella, R. S., & Baumgartner, L. M. (2007). *Learning in adulthood* (3rd ed.). San Francisco, CA: Jossey-Bass.

O'Shea, E. (2003). Self-directed learning in nurse education: A review of the literature. *Journal of Advanced Nursing, 43*(1), 62–70.

Rogers, C. R. (1961). *On becoming a person.* Boston, MA: Houghton-Mifflin.

Ruchala, P. (2013). Young and middle adults. In P. A. Potter, A. G. Perry, P. A. Stockert, & A. M. Hall (Eds.), *Fundamentals of nursing* (8th ed., pp. 157–170). St. Louis, MO: Mosby Elsevier.

Santrock, J. W. (2014). *A topical approach to life-span development* (7th ed.). Boston, MA: McGraw-Hill.

7

The Older Learner

OBJECTIVES

Upon completion of this chapter, you will be able to do the following:

- Discuss ageism and the subjective experience of the older client.
- Describe the psychosocial stages, developmental tasks, and physiologic changes that are characteristic of late adulthood and affect teaching and learning.
- List health education topics for clients in late adulthood related to psychosocial stages, developmental tasks, and normal physiologic changes.
- Identify common chronic diseases of older adults and their implications for health education.
- Describe the importance of cultural assessment before teaching the ethnic elderly.
- Identify the implications of nutritional status on teaching and learning.
- Identify the teaching and learning implications of working with clients with special needs, individuals, families, groups and communities, and health team members.

KEY TERMS

ageism	old old adult	psychosocial stage
cognitive functioning	physiologic change	visual acuity
developmental task	presbycusis	young old adult
frail elderly	presbyopia	

INTRODUCTION

Because people are living longer and healthier, you will encounter older clients in virtually every healthcare and community setting. Older clients, like their younger counterparts, also are lifelong learners and have many lived experiences and much wisdom to share. The focus of this chapter is on providing health education to older adult clients. We do this by first looking at the concept of ageism that permeates U.S. culture. We then address the psychosocial stages, developmental tasks, and normal physiologic changes that are characteristic of late adulthood and their implications for teaching and learning. Some older adult clients have special needs that nurses will encounter in their role as educators. It is common, for example, for clients to have one or more chronic diseases. Also, **cognitive functioning,** an important consideration for all clients, is discussed as it relates to memory and medications. The chapter concludes with a discussion of the nutritional needs of older learners and the ethnic elderly and aging.

We define older adult learners as those who are age 65 years and older. This group numbered 41.4 million in 2011; which meant that one in every eight persons in the United States (13.3% of the population) was an older American. This age group is projected to increase to 79.7 million in 2040, according to the most recent year for which data are available (Administration on Aging [AOA], 2012). As the baby boomer generation (those born between 1946 and 1964) reaches age 65, which began in 2011, the number of older Americans will substantially increase.

In 2011, 21% of those aged 65 years and older were members of racial or ethnic minority populations: 9% were African Americans, 7% were Hispanic, 4% were Asian or Pacific Islanders, less than 1% were American Indians or Native Alaskans, and 0.6% were identified as two or more races. This population is expected to increase from 21% of the population in 2011 to 28% in 2030 (AOA, 2012).

The older population itself is increasingly getting older. In 2011 people aged 65 years and older represented 13.3% of the population and are expected to grow to 21% by 2040. The population of people aged 85 years and older is projected to triple from 5.7 million to 14.1 million in 2040. Those reaching age 65 years can expect to live an additional 20.4 years for women and 17.8 years for men. Gender differences are present in the older population. In 2011 the ratio of women to men was 131 women for every 100 men. At age 85 years and older, this ratio increases to 203 women for every 100 men (AOA, 2012). These data suggest that aging is increasingly a women's issue.

AGEISM

Ageism is a term used to denote discrimination against the elderly. Although fascination with youth in the United States is waning, this country still lacks a culture that values everyone regardless of age or ethnic background. As a nurse you will be working with older clients, so it is important that you examine your attitudes about aging. How you see older clients wittingly or unwittingly influences how you react and treat them. This, in turn, influences how they see and value themselves. This means confronting the myths and stereotypes about the elderly that research and experience have demonstrated are not true. For example, some people believe that many elderly are confused, lonely, and generally in poor health, none of which is true. Many older adults live alone or with family members, have sufficient financial resources, and are in generally good health (Korem, 2013).

Health promotion and disease prevention for older adults is just as important as it is for all other age groups, including children. Health promotion activities, such as regular exercise, proper nutrition, cessation of smoking and other harmful health habits, are effective in improving the quality of health among older adults regardless of their age. A person is never too old to improve his or her health by changing poor habits to health-promoting ones. Health promotion topics are fruitful areas for health education, and they enrich the quality of life regardless of age (Blais, 2014).

PSYCHOSOCIAL STAGES, DEVELOPMENTAL TASKS, AND PHYSIOLOGIC CHANGES OF LATE ADULTHOOD

The older population is increasing rapidly and has the longest developmental time span of any age group (Santrock, 2014). How people age is an individual process and varies greatly as people grow older. In addition to normal physiological aging and genetics, other factors influence aging. These factors include the environment, economic circumstances, culture, lifestyle, and psychosocial variables. Each client must be assessed in terms of his or her unique circumstances and functional abilities. For example, some older learners may be cognitively competent and active in their daily lives, while others may be cognitively challenged and need assistance with the activities of daily living. Some older adults participate in walking and hiking activities, while others are more sedentary and limited in their physical abilities.

Because of this rapidly increasing population of older adults, demographers divide this age group into two time periods: **young old adults** (aged 65 to 84 years) and **old old adults** (aged 85 years and older). In this section we address the psychosocial stages, developmental tasks, and physiological changes of the young old adult and the old old adult. In practice, each client is unique and deserves individual assessment and evaluation.

Psychosocial Stages

We view the psychosocial stages through the work of Erik Erikson (1963, 1982). The eighth developmental stage that he identified is ego integrity versus despair. In this stage individuals engage in a life review. They evaluate the meaning of their lives, their accomplishments and failures, and their satisfactions and disappointments. It is a time of reflection, evaluation, interpretation, and often reinterpretation of their experiences. Many look back with satisfaction, knowing they have done their best in spite of failures (integrity), whereas others look back with regret and see themselves as failures (despair). This stage holds the potential for growth, understanding, and the development of wisdom (Balakas, 2013; Santrock, 2014). Wisdom is the positive growth that comes from life's experiences and results in deeper insights, perceptions, and judgments.

Because the life span for humans continues to lengthen, Erikson and his wife, Joan, further explored the 80- to 90-year-old age group and added a ninth stage by enhancing their eight stages. They reversed the order of each of the previous eight stages and added to the positive aspect as follows:

1. Basic mistrust versus trust: Hope
2. Shame and doubt versus autonomy: Will
3. Guilt versus initiative: Purpose
4. Inferiority versus industry: Competence
5. Identity confusion versus identity: Fidelity
6. Isolation versus intimacy: Love
7. Stagnation versus generativity: Care
8. Despair and disgust versus integrity: Wisdom

Placing the negative before the positive emphasizes how the negative aspects of each stage may potentially affect individuals in this age group. Physiologic aging changes occurring during this time result in daily difficulties and reevaluations. It is the final life cycle stage when individuals must come to terms with declining independence, loss of control, and weakening self-esteem and confidence. Individuals who successfully deal with the negative aspects of this stage move on to gerotranscendence; that is, rising above the negative and celebrating the life that remains (Erikson & Erikson, 1997).

Robert Peck (1968) expanded upon Erikson's final developmental stage of the older adult, ego integrity versus despair. Peck stated that this final stage is divided into three additional tasks: ego differentiation, body transcendence, and ego transcendence. The first task, ego differentiation, is for the older person to develop satisfaction from the self as a person, rather than from an occupation role or a parent. The second task, body transcendence, is to adjust to the physical declines of aging, rather than becoming absorbed in health problems or physical limitations imposed by aging. The third task, ego transcendence, is to have satisfaction when reflecting on one's life and accomplishments rather than dwelling on the prospect of death.

Maslow's hierarchy provides another framework for viewing the importance of individual needs. It is a theory of motivation that applies to the elderly. At certain times in the older person's life, basic needs, such as nutrition, may be the most important, whereas at other times the same individual may be engaged in self-actualization. It is important to assess each individual to determine present needs.

This is also a time of adjusting to transitions and new social roles. With longer lives, adults experience more losses, transitions, and adjustments to new social roles. Major losses include retirement, financial status, and possibly health. Social roles, relationships, and networks also change. The most difficult losses are usually related to the death of loved ones and friends (Korem, 2013). Your role as an educator in working with older adults is to help them successfully accept, adapt, and adjust to these psychosocial stages.

Developmental Tasks

Developmental tasks refer to the issues and problems that older adults face in living, including their changing social roles. Knowing about these tasks helps you understand the life stage clients are in and the common issues they face.

In late adulthood many clients are adjusting to retirement and may use this time to explore new interests and find new activities. Many clients want to continue employment because it gives meaning to their lives. Others continue employment because of difficult economic times. Financial stress is particularly difficult to deal with when resources are limited or insufficient to meet daily needs. Declining financial resources may require a change in the living situation to which the individual must adjust. If clients are receiving a pension, Social Security, or welfare, they have to learn about that system and how to navigate it. The same is true with navigating Medicare and Medicaid (Knowles, 1990).

Many retired adults expand their interests and hobbies during this time and find satisfaction in volunteer work. Many want to be useful and associate with like-minded individuals. The death of a spouse or significant other will require an adjustment in living. Roles change in retirement, and new ones have to be negotiated with the spouse or significant other, children, and grandchildren (Knowles, 1990; Santrock, 2014).

As the educator, you need to be tuned in to clients' changing social roles. Retirement, for example, is a major lifestyle rearrangement for both men and women. For those who have identified themselves by their work without developing strong interests in other areas, retirement may be particularly difficult. These individuals may experience feelings of dependency, powerlessness, and helplessness. For clients about to retire or who are having difficulty adjusting to retirement, encourage them to gradually disengage from the work role. Help them identify

FIGURE 7-1

Many Older Adults Lead Active, Productive Lives

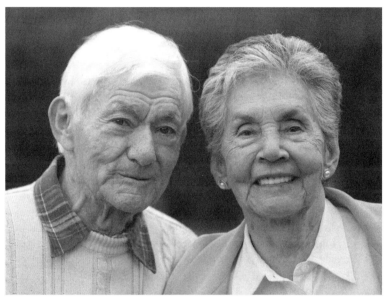

© Andresr/ShutterStock, Inc.

other areas of interest and activities to pursue. Do not overlook the effect on the spouse when one marriage partner retires. Many wives comment about the adjustments they have to make when their spouse retires and begins following them around the house all day.

Physiologic Changes that Affect Teaching and Learning

Older adults experience an increasing number of **physiologic changes** during this time; however, there is considerable variability in the rate and nature of these changes. Adults aged 65 to 84 years are increasingly healthier when compared with previous generations, and they can lead active, productive lives **(Figure 7-1)**. They have substantial potential for physical strength and fitness and retain much of their cognitive capacity. Adults aged 85 years and older are more **frail** and show a greater loss in cognitive skills. They also experience a decline in general health and well-being (Santrock, 2014). In evaluating the physiologic changes that occur with aging, it is important to distinguish between normal aging and pathologic processes. This section covers those physiologic changes that most affect teaching and learning. More complete information is found in medical–surgical textbooks. A chart of physical changes associated with aging by system is found in Appendix B.

The impact of biologic aging is evident in every body system and in the person's general appearance. While genetics is something that cannot be controlled, health habits and choices can be. Good health habits, preventive measures, and lifestyle patterns such as rest, exercise, nutrition, and stressors greatly affect the health of every individual. In the older person, the long-term accumulated effects of these patterns become more obvious. In this section we highlight some physiologic changes and pathophysiologic problems that occur with aging and how they affect teaching and learning.

Appearance

The most obvious signs of aging are seen in the skin. Wrinkling and sagging skin, thinning and graying hair, dryness, and pigmentation changes are common. Many skin changes are caused by exposure to sunlight, a problem that is addressed in much of health education today. Clients with diabetes or cerebral vascular accidents have decreased sensation and must be taught to prevent burns from heating pads, bathing, and cooking (Eliopoulos, 2014). The appearance of the body changes and alters the contours of earlier years. Body mass diminishes from the face and extremities and increases in the trunk, abdomen, and hips.

Musculoskeletal System

In the musculoskeletal system, muscle mass and strength diminishes, bone mass declines, and degenerative joint changes can occur. Almost 30% of muscle mass is lost by the 70s. Older adults who regularly exercise retain more bone, muscle mass, and muscle tone compared to inactive individuals, providing an excellent opportunity for health education. There is a progressive loss of height, especially among women because of osteoporosis, which is demineralization of the bones (Roberts, 2014). Expect clients to fatigue more easily than younger ones. Their movements may be slower and more rigid. Taking frequent breaks and allotting sufficient time help compensate for this. Older clients are more comfortable sitting in padded chairs with arms.

Cardiovascular System

Cardiovascular changes occur with aging, as evidenced by a decrease in cardiac output, abnormal increases in systolic or diastolic blood pressures, and weak peripheral pulses, particularly in the lower extremities. Hypertension, if present, can lead to serious health problems such as heart failure, stroke, renal failure, coronary heart disease, and peripheral vascular disease. Collagen in the heart muscle increases and elastin decreases, affecting myocardial contractility. The heart valves become thickened and fibrotic from lipid accumulation and degeneration of collagen; fibrosis of the aortic and mitral valves is most frequently affected. The coronary blood flow decreases significantly. The number of pacemaker cells in the sinoatrial node, and conduction cells in the atrioventricular node, the bundle of His, and bundle branches also decrease, which may result in conduction problems. Atherosclerosis and arteriosclerosis are common in the arterial walls, diminishing elasticity and vasomotor tone. Total peripheral resistance is increased, which results in an increase in blood pressure. These changes result from disease, environmental factors, lifetime health behaviors, and aging; they are not caused by aging alone. As a result, the older adult is less able to respond to physical and emotional stress (Disabatino & Bucher, 2014). Factors such as obesity, diet, activity, and habits have been implicated as etiologic factors, all of which have implications for nurses as educators, particularly among younger adults.

Respiratory System

Lung function decreases as respiratory muscle strength and mobility of the ribs declines. Osteoporosis is often present, leading to dorsal kyphosis, a curvature in the thoracic spine. The anteroposterior diameter of the thorax increases, giving the chest a barrel-shaped appearance. The number of functional alveoli decreases, resulting in an increase in residual volume (the amount of air remaining after maximum expiration). The alveoli are less elastic and relatively more fibrous, which decreases the older person's ability to engage in physically taxing activities. Dyspnea may be evident on little exertion or stress (Eisel, 2014). With these respiratory changes, clients may fatigue easily and need their learning activities adjusted to their abilities.

Changes in the musculoskeletal, cardiovascular, and respiratory systems affect the older client's energy level, strength, and speed. Endurance certainly may be affected, but another influential variable is the person's usual activity level. Older people who lead very active lives tend to have remarkable endurance. They may be able to do a sustained activity familiar to them better than a younger individual who has less practice. Maintaining the functional ability of older adults—that is, maintaining their ability to live independently and perform the activities of daily living—is enhanced with regular exercise. Exercises also can reverse or slow declines in age-related motor performance (Fahlman, Topp, McNevin, Morgan, & Boardley, 2007). Nurses can encourage older adults to participate in exercises by teaching the benefits of a regular program. Ask older clients if they have noticed a decline in their strength and motor functioning. This focuses their attention on the topic, after which you can explain how exercise limits or reverses a decline, retains their independence, and maximizes their ability to engage in the activities of daily living (Schneider, Eveker, Bronder, Meiner, & Binder, 2003).

Exercise improves strength and endurance of people at all ages, including those who reside in nursing homes. Fahlman and colleagues (2007) found that a structured exercise program for older adults with limited functional ability increased their strength and endurance. For example, nursing students led older clients at senior centers in an exercise program. It was a lively activity, enjoyed by students and participants. If you are working with institutionalized clients, take into consideration their current rest and exercise routine when deciding on the best time to initiate teaching. Clients learn better when they are well oxygenated by an invigorated circulatory system and when they are rested enough to have the extra energy needed to focus on learning. Weinrich, Boyd, and Nussbaum (1989) recommend low-impact exercises for the elderly, during which their feet do not leave the floor. They also recommend slowing the speed of exercise and increasing the warm-up and cool-down time. As educators, focus on helping older clients retain as much physical strength and agility as possible.

Gastrointestinal–Urinary Systems

Bowel and bladder problems increase with age. Bowel motility decreases, resulting in constipation. Bladder capacity decreases and can result in urinary incontinence. To address bowel changes, nurses should teach clients the benefits of drinking adequate fluids, eating sufficient roughage, and getting regular exercise. Some medications have an effect on intestinal motility and need further evaluation. To address bladder changes, nurses should identify the cause of the incontinence, work with clients to establish a regular voiding schedule, and teach pelvic floor or Kegel exercises (Blais, 2014). Bladder capacity and urinary incontinence are conditions to be aware of when planning learning activities. Providing frequent breaks may be necessary.

Neurologic System

Functional changes in the neurologic system occur with aging. Neuron loss occurs, affecting the function of chemical substances (epinephrine and acetylcholine) that enhance or inhibit nerve impulse transmission. Degenerative changes in myelin can interfere with nerve conduction. Voluntary reflexes are slower, and the older person's ability to react quickly to stimuli is slowed (Lueckenotte, 2009). In addition to vision and hearing changes, other aging-related neurologic changes include decrease in memory, taste, smell, vibration and position sense, and muscle strength (Olson, 2014).

Some clients have benign essential tremors that affect their upper extremities, head, and voice, a condition commonly seen in older adults. Tremors also may be associated with pathology such as Parkinson's disease or with side effects of drugs (Millsap, 2007). The presence of tremors affects the type of learning activities in which these clients can successfully engage. Fine hand movements in manipulating equipment or writing tasks are difficult for these clients, so other learning activities should be selected.

Sensory Changes

Sensory changes have an effect on the lifestyle of older clients. The most important sensory changes affecting teaching and learning are vision and hearing impairments. Diminished functional ability in either or both interferes with the older client's ability to communicate orally and in writing. This leads to social isolation as clients avoid the strain of hearing a muted or indistinguishable conversation, embarrassment associated with responding inappropriately to comments of others, or diminished mobility associated with loss of vision. All senses may be affected by aging, but vision and hearing are the most important to consider as you plan health education. Because of this, we address the functional declines in vision and hearing in greater depth and discuss how to use this information to adapt health education to the abilities of older clients.

Sensory Changes: Vision

In 2010 vision trouble affected 14% of the older population (13% of men and 15% of women). Among people aged 85 years and older, 23% reported trouble seeing (AOA, 2012). The lens loses its ability to accommodate as it becomes less elastic, larger, and denser, resulting in a condition called presbyopia (farsightedness). The increased density plus the accumulation of loosened degenerative cells on the iris, cornea, and lens capsule result in increased scattering of light and sensitivity to glare. The lens becomes progressively yellowed and opaque, resulting not only in **visual acuity** difficulties, but also in the inability to discriminate blues and greens. This is attributed to the decreased ability of the aging, yellowed lens to filter the shorter wavelengths of light (violet, blue, and green). It is easier for older clients to distinguish among warm colors, such as yellow, orange, and red (Linton, 2007). The use of these colors in teaching materials makes it easier for clients to distinguish them.

When teaching older clients, sit or stand in front of them so they have a full view of you. Clients should be able to see your face and mouth as you talk (Lueckenotte, 2009). If you are using visual aids, consider the impact of colors. For example, a color with a longer wavelength, such as yellow, printed on a white background would not be easy for older eyes to see because there is insufficient contrast between the two colors. A thick black outline surrounding the yellow material would improve readability. Even more effective is a background color, such as light blue, that contrasts with deep yellow lettering outlined in black.

We now examine functional visual changes (visual acuity, glare, dark and light adaptation, and loss of peripheral vision) that affect the teaching and learning process.

Visual Acuity

Virtually everyone will have visual difficulties related to the aging process, regardless of sex, race, ethnicity, or socioeconomic status. Many older adults wear glasses for reading or distance vision because of decreased visual acuity. Watch older clients for signs of difficulty. Note how clients read. How close do they hold a book to read? How much reading do they do? If institutional clients wear glasses, be sure they have them on and the lenses are clean to view your instructional materials. Older clients with presbyopia hold their reading materials at arm's length to focus clearly on the print. Symbols, letters, and objects that are small are more difficult to distinguish from one another. Diminishing ability to discriminate between stimuli is evident among older clients in terms of the size of words and pictures and their intensity and color. Small images, which project shorter light waves into the eye, are harder to distinguish, as are crowded or softly colored images. Larger and more intensely colored print is easier to see. There is enough of the image getting through the nerve pathways for clients to fill in the missing parts. Allowing space between each of the letters also helps.

This is harder to read for a person with aging eyes because the print is fine and there is a lot of it.

This print is easier to read.

Glare

Glare is a serious problem for older clients. It affects their ability to drive at night by leaving them virtually blind in its presence. Glare may come from a variety of sources, such as reflections off windows and shiny floors. Linton (2007) recommends soft incandescent lighting rather than fluorescent lighting to minimize glare. Sheer curtains or rugs can also help reduce glare. If you become involved with the production of instructional materials, avoid using slick, shiny, white paper, which is more likely to produce glare. If you are arranging lighting for elderly clients, make the light brighter but not glaring.

Dark and Light Adaptation

It takes longer for the eyes of older clients to adapt to dark and light. It takes more time for their eyes to adjust if the room is darkened for a DVD, video, or slide show. Plan for this extra time as you prepare the teaching plan. When you turn the lights back on, clients need extra time to readjust their vision. Because pupils become smaller when the lights are turned on, less light is reaching the retina; thus, extra lighting is required (Linton, 2007). If you are using a physical model or object in teaching, consider placing high-intensity lighting on it. This increases the visibility of the model or object, which is preferable to increasing the light in the entire room. The level of intensity, however, needs to be balanced to avoid glare, which older eyes are more sensitive to.

Loss of Peripheral Vision

With the loss of peripheral vision, older clients are unaware of people and learning activities outside of their line of central vision. This may interfere with how your clients relate to others if you are teaching a group. They may not be aware of others sitting next to them or objects located in their peripheral visual fields. As a result they may appear to lack social interaction skills or appear clumsy if they spill something or knock something over. They may not be able to see an object that you may refer to that is outside of their visual field. Do your best to stay in the clients' line of central vision when teaching to address this condition.

Sensory Changes: Hearing

Some degree of hearing loss caused by changes in the inner ear or tympanic membrane inevitably accompanies the aging process. In 2010, 46% of older men and 31% of older women aged 65 years and older reported trouble hearing. The percentage of older Americans with trouble hearing was higher for people aged 85 years and older (59%) than for people aged 65–74 years (31%) (AOA, 2012). Presbycusis is associated with aging and is the most common type of hearing loss. It begins in young adulthood and becomes evident usually after age 50 years. Initially high-pitched sounds beyond the range of human speech are lost. Because these sounds have little functional significance, the individual is unaware of the loss. As the client ages, the loss eventually involves the sounds in the middle and lower ranges. It becomes problematic for clients when higher sounds are missed and only lower sounds are heard. Words sound distorted and conversations are difficult to understand, especially in the presence of background noise (Linton, 2007).

With high-tone hearing loss, it is more difficult for clients to discriminate among consonants, such as *s, t, f, g, ch, sh, z,* and *th,* which have high frequencies. Clients with presbycusis have difficulty distinguishing among phonetically similar words. Words are distorted and sentences make little sense. A sentence such as "I think he should go to the store" might be interpreted as "I wish we could go to the show." As hearing loss progresses, explosive consonants, such as *b, d, k, p,* and *t,* also become distorted (Miller, 1990).

Clients with presbycusis need more time to process information. Rapid speech is difficult for older clients to understand. If you speak rapidly, remember to slow down when you teach older clients. Lower your pitch and speak more slowly and loudly. Face clients when you speak so they can see you. They may lip read to fill in what they do not hear. Reduce any background noise or move to a quiet room. If clients wear hearing aids, be sure they are operational, in place, and turned on with sufficient volume (Lueckenotte, 2009).

Older clients in a group setting may not want to participate or answer questions for fear of appearing foolish. Hearing loss affects self-confidence and may lead to social isolation. Uninformed healthcare providers may assume that a hard-of-hearing client is demented. Consider the example of a woman who was attempting to communicate with her elderly mother-in-law. "My mother-in-law does not pay attention to anything I say. Even if I practically shout at her it does no good. But let my husband come in the room and just talk to her in a normal voice, and she hears every word he says." The nursing student responded with sensitivity to what may be symptoms of a family conflict. She explained the facts about sound waves to the woman and explained that a woman's voice is likely to contain higher sound frequencies. If she raises her voice in an effort to be heard, it is likely that she also raises the pitch. Tension also results in a rise in voice pitch. If the relationship already suffers from tension, it is likely that the voice with which the woman begins to speak is already higher than her relaxed voice. These factors make her speech less intelligible to an aging person whose hearing is diminishing. The man who casually comes into the room is likely to speak in a lower-pitched voice, which has a longer wavelength.

Suspect hearing loss if older clients give inappropriate responses to questions, are unable to follow oral directions without cues, or frequently ask you to repeat a message. If clients watch you closely, turn their ear toward you, get unusually close to you, do not respond to loud environmental noises, speak too loudly or inarticulately, speak in a monotone voice, or avoid group settings, you should suspect hearing impairment (Miller, 1990). Remember, however, that not all older clients are hard of hearing. It is distressing for older persons to be spoken to as if they are deaf when they are not.

Physiologic Aging Changes and Teaching–Learning Topics

Older adults experience many biologic and psychosocial changes in their lives and need different levels of help adapting to these changes. They are dealing with faltering health, decreasing strength, and biologic changes that alter or limit their activities. They are adjusting to losses, adapting to changing living circumstances, and changing their self-image. They may be enriching their lives by expanding their knowledge, developing new interests, and learning new skills. This is a time rich with opportunities for nurses to recognize unspoken and unmet needs and to take opportunities to provide health education. We now look at how this information helps you to promote, retain, and restore the health of older clients (**Table 7-1**).

Promote and Retain Health

The focus of promoting health is on prevention, whereas the focus of retaining health is on maintaining one's present health status, assuming it is satisfactory. Clients are never too old to start an exercise program, improve their diet, and change unhealthful habits. **Table 7-2** lists suggested topics that are appropriate for older learners to promote and retain health (Hall, 2009; Lueckenotte, 2009). These suggestions are not all-inclusive and must be adapted to the circumstances of the individual client.

Restore Health

Restoration of health for older adults refers to people who are experiencing an acute or chronic illness or disability. The purpose of health education is to help clients understand the nature of their health problem, the treatment regimen, and how to deal with the limitations imposed by health problems, disabilities, or injuries. This involves not only working with the client but also with family members and caretakers. **Table 7-3** suggests topics related to the restoration of health (Baker & Heitkemper, 2014; Hall, 2009; Lueckenotte, 2009).

TABLE 7-1

Selected Physiologic Aging Changes and Teaching–Learning Implications

Physiologic Changes	*Teaching–Learning Implications*
Musculoskeletal: • Muscle mass and strength diminish • Bone mass declines • Degenerative joint changes • Loss of height • Demineralization of bone	• Expect slower movements when teaching exercises • Observe for fatigue with physical activities and adjust accordingly • Take frequent breaks • Allow sufficient time for activities that involve movement • Provide comfortable seating • Increase warm-up and cool-down times
Cardiovascular: • Decrease in cardiac output • Orthostatic hypotension • Abnormal increases in systolic or diastolic blood pressure • Decreased coronary blood flow • Arthrosclerosis and arteriosclerosis common • Conduction problems (atrial fibrillation)	• Select activities based on client energy level, endurance, and speed • Select teaching times in midmorning when energy levels are high • Spread teaching sessions over several days rather than one lengthy session • Move slowly when rising from a sitting position • Adjust pace of activities based on client feedback
Respiratory: • Lung function decreases • Mobility of ribs declines • Functional alveoli decrease in number	• Base activities on the level of exertion tolerated by the client • Encourage clients to maintain the highest level of functional abilities • Use oxygen safely if prescribed
Gastrointestinal and urinary: • Bowel motility decreases (constipation) • Urinary bladder capacity decreases (incontinence)	• Provide frequent breaks • Provide liquids • Avoid embarrassment
Neurological: • Benign essential tremor common • Cognitive slowing • Decreased sensitivity to stimuli • May have decreased blood flow to brain	• Allow additional time for teaching and learning • Adapt pace of teaching • Focus on essential information based on client interest • Repeat and reinforce important concepts • Reduce background noise and environmental distractions • Relate new information to current knowledge • Emphasize concrete rather than abstract information • Attend to nonverbal cues regarding comfort and questions • To evaluate learning ask clients to demonstrate skills

(continues)

TABLE 7-1

Selected Physiologic Aging Changes and Teaching–Learning Implications (Continued)

Physiologic Changes	Teaching–Learning Implications
Sensory changes, vision: • Decreased visual acuity • Sensitivity to glare • Decreased depth perception • Presbyopia or cataracts • Decreased adaptation to dark and light • Loss of peripheral vision • Poor night vision • Decreased ability to discriminate colors	• Evaluate client's reading ability • Select instructional materials with large print • Use warm colors such as orange or red in printed materials • Stand in client's line of central vision • Choose age-appropriate positive images for instructional materials • Provide sufficient lighting and reduce glare • Allow time for vision adaptation from dark to light • Encourage the use of corrective lenses or magnifying glass
Sensory changes, hearing: • Hearing acuity decreases (presbycusis) • Loss of high-pitched sounds • Distracted by background noise • Difficulty discriminating consonant sounds such as *s, t, f, g, ch, sh, th,* and *z*	• Speak slower and slightly louder • Use words that are familiar and avoid medical terms • Lower the pitch of your voice • Let clients see your face and mouth • Select a quiet place for teaching • Repeat frequently as necessary • Confirm that clients have heard you by having them teach back the information

TABLE 7-2

Suggested Topics to Promote and Retain Health

Nursing Assessment	Health Education Topics
Biologic aging	• Knowing normal age-related body changes • Knowing age-related changes to body system of interest
General health habits	• Eating well-balanced, nutritious diet • Maintaining adequate hydration • Practicing oral hygiene and dental care • Knowing benefits of exercise program • Coping effectively with physical and mental stress • Visiting regularly with healthcare providers • Participating in meaningful activities
General living conditions	• Maintaining home cleanliness • Evaluating need for mechanical aids to assist in activities of daily living • Making lifestyle adjustments • Preventing accidents and falls • Creating safe home environment (slip-resistant rugs, night-lights, nonskid adhesive strips in tub and shower, handrails on steps, grab bars in bathrooms, smoke detectors, etc.)

(Continues)

TABLE 7-2

Suggested Topics to Promote and Retain Health (Continued)

Nursing Assessment	Health Education Topics
Disease and illness prevention	• Avoiding risk factors (smoking, alcohol, etc.) • Modifying behavior to avoid risk factors • Obtaining immunizations (flu, pneumonia) • Having regular physical examinations • Screening procedures (mammograms, cholesterol, vision, hearing, blood pressure, blood sugar) • Knowing medications • Maintaining medication regimen and medication safety • Recognizing symptoms of depression
Sexual habits	• Preventing sexually transmitted diseases • Knowing mode of disease transmission • Knowing partner's sexual history and practices • Using safe sexual practices • Recognizing symptoms
Community services	• Knowing about community luncheon sites • Knowing community senior center services • Knowing county and state government senior services

TABLE 7-3

Suggested Topics to Restore Health

Nursing Assessment	Health Education Topics
Acute illness	• Knowing nature and cause of the health problem or disability • Common conditions: Urinary tract infections, fluid and electrolyte imbalance (hyponatremia, dehydration), pneumonia, hip fracture, dysrhythmias • Understanding diagnostic tests • Supporting and explaining treatment regimen • Orienting to hospital and clinic environment and routines • Adapting to lifestyle changes
Chronic illness	• Knowing nature and cause of the health problem or disability • Common conditions: Hypertension, cardiovascular disease, stroke, diabetes mellitus, cancer, arthritis • Understanding diagnostic tests • Supporting and explaining treatment regimen • Using physical, occupational, and speech therapies • Managing exacerbations and remissions • Preventing complications • Adapting to lifestyle changes • Adapting home environment • Identifying and using self-help devices • Supporting continued provider supervision

(continues)

TABLE 7-3	

Suggested Topics to Restore Health (Continued)

Nursing Assessment	Health Education Topics
Disability	• Assessing strengths and limitations of disability • Managing activities of daily living • Building on abilities • Identifying and using self-help devices
Accidents	• Knowing nature of injury sustained and impact on function • Managing activities of daily living • Building on abilities • Assessing rehabilitation issues • Preventing accidents and injuries • Maintaining safe home environment (slip-resistant rugs, night-lights, nonskid adhesive strips in tub and shower, handrails on steps, grab bars in bathrooms, smoke detectors, etc.)
Community services	• Knowing about community luncheon sites • Knowing community senior center services • Knowing county and state government senior services

WORKING WITH CLIENTS WITH SPECIAL NEEDS

Chronic Diseases

Chronic diseases are not a part of normal aging; however, the prevalence of chronic disease is higher among older adults. The increasing number of older Americans means that more of them need services from the healthcare system. People aged 65 years and older are less likely to have as many acute conditions as younger people; however, they are more apt to have at least one chronic condition for which they likely require assistance. Many have multiple chronic conditions. In 2009–2011 the most frequently occurring conditions among older persons were as follows: diagnosed arthritis (51%), all types of heart disease (31%), any cancer (24%), diagnosed diabetes (20% in 2007–2011), and hypertension (high blood pressure) or taking antihypertensive medications (72% in 2007–2010) (AOA, 2012). Other common chronic diseases are asthma, bronchitis, emphysema, depression, vision loss, and hearing impairment.

Race and ethnic differences play a role in these conditions. For example, racial and ethnic groups have higher rates of hypertension, tend to develop hypertension at an earlier age, and are less likely to undergo treatment to control their high blood pressure. Obesity continues to be higher for African American and Mexican American women. People of diverse racial, ethnic, and cultural heritage are less likely to get regular medical checkups, receive immunizations, and be routinely tested for cancer when compared with the majority of the U.S. population (National Center for Cultural Competence, 2003).

Teaching older clients how to adapt to chronic diseases is a major theme in working with them. The causes of chronic diseases are multiple and are frequently related to lifestyle. Chronic diseases develop slowly over time. Older clients may not understand their illness, especially if it is characterized by exacerbations and remissions. Clients with chronic diseases may experience depression, which further compounds their ability to function. The depression may be related to the disease and the disability it inflicts or the many losses that older adults experience at this time in their lives. Working with older clients who have chronic diseases challenges you as the educator. Determine how well they understand their disease and the degree to which they are willing to adhere to the prescribed treatment. Clients need to be educated about how to prevent and manage crises, manage the therapeutic regimen, and control symptoms. They also need to know how to organize their time, prevent social isolation, and have a normal lifestyle and inter-actions with others despite disease. Refresh your memory about specific chronic diseases so you can answer questions that older clients may have.

Teaching related to general health is a fruitful area for educating older clients about health. General health measures are instrumental in improving health status and helping clients feel better. Consider teaching the virtues of exercising regularly, improving nutritional intake, con-trolling weight loss or gain, getting adequate rest, managing stress, and cooperating with the medical regimen. We have enjoyed teaching these topics, especially classes about exercises, to older clients during their noon meal at community lunch sites for senior citizens. The exercises we taught were suitable to the age of the clients and involved simple range-of-motion exercises. The clients perked up and began to smile and interact with one another in a way they had not before. Many said they felt better as a result of the classes.

Alcohol continues to be an underestimated and hidden problem for older adults. A national survey in 2008 found that about 40% of adults aged 65 years and older drink alcohol. Alcohol detoxification and excretion from the older body is less efficient than in younger counterparts and can lead to accidents, nutritional deficiencies, and damage that affect all body systems. Heavy drinking can make health problems worse, including diabetes, high blood pressure, congestive heart failure, liver problems, osteoporosis, memory problems, and mood disorders. Alcohol use and some prescription and over-the-counter medications are synergistic or incom-patible. Medications that can interact badly with alcohol include aspirin, acetaminophen, cold and allergy medicine, cough syrup, sleeping pills, pain medication, and anxiety or depression medicine (National Institute on Alcohol Abuse and Alcoholism, n.d.). Older adults need to be aware of these facts and should be taught to carefully regulate and monitor their alcohol consumption.

The following experience illustrates how one nursing student made a significant difference in the life of an 87-year-old client, Mrs. Green. She is a widow who was happily married with two children, both of whom have now died. She has two granddaughters who live in different cities and do not visit. When Mrs. Green was younger, she was a supervisor in a large corpo-ration and had an active social life. Through the aging process, she has become isolated. She has arthritis, which limits her activity, and cataracts, which limit her sight. These problems, along with a few other physical ailments, have contributed to her becoming a shut-in. At first Mrs. Green was hesitant to let the nursing student come to her home. Previously she had some unfortunate experiences with physicians and had not been seen by anyone for more than 2 years. Her failing vision had contributed to a fear of strangers, and arthritis had kept her from going out of the house. With some coaxing, and because she was having abdominal pain that she wanted to have treated, she let the nursing student come to her home.

When the nursing student arrived, Mrs. Green was pleasant but cautious. The student conducted a health history and physical assessment. Through a telephone consultation with the clinic physician, Mrs. Green was diagnosed as having a flare-up of an old ulcer, and appropriate medication was prescribed. The student returned weekly and, within a month,

Mrs. Green learned to trust the nurse. Each week they discussed Mrs. Green's vision and, if it could be improved, how she would be able to continue taking care of herself. At first Mrs. Green was determined never to see a doctor again, but after a few weeks she made an appointment, arranged for a ride, and went to see an eye surgeon. A short time later she had surgery to remove a cataract. The surgery made a big difference. When the nursing student made her next visit, she found Mrs. Green was a different person. Mrs. Green did not talk about any of her health problems; rather, she chatted about current events and other interesting topics. Mrs. Green was joyous about the difference the surgery had made in her sight. She had changed from being a lonely, fearful person to being outgoing and cheerful. She still is a shut-in because of her age and arthritis, but she no longer lives in a world of haze. Mrs. Green is less isolated now. She is safer and will be able to live in her own home longer.

Finally, never assume that older adults are not interested in sex. Many individuals continue to be sexually active beyond the expectations and imaginations of their younger counterparts. Health education about sexuality in later years generates more interest than you might anticipate, even though many older adults were raised to not talk about sex. Keep in mind that elders with chronic diseases may need additional health education about meeting their needs (Kautz & Barnett, 2014). Consider the example of a 70-year-old female client seen in an outpatient clinic. She came in for her routine checkup and renewal of her prescription for vaginal Premarin (estrogen). She exercised regularly, ate nutritious meals, and maintained a long-standing sexual relationship with a 50-year-old man.

Social support networks are important for older adults. People who maintain relationships with others and remain active and involved with group activities fare better in terms of health and happiness. Self-help and peer support groups are also beneficial when clients are dealing with specific health problems. Your role as an educator is to foster these support networks.

Cognitive Functioning

Cognitive changes in the aging brain have been the topic of research and medical discussion with few definitive conclusions. Although there are age-related changes in brain composition, cells, and synapses, they do not necessarily affect thinking and cognition. The cognitive abilities of most healthy older adults show no noticeable evidence of decline (Baker & Heitkemper, 2014; Blais, 2014). Current research from longitudinal studies shows that some cognitive (thinking) functions decline with age, but other cognitive processes function at very high levels well into the later years. The decline that does occur is not as drastic as previously believed, and individuals can compensate for the decline in ways that are not noticeable (Bjorklund & Bee, 2008). It is a common misperception that older adults become cognitively impaired as they age; that is, that they become confused, forgetful, and unable to manage their affairs. This is a myth because cognitive impairments are not part of normal aging. Keep in mind that most healthy older adults live without cognitive difficulties. Those who do show signs of mild cognitive impairment (MCI) should be evaluated by a physician. MCI is characterized by memory loss, language difficulties, and impairments in judgment and reasoning due to pathologic processes (Blais, 2014). MCI does not affect the individual's ability to carry out activities of daily living (Alzheimer's Association, 2014). MCI may increase the risk of later progressing to dementia, but some people with MCI never get worse and a few eventually get better (Mayo Clinic, 2012). Dementia and Alzheimer's disease are more serious conditions that require physician evaluation and treatment.

Older learners may lose some ability to concentrate on more than one task at a time, may be slower to process information, and may need more time to learn and process information (Eliopoulos, 2014). You can help clients concentrate by having them focus on only one task at a time, beginning with the most important. Clients may need more time to process information, so speak slowly and seek feedback that indicates they follow your instruction and understand the message. Use multiple instructional materials to augment your message, focus clients' attention, and reinforce your message. If the information is new, clients may need additional time to absorb it. Repetition facilitates learning.

Memory

If learning is the process of acquiring new knowledge, then memory is the process of retaining that knowledge over time. When memory falters or is lost completely, it is frustrating, particularly to the elderly. Memory is the "ability to retain or store information and retrieve it when needed" (Bjorklund & Bee, 2008, p. 107). Short-term memory loss is more commonly seen with aging than long-term memory loss. Short-term memory refers to remembering events in the recent past, whereas long-term memory refers to distant events (Williams & Mees, 2014). There is great variation in cognitive functioning among individuals as they age because people do not follow a predictable pattern.

The causes of memory loss are many. They include physiologic causes, such as cerebrovascular changes and pathologic causes like disease or trauma, which cause a loss of neural cells. Psychosocial issues can lead to stress, depression, and social isolation (Williams & Mees, 2014). When older clients become aware of memory slippages, they often incorrectly conclude that something is wrong with their brain or that they are losing their mind. Believing that, they become fearful and anxious, which can interfere with the learning process and create a self-fulfilling prophecy. Memory loss does not necessarily mean brain disease because there are many causes of memory loss. Older clients may need to be reminded about the many memory tasks that they perform daily that are accurate and important (Bjorklund & Bee, 2008).

An important variable in memory and learning is the attitude of both clients and nurses. Your message and the client's internal messages (self-talk) matter. Clients may be aware of short-term memory deficits and become discouraged. It may be true that older clients cannot learn as much or as fast as when they were younger. However, older clients can learn when they set the pace of learning to suit their current ability. It also helps when they develop memory aids themselves. You help older clients learn better when you break up the material to be learned into sensible portions and deliver it at a slower pace with adequate space between units.

The following example is a description of the memory problems experienced by a 90-year-old woman who came out of retirement at 75, left her home in Colorado, and went to Alaska to teach children in a completely new, remote, and harsh environment. The woman offers nurses the following description and advice: "I go to get something in a room and when I get there, I have forgotten what I needed to get. I forget lists (in my head), and even three items can be troublesome. I cannot recall names of places, people, and things when I need the information, especially if I am in a mildly stressful situation. I leave out an item in a familiar recipe. I forget to turn off the stove under cooking pots so a timer is a must. Sequential directions are easily confused or omitted. Did I take my medication or not? Give me short, specific instructions. Repeat the instructions. Give me a hands-on demonstration of a procedure."

In addition to the preceding client's advice, we recommend that you encourage clients to use written lists and reinforce memory compensation devices like the timer on the stove. Color-coding medication with colored dots is helpful; for example, put blue dots on the medicine container that is taken at both breakfast and supper. A calendar is very helpful for remembering important appointments. Poems help, too. A woman complained to the nurse that she became confused when she stepped off the elevator to visit the doctor because elevators on opposites sides would take her to the correct floor. When she stepped off the elevator, she would forget which way to turn. She finally solved the problem by noting sunlight streaming in one window. She now tells herself, "Turn to the light and then to the right."

We recommend that you encourage older clients to make a record of important information and keep it in a brightly colored folder: name of doctor, name of insurance, important identification numbers, names of medications, and important people's phone numbers. Clients should also place questions that occur between visits to the doctor or you in this folder.

Interest is an important variable affecting memory and aging. "I remember what I want to remember" one elderly client said. Help clients find a reason for making the effort to learn. Fear, for example, was the motivator for a 96-year-old gentleman who was learning to walk again after a severe accident. The nurses caring for him remarked on his willpower. He replied, "It is not willpower. If I don't keep trying to walk, you will put me in one of those 'places.'" He wanted to remain in his own assisted-living apartment and not be placed in a nursing home.

Interest is closely related to attention. To assess a client's present level of cognitive competence, ask the following questions: "How well do you pay attention? What activities help you pay attention? How well do you concentrate?" A good way to foster attention is to involve several senses. For example, establish eye contact with American or western European clients. Eye contact indicates that they are probably listening attentively. Some clients have hearing deficits, so ask them to restate a message you have given. If the client is willing to repeat the message back to you, you will learn how the client has understood the message, the modality through which the client learns most easily, and the pace that suits the client. "I see what you mean," may indicate that the client is a visual learner. "I get it," may signify a tactile learning style. "I hear you" may indicate the client is an auditory learner.

Most people learn more easily and remember better from visual presentation, and visual aids are widely available for educational purposes. To be sure that the visual channel would be helpful to an individual client, assess the visual cues the client pays attention to. You might take the initiative to point out characteristics that are apparent; for example, "Notice that this little pill is red and round, whereas that one is long and green." If the client is an auditory learner, search for auditory cues to enhance learning, such as "Let me spell it for you." or "The name of the pill is Lanoxin, like Lenox china." Clients who are tactile learners can benefit from activities that involve touching or otherwise manipulating the materials. For example, you could give a set of instructions to the client for them to hold during the teaching session, or you could obtain a model (such as a heart) or the actual object (a pill) under discussion for the client to manipulate.

Other senses, such as taste and smell, may be incorporated as appropriate. If the medicine is liquid, it may have a distinctive odor. If a wound is being dressed or a discharge needs to be monitored, smell can be an important clue to the progression of healing and to a warning sign of necrosis or infection. The involvement of several senses raises the likelihood that learning will occur.

Memory often works through association. To help clients remember a new idea, help them find ways to associate it with ones they already have, or help them organize the new information into a gestalt that makes sense for them as individuals. Logical connections are helpful, but imaginative association is usually stronger. The preceding example of associating Lanoxin with Lenox china illustrates this.

Memory is enhanced by arousal. We are more apt to remember events to which we have attached emotions. Events associated with pleasant, aggravating, or frightening emotions seem to have a higher likelihood of being recalled. You may be able to say or do something amusing as a way to help them remember an event or bit of instruction. For example, to help elderly clients living in a high-rise facility improve their appearance, a nursing student dressed in mismatched garments with conflicting colors and excessive jewelry. The clients found it very amusing but understood the message.

"Do you understand?" is a tricky question and reveals only if the client acts cooperatively. Not all clients are assertive; many older clients try not to bother busy nurses. When they are feeling overloaded, clients may hide their feelings of ignorance, smile politely, and agree when they are asked this question. This type of response (with a half-hearted yes or a smile and a nod) may feel satisfying to a nurse who is very busy, but it is deceptive. When asked for specific feedback, the nurse may discover that the client understood very little. Eliciting this information is done by asking the client, "Tell me what you understand by what I said." Deception is also common whenever there is a perceived difference in status, such as between nurses and clients. Clients may not want to acknowledge they do not understand what the nurse said to avoid disappointing the nurse. Sometimes it may be necessary to check with the client's spouse to see if the client understands and to learn how the client is doing.

Medication and Cognitive Functioning

Medications can interfere with cognitive functioning. Antimisiaris & Cheek (2014) cited surveys of older adults that found many take an average of five to six medications per day and noted that the number of prescriptions per person increases with age (Korem, 2013). Taking multiple medications is known as polypharmacy, which increases the risk of undesirable side effects and interactions among the medications. When asked what medications they take, clients vary in their reliability as historians. Nurses also vary in their interviewing skills and the amount of thought they give to clients' answers. It was common for clients seen in a well oldster clinic to list only their prescribed medications. They routinely omitted herbs and over-the-counter medications, such as vitamins, laxatives, and pills taken for headache or upset stomach. They also did not mention medications prescribed by other doctors because they did not want to seem dissatisfied with the present providers. When working with older clients, teach them how drugs affect them, how multiple drugs can have untoward interactions in the body, and how to take drugs safely.

Nutrition

Sufficient food intake and adequate nutrition are important to maintaining health and preventing disease in older adults. Nutritional status is enhanced if sufficient food and adequate nutrition have been a pattern throughout life. Many factors affect nutrition in older adults, including age-related biologic changes, food preferences, financial status, lifestyle, medications, and presence of chronic disease. For healthy eating guidelines, review MyPlate for Older Adults, prepared by the Jean Mayer USDA Human Nutrition Research Center on Aging at Tufts University (TuftsNow, 2014). It replaces the Modified MyPyramid for Older Adults. The guidelines recommend that older adults meet the same nutritional requirements as their younger counterparts, even though their calorie needs and physical activities decline with age. Several daily servings of fruits and vegetables that are high in vitamins and minerals are recommended. Whole, enriched, and fortified grains are recommended for their fiber content. Limited foods include those that are high in trans fat and saturated fat and those with added salt and sugars. The food intake of older adults should follow those guidelines, and older adults should continue engaging in regular physical activities to maintain a desirable body weight. Proper nutrition is a broad topic that provides many opportunities for nurses to educate clients and their families.

Nutrition affects memory. The body is dependent on many nutrients to manufacture the neurotransmitters that are essential to learning. The B vitamins are essential ingredients in this process. Iron is essential for the transmission of oxygen to the brain, and water is vital to every metabolic process in the body. Many older adults who live alone do not eat a balanced diet. They may lack motivation to prepare nutritious meals and may benefit from community programs such as Meals on Wheels or those offered at community senior centers.

Many older adults are also dehydrated and do not consume enough liquids daily. This occurs because of physiologic changes and decrease in thirst sensation. Some older people tend to drink less in an effort to avoid the inconvenience or embarrassment of needing to empty their bladders more often. This problem of self-imposed dehydration may be exacerbated by a subculture among the older generation that considers bodily functions or attention to them as taboo. If clients are not properly hydrated, their health is endangered and their ability to learn will be impaired (Eliopoulos, 2014).

Although more Americans value fitness, many older adults do not see the connections among exercise, cardiorespiratory functioning, and an oxygenated, nourished brain. Give clients information and choose a time to teach when they are more invigorated, such as when they are sufficiently rested and have the energy to learn so they are sufficiently stimulated to pay attention.

Ethnic Elderly

Ethnic groups may view aging differently than the dominant white culture. Of the five major cultural groups in the United States, all show greater respect and reverence for the elderly when compared with the dominant culture (Purnell, 2013). For example, the elderly in the dominant culture are expected to live apart from their adult children and maintain their independence as long and as much as possible. The elderly in the African American culture enjoy closer family ties with the extended family than occurs in the dominant culture. The elderly in the Hispanic culture are respected and often live with large, extended families. Elderly Asians enjoy a high level of respect in the family, which increases as they age. The adult children are expected to take care of their aging parents. Elderly people in American Indian cultures enjoy a very high level of honor and respect for their accumulated knowledge and wisdom (Schmall, as cited in Wallace, 2006).

As with any age group, there is great diversity of beliefs and values among the elderly, both across ethnic groups and within any one ethnic group. A variety of factors affect how ethnic elders approach health care, including cultural beliefs, social supports, socioeconomic status, and cultural values. Nurses often are the first healthcare provider to have direct contact with elders and need to expand their expertise in interacting and caring for older persons. This includes being educated on the progression of normal aging and staying abreast of research to provide culturally competent care. It is essential that you conduct a thorough cultural assessment to identify the health beliefs and values of the older client, family, or group that you are teaching. To avoid stereotyping, ask if there is a cultural or ethnic group with which elders identify and what their beliefs are about health and illness (Eliopoulos, 2014). Your cultural assessment will identify the health practices of the client and the degree to which the client believes in and adheres to folk practices and Western health practices.

Clients who are immigrants or first-generation residents in the United States may adhere more strongly to the health beliefs and practices of their primary cultural affiliation. These immigrants, who may have come to the United States to join their children, have the unique challenge of relocating to a new culture and language late in life. The nurse as educator should be aware that the inability of elders to acculturate may play a part in the lack of adherence to recommended health measures. Other ethnic elderly clients who have lived a lifetime in the United States are more likely to have become assimilated into U.S. culture, to have had some experiences with the nation's healthcare system, and to have better knowledge of its health practices. By assessing health beliefs, values, and practices, you can tailor your health teaching to the individual client.

Language may be a barrier in communicating with the ethnic elderly. The client may speak little or no English. In that case, it is better to use a qualified interpreter rather than a family member, especially when the topic is sensitive.

In providing health education, be sure your message is realistic in terms of the client's diagnosis, living situation, support network, educational background, and financial resources. For example, teaching an elderly Hispanic woman with diabetes about the importance of a daily intake of fresh fruits and vegetables may be meaningless if she has limited financial resources. Her situation could be compounded if she cannot drive and her family lives far away. It is also important to know that diabetes affects an estimated one-third of older Hispanics, and the risk of depression among elders with diabetes is 30% higher when compared to elders without diabetes (Strunk, Townsend-Rocchiccioli, & Sanford, 2013).

A holistic approach to assessment may alter your teaching approach. For example, an elderly African American woman who has been on medication for hypertension for several years is found to have elevated blood pressure. After a lengthy discussion with the client, the nurse learns that the client had not been taking her medication. Because of her limited financial resources and the fact that her symptoms were not bothering her, she felt it was not necessary to take her medications. The nurse as educator needs to be aware that a misconception in the African American population about hypertension and its treatment is that hypertension is an episodic condition rather than a chronic illness (Middleton, 2009). Establishing a trusting, ongoing relationship influences adherence to a treatment plan. By correcting misconceptions the nurse can establish a relationship centered around providing culturally sensitive care. In this case the elder could also be referred to a social worker to address financial issues.

If an elderly client is undergoing treatment for a current health problem, inquire about what he or she is doing to treat it. The client may be engaging in a folk practice designed to ameliorate the condition. Listen carefully to the client's self-care practices and determine if these practices are helpful, neutral, or harmful; that is, if they should be preserved, accommodated, or restructured (DeRosa & Kochurka, 2006). Unless the practice is harmful, be supportive of it and view it as an adjunct to your nursing and medical interventions. Remember that the mind has a profound influence on health and healing, and we do not fully understand the extent of its influence. If clients' practices provide them with meaning and give them a sense of participating in healing, then the practices deserve our respect, not disdain.

WORKING WITH FAMILIES

Older clients, as with their younger counterparts, value their privacy and do not wish to be overly dependent on their adult children. Often family members or friends will need to be involved with the older person's care, and it is to them that you direct your health teaching. When this is necessary, be sensitive to the privacy concerns clients may have. Be respectful and avoid embarrassing elderly clients by sharing unnecessary information about them with others. When you teach family members or friends, reveal only the information that is essential for understanding the health message. If clients live alone and need assistance from family members or friends, identify the care needs and arrange mutually agreeable times for them to visit. If clients live with family, meeting the clients' care needs requires working around the family's employment and other routines.

WORKING WITH GROUPS AND COMMUNITIES

Senior citizen sites, community gathering places like senior lunch programs, and long-term care facilities provide opportunities for health education. Everyone is invited to participate and many will do so if for no other reason than to enjoy companionship with like-minded individuals. This is also an opportunity to encourage team members to attend so they can update their knowledge about your health topic.

When you are presenting health education information to groups of older adults, be sure to make it lively and interesting. Announce your presentation in advance and give it an interesting and catchy title that will capture their attention. The institution where you teach can help advertise your presentation in advance. If possible, use teaching strategies that encourage active participation, such as asking questions and waiting for responses and engaging clients in small group or short dyad learning activities. Your presentation will be more interesting and remembered longer if the attendees are active participants. Clients like to be given written materials that they can read in privacy on their own. Brochures and handouts also reinforce your teaching.

WORKING WITH HEALTH TEAM MEMBERS

As the number of older adults increases, there is a corresponding need for caregivers to provide healthcare services, whether in long-term care facilities or assisted living residences. Providing these services is a growth industry in the United States. Many of today's caregivers have little formal training for their roles and responsibilities, especially in long-term care facilities in which the primary caregiver is a certified nursing assistant. Certified nursing assistants are supervised by a registered nurse; however, the ratio is often unbalanced and the supervisor may be overloaded. Medicare and many states require that nursing assistants and other care providers undergo training. Because of this, there are multiple opportunities for you to provide health education for these valuable team members.

As with teaching adult learners, you must begin by knowing the provisions of the nurse practice act in your state and know the scope of practice for each team member: nursing

BOX 7-1

Evidence-Based Nursing Practice

Crumlish, C. M., & Magel, C. T. (2011). Patient education on heart attack response: Is rehearsal the critical factor in knowledge retention? *MEDSURG Nursing*, 20(6), 310–317.

Purpose: Explore a means to reduce delay in responding to heart attack by improving knowledge of the accurate signs and symptoms and the appropriate response in adults aged 55 years and older.

Method: Community-based quasi-experimental study with assignment (cluster randomized trial) comparing basic heart attack education (control group) to basic heart attack education with rehearsal (treatment group) targeted toward community-dwelling older adults. The educational program was the National Heart, Lung, and Blood Institute Heart Attack Awareness Campaign Act in Time to Heart Attack Signs with pretest and posttest cardiac quizzes.

Results: Knowledge of the signs and symptoms of a heart attack and the appropriate steps to take significantly improved in the intervention group (treatment) between pretest and posttest. However, the improvement was not sustained after a 6-month interval. Recommend that modifications be made to interventions to facilitate retention of knowledge over time and provide periodic poststudy reminders to study participants.

assistant, licensed practical nurse, and registered nurse. You must also know the general policies and practice guidelines of your employer. Long-term care institutions may or may not have in-service education departments to provide continuing education for employees. If such a department is available, you can work with the staff to identify the education needs of the team members and plan for appropriate health education.

If no such department is available, it becomes your responsibility to provide health education to your health team members. In this case, you should first assess their learning needs. You can identify these as you work with health team members and become familiar with their capabilities and deficiencies. While assessing team members, remember the three learning domains—cognitive, affective, and psychomotor—and consider in which domain the team member needs health education. For example, does the team member lack knowledge about the client's medical and nursing diagnoses and the rationale for treatment (cognitive domain)? Does the team member's attitude show a lack of understanding or compassion toward clients (affective domain)? Does the team member know how to safely and accurately perform a needed nursing care procedure (psychomotor domain)? After you have determined the learning domain in which health education is needed, you can plan appropriate teaching strategies to address those needs. Your next focus will be to determine whether the content to be taught can be done informally on the job or if the team member needs formal teaching away from the nursing unit. After teaching, you need to assess the effectiveness of your teaching.

SUMMARY

Because of the growing number and ethnic diversity of aging Americans, teaching and learning among this population are increasingly important. Older clients are different from younger and middle-aged clients in ways that significantly affect the planning and implementing of health education. Significant variables include psychosocial stages, developmental tasks, and physiologic changes associated with aging. Clients must be assessed individually to identify their particular characteristics and to plan health education that meets those needs. Suitable health education topics for assisting clients to promote, retain, and restore health were identified.

Chronic disease is present in many older clients and affects teaching plans. Many clients simply need more information about the nature of their chronic disease and how they can lessen its effect and work cooperatively with the physician to implement the treatment plan. Some clients have nutritional deficiencies that affect learning and are addressed through health education.

Although researchers are not in agreement about the causes and extent of memory changes, many older individuals and their associates are aware of problems with short-term memory. Fortunately a number of promising and tested remedies are available to the interested older individual. The nurse who is helping older clients learn information, attitude changes, or skills to promote health can make use of research. As the educator, you can adapt learning theories and principles to enhance older clients' chances of success.

EXERCISES

Exercise I: Ageism

Purpose: Develop awareness of your own attitudes toward the elderly.
Directions: Debate the proposition that ageism negatively affects healthcare services given to the elderly.

1. Divide into two groups, with each group taking opposing sides of the issue. Take 15 minutes to prepare your comments.
2. Reconvene as one group and debate the proposition.

Exercise II: Teaching Older Adults

Purpose: Identify suitable health education topics for older adults.
Directions: Divide into three groups and discuss the following client situations, all seen in a well-oldster clinic. Identify what health education topics are important to discuss with each client. Reconvene as a class and share your findings.

1. A thin 80-year-old woman presents with a chief complaint of multiple subjective symptoms. Her objective findings included low sodium and chloride, elevated calcium, dry eyes and mouth, and other evidence of dehydration. She has a history of chronic obstructive pulmonary disease, long-standing alcoholism, osteoarthritis, and kyphosis.
2. An obese 65-year-old man has a chief complaint of increased hunger, thirst, and fatigue. He was diagnosed with adult onset diabetes mellitus and appears motivated to learn better self-care and self-management. His blood glucose was 240 mg/dL (65 to 99 is normal). He is employed at a local cafeteria where he eats two meals per day.
3. A slightly obese 85-year-old woman presents with a chief complaint of constipation that has been a problem off and on for the past year. Subjectively she complains of periodic abdominal discomfort. Her objective symptom includes a slightly distended abdomen.

Exercise III: Impact of Aging Physiology on Teaching and Learning

Purpose: Analyze the implications of aging physiology on teaching and learning.

Directions: Divide into small groups and discuss how the age-related changes in the following body systems affect teaching and learning:

1. Musculoskeletal system
2. Cardiovascular system
3. Respiratory system
4. Neurologic system
5. Sensory changes in vision and hearing

List teaching and learning strategies for dealing with each change you identify:

■ Describe how the physiologic changes that occur with aging affect teaching and learning with older adults.

■ Give an example of an older client that you have worked with and how you adapted teaching to the client's physiologic changes.

■ Describe what accommodations you have made when teaching a client with the following special needs:
   ● Chronic disease
   ● Cognitive functioning
   ● Nutrition
   ● Ethnic elderly

REFERENCES

Administration on Aging. (2012). A profile of older Americans: 2012. Retrieved from http://www.aoa.gov/AoARoot/Aging_Statistics/Profile/index.aspx

Alzheimer's Association. (2014). Mild cognitive impairment. Retrieved from http://www.alz.org/dementia/mild-cognitive-impairment-mci.asp

Antimisiaris, D., & Cheek, D. J. (2014). Polypharmacy. In K. L. Mauk (Ed.), *Gerontological nursing* (3rd ed., pp. 417–454). Burlington, MA: Jones & Bartlett Learning.

Baker, M. W., & Heitkemper, M. M. (2014). Chronic illness and older adults. In S. L. Lewis, S. R. Dirksen, M. M. Heitkemper, & L. Bucher (Eds.), *Medical–surgical nursing: Assessment and management of clinical problems* (9th ed., pp. 61–78). St. Louis, MO: Mosby Elsevier.

Balakas, K. (2013). Developmental theories. In P. A. Potter, A. G. Perry, P. A. Stockert, & A. M. Hall (Eds.), *Fundamentals of nursing* (8th ed., pp. 130–138). St. Louis, MO: Mosby Elsevier.

Bjorklund, B. R., & Bee, H. L. (2008). *The journey of adulthood* (6th ed.). Upper Saddle River, NJ: Pearson Education.

Blais, K. (2014). Older adult. In C. L. Edelman, E. C. Kudzma, & C. L. Mandel (Eds.), *Health promotion throughout the life span* (8th ed., pp. 591–620). St. Louis, MO: Elsevier Mosby.

Crumlish, C. M., & Magel, C. T. (2011). Patient education on heart attack response: Is rehearsal the critical factor in knowledge retention? *MEDSURG Nursing, 20*(6), 310–317.

DeRosa, N., & Kochurka, K. (2006). Implement culturally competent healthcare in your workplace. *Nursing Management, 37*(10), 18–26.

Disabatino, A. J., & Bucher, L. (2014). Nursing assessment cardiovascular system. In S. L. Lewis, S. R. Dirksen, M. M. Heitkemper, & L. Bucher (Eds.), *Medical–surgical nursing: Assessment and management of clinical problems* (9th ed., pp. 686–708). St. Louis, MO: Elsevier Mosby.

Eisel, S. J. (2014). Nursing assessment respiratory system. In S. L. Lewis, S. R. Dirksen, M. M. Heitkemper, & L. Bucher (Eds.), *Medical–surgical nursing: Assessment and management of clinical problems* (9th ed., pp. 475–496). St. Louis, MO: Elsevier Mosby.

Eliopoulos, C. (2014). *Gerontological nursing* (8th ed.). Philadelphia, PA: Wolters Kluwer Health/ Lippincott Williams & Wilkins.

Erikson, E. H. (1963). *Childhood and society* (2nd ed.). New York, NY: W. W. Norton.

Erikson, E. H. (1982). *Life cycle completed: A review.* New York, NY: W. W. Norton.

Erikson, E. H., & Erikson, J. M. (1997). *The life cycle completed.* New York, NY: W. W. Norton.

Fahlman, M. M., Topp, R., McNevin, N., Morgan, A. L., & Boardley, D. (2007). Structured exercise in older adults with limited functional ability. *Journal of Gerontological Nursing, 33*(6), 32–39.

Hall, A. M. (2009). Client education. In P. A. Potter & A. G. Perry (Eds.), *Fundamentals of nursing* (7th ed., pp. 361–383). St. Louis, MO: Mosby Elsevier.

Kautz, D. D., & Barnett, L. (2014). Sexuality. In K. L. Mauk (Ed.), *Gerontological nursing* (3rd ed., pp. 793–808). Burlington, MA: Jones & Bartlett Learning.

Knowles, M. S. (1990). *The adult learner: A neglected species* (4th ed.). Houston, TX: Gulf.

Korem, K. (2013). Older adults. In P. A. Potter, A. G. Perry, P. A. Stockert, & A. M. Hall (Eds.), *Fundamentals of nursing* (8th ed., pp. 171–191). St. Louis, MO: Mosby Elsevier.

Linton, A. D. (2007). Age-related changes in the special senses. In A. D. Linton & H. W. Lach (Eds.), *Matteson and McConnell's gerontological nursing concepts and practice* (3rd ed., pp. 600–627). St. Louis, MO: Saunders Elsevier.

Lueckenotte, A. (2009). Older adult. In P. A. Potter & A. G. Perry (Eds.), *Fundamentals of nursing* (7th ed., pp. 191–214). St. Louis, MO: Mosby Elsevier.

Mayo Clinic. (2012). Mild cognitive impairment (MCI). Retrieved from http://www.mayoclinic.com/ health/mild-cognitive-impairment/DS00553

Middleton, J. L. (2009). A proposed new model of hypertensive treatment behavior in African Americans. *Journal of the National Medical Association, 101*(1), 12–17.

Miller, C. A. (1990). *Nursing care of older adults.* Glenview, IL: Scott, Foresman/Little, Brown Higher Education.

Millsap, P. (2007). Neurological system. In A. D. Linton & H. W. Lach (Eds.), *Matteson and McConnell's gerontological nursing concepts and practice* (3rd ed., pp. 406–441). St. Louis, MO: Saunders Elsevier.

National Center for Cultural Competence. (2003). Policy Brief 1 Rationale for Cultural Competence in Primary Care. (n.d.). Retrieved from http://nccc.georgetown.edu/documents/Policy_Brief_1_2003. pdf http://www11.georgetown.edu/research/gucchd/nccc/resources/cultural6.html

National Institute on Alcohol Abuse and Alcoholism. (n.d.). Older adults. Retrieved from http://www. niaaa.nih.gov/alcohol-health/special-populations-co-occurring-disorders/older-adults

Olson, D. W. (2014). Nursing assessment nervous system. In S. L. Lewis, S. R. Dirksen, M. M. Heitkemper, & L. Bucher (Eds.), *Medical–surgical nursing: Assessment and management of clinical problems* (9th ed., pp. 1335–1355). St. Louis, MO: Elsevier Mosby.

Peck, R. C. (1968). Psychological developments in the second half of life. In B. Neugarten (Ed.), *Middle age and aging* (pp. 88–92). Chicago, IL: University of Chicago Press.

Purnell, L. D. (2013). *Transcultural health care: A culturally competent approach* (4th ed.). Philadelphia, PA: F. A. Davis.

Roberts, D. (2014). Nursing assessment musculoskeletal system. In S. L. Lewis, S. R. Dirksen, M. M. Heitkemper, & L. Bucher (Eds.), *Medical–surgical nursing: Assessment and management of clinical problems* (9th ed., pp. 1489–1504). St. Louis, MO: Elsevier Mosby.

Santrock, J. W. (2014). *A topical approach to life-span development* (7th ed.). Boston, MA: McGraw-Hill.

Schneider, J. K., Eveker, A., Bronder, D. R., Meiner, S. E., & Binder, E. F. (2003). Exercise training program for older adults. *Journal of Gerontological Nursing, 29*(9), 22–31.

Strunk, J. A., Townsend-Rocchiccioli, J. T, & Sanford, J. T. (2013). The aging Hispanic in America: Challenges for nurses in a stressed health care environment. *MEDSURG Nursing, 22*(1), 45–50.

TuftsNow. (2014). MyPlate for older adults. Retrieved from http://now.tufts.edu/news-releases/tufts-university-nutrition-scientists-unveil

Wallace, M. (2006). Older adult. In C. L. Edelman & C. L. Mandle (Eds.), *Health promotion throughout the life span* (6th ed., pp. 571–598). St. Louis, MO: Mosby.

Weinrich, S. P., Boyd, M., & Nussbaum, J. (1989). Continuing education: Adapting strategies to teach the elderly. *Journal of Gerontological Nursing, 15*(11), 17–21.

Williams, K., & Mees, K. (2014). Therapeutic communication with older adults, families and caregivers. In K. L., Mauk (Ed.), *Gerontological nursing* (3rd ed., pp. 97–121). Burlington, MA: Jones & Bartlett Learning.

8

The Culturally Diverse Learner

INTRODUCTION

This chapter examines the role of **culture** in the process of client education. Culture is defined as "the totality of socially transmitted behavioral patterns, arts, beliefs, values, customs, lifeways, and all other products of human work and thought characteristic of a population of people that guide their world view and decision-making" (Purnell, 2013, p. 6). **Cultural factors** include beliefs, values, moral principles, habits, dress, language, rules for behavior, economics, politics, dietary practices, and health care (Burchum, 2002). Not only do cultural factors relate to race and ethnicity, but also to behaviors and beliefs characteristic of particular social, ethnic, disabled, age, and gender groups. **Ethnicity** is identity with or membership in a particular racial, national, or cultural group and observance of that group's customs, beliefs, and language.

Knowledge of culture is a critical element in the process of delivering health education. All cultural and ethnic groups hold concepts related to health and illness and associated practices for maintaining well-being or providing treatment when it is indicated. The perception of health and illness is **enculturated** into members of a cultural group. In addition, the individual's socioeconomic, educational, geographic, religious, and other factors shape their cultural and ethnic health beliefs. Over time **acculturation** may occur, which means that members of a group modify or give up traits from the culture of origin as a result of contact with another culture. Demographic changes anticipated over the next decade magnify the importance of addressing racial and ethnic disparities in health care.

CHARACTERISTICS OF CULTURALLY DIVERSE LEARNERS

Shifting Demographics

The U.S. Census Bureau reports that the population of the United States is more racially and ethnically diverse than ever before. The majority population of English-speaking whites is giving way to a new influx of immigrants with many different cultures and ethnic backgrounds. Minorities made up 37% of the U.S. population in 2013 but will comprise 57% of the population in 2060. It is projected that the U.S. population will continue to be older and more racially and ethnically mixed (U.S. Census Bureau, 2012). This change is not occurring only in the United States. Demographics changes are occurring in many countries worldwide (Flowers, 2009). As a result of this multicultural phenomenon, the **cultural competence** of nurses is becoming more critical to ensure positive outcomes for an increasingly diverse client population. Nurses must also realize that addressing cultural diversity goes beyond knowing the values, beliefs, practices, and customs of African Americans, Asians, Hispanics/Latinos, and American Indians/Native Alaskans. In addition to racial classification and national origin, there are many other facets of cultural diversity. "Religious affiliation, language, physical size, gender, sexual orientation, age, disability (both physical and mental), political orientation, socioeconomic status, occupational status and geographical location are but a few of the faces of diversity" (Campinha-Bacote, 2003, p. 1).

It is important not to stereotype people of different cultures, but to cultivate an appreciation for individual cultural variations. Andrews notes that having an understanding of culture, either your own or others, does not necessarily bring about respect and understanding: "Nursing students, nurses, and other health care providers must have positive experiences with members of other cultures and learn to genuinely value the contributions all cultures make to our multicultural society" (2012, p. ix).

Healthcare Disparities

The health and life expectancy of Americans are improving, but racial and ethnic minorities have not benefited equally from this progress. Complex sociologic, cultural, political, and economic factors account for this. A major concern is that even those diverse clients with equivalent access to the healthcare system receive lower-quality care than white patients for many medical conditions (Smith et al., 2007). These differences in health disparities were revealed in the 2002 Institute of Medicine report, *Unequal Treatment: Confronting Racial and Ethnic Disparities in Health Care.* Despite improvements in the overall health status of the U.S. population in the past few decades, disparities in health status among ethnic and racial minorities continue to be a serious local and national health challenge. Populations with health disparities have increased incidence of diseases, as well as morbidity and mortality, when compared to the general population. Because of this, eliminating health disparities is one of the most important priorities of Healthy People 2020 (U.S. Department of Health and Human Services, 2010). The issue of disparities in health status continues to be one of importance to healthcare providers. Experts have also noted that without new and more effective interventions, health disparities will be difficult to eliminate and may become an even larger problem as racial and ethnic minorities become a greater proportion of the U.S. population (Smith et al., 2007). To meet the needs of culturally diverse groups, nurse educators must engage in the process of becoming culturally competent.

CULTURAL COMPETENCE

Definition

Campinha-Bacote defines cultural competence as "the process by which the health care professional continuously strives to achieve the ability and availability to effectively work within the cultural context of a client (individual, family, community)" (1998, p. 6). This process requires nurses to see themselves as *becoming* culturally competent, rather than *being* culturally competent. Cross, Bazron, Dennis, and Isaacs (1989) further describe cultural competence as a developmental process that evolves over an extended period of time that includes both individuals and organizations at various levels of awareness, knowledge, and skills along the cultural competence continuum. Practicing cultural competence brings about the practice of **culturally competent care** that is considered to be "the knowledge, skills, and attitudes required to provide quality clinical care to patients from different cultural, ethnic, and racial backgrounds" (Harvard Medical School, 2009). The American Nurses Association recognizes the need to provide culturally competent care. It states in the association's code that nurses should "practice with compassion and respect for the inherent dignity, worth and uniqueness of every individual" (2001, p. 4).

Campinha-Bacote Cultural Competence Model

Campinha-Bacote's model, the Process of Cultural Competence in the Delivery of Health Services, includes the components of cultural desire, cultural awareness, cultural knowledge, cultural encounters, and cultural skill (conducting culturally sensitive assessments) (Campinha-Bacote, 2002). Because cultural competence is an important attribute of the nurse as educator, the five key concepts of the model are described further.

Cultural desire is the most critical concept of cultural competence because it is the nurse's desire that brings about the entire process of cultural competence. This desire must come from the nurse wanting to engage in becoming culturally competent, not from having to participate in the process. The nurse takes a humble approach to client differences and, as educator, examines her or his personal motivation to work with clients of different cultures. In this important first step, the nurse as educator asks, How will I develop the willingness and patience to work with clients who are different from me?

Cultural awareness is the self-examination and in-depth exploration of one's own cultural background. This process involves the recognition of the nurse's biases, prejudices, and assumptions about individuals who are different. This means examining past experiences and considering how to handle biases and assumptions. The nurse asks the question, How will I develop the skill to be objective and open to cultural differences?

Cultural knowledge is the process of seeking and obtaining a sound educational foundation about diverse cultural and ethnic groups. Obtaining cultural knowledge about the client's health-related beliefs and values involves understanding how clients interpret their illnesses and how their view of the world guides their thinking, doing, and being. It is in this part of the model that stereotyping is addressed. Campinha-Bacote states that "no individual is a stereotype of one's culture of origin, but rather a unique blend of the diversity found within each culture, a unique accumulation of life experiences, and the process of acculturation to other cultures" (2003, p. 7). The nurse as educator makes a commitment to learning about other cultures and to grow and evolve in that knowledge.

Cultural encounter is the process that encourages the nurse to directly engage in face-to-face interactions with clients from culturally diverse backgrounds. Interacting with clients from diverse cultural groups has the potential to refine or modify nurses' beliefs about cultural groups and aids in preventing stereotyping. It is important to note that interacting with only three or four members from a specific ethnic group does not make one an expert on the cultural group, but these encounters give the nurse as educator valuable experiences to draw from. As the nurse approaches the role of educator, it is advisable to look for opportunities to expand knowledge of other cultures either locally or even internationally.

A final component of Campinha-Bacote's model, cultural skill, is the ability to collect relevant cultural data regarding the client's presenting problem and accurately performing a culturally based physical assessment. Cultural assessment is defined as "a systematic, comprehensive examination of individuals, families, groups, and communities regarding their health-related cultural beliefs, values and practices" (Campinha-Bacote, 2002, p. 184). As part of achieving cultural skill, a variety of more in-depth cultural assessment tools are presented here. These tools should be selected and used to meet the specific needs of the learning situation. The nurse as educator should be aware that the way these tools are implemented through the nurse–client interaction is important. Cultural skill brings all the knowledge from the components of the model together to create culturally competent client interaction.

Cultural Assessment Models

Andrews/Boyle Transcultural Nursing Assessment Guide for Individuals and Families

Andrews and Boyle (2012) offer an extensive in-depth assessment tool titled the Andrews/Boyle Transcultural Nursing Assessment Guide for Individuals and Families. The major categories in this guide include cultural variations and cultural aspects of the incidence of disease, communication, cultural affiliations, cultural sanctions and restrictions, developmental considerations, economics, health-related beliefs and practices, kinship and social networks, nutrition, religion and spirituality, and values orientation. The guide focuses on a holistic cultural approach to the health history and the physical examination.

Leininger's Sunrise Model

The Sunrise Model is part of Leininger's Theory of Cultural Care Diversity and Universality and includes seven assessments of culturally congruent nursing care. They include a holistic approach that looks at cultural values and lifeways; religious, philosophical, and spiritual beliefs; economic factors; educational factors; technological factors; kinship and social ties; and political and legal factors (Leininger, 1991).

Purnell's Model for Cultural Assessment

Purnell's Model for Cultural Assessment includes domains of culture for assessing ethnocultural attributes of individuals, families, or groups (Purnell, 2013). The 12 domains are inhabited localities and topography, communication, family roles and organizations, workforce issues, bicultural ecology, high-risk behaviors, nutrition, pregnancy and childbearing practices, death rituals, spirituality, health practices, and healthcare practitioners. The strength of this model includes the domain of bicultural ecology that identifies specific physical, biologic, and physiologic variations in ethnic and racial origins. This is a source of information on cultural variations in physical assessment for nurses as educators.

Giger and Davidhizar's Transcultural Assessment Model

Giger and Davidhizar's Transcultural Assessment Model consists of six cultural phenomena that go across all cultures and that affect nursing care. They are communication, space, social organization, time, environmental control, and biological variations (Giger & Davidhizar, 2008). The model applies these concepts to 23 specific cultural groups that are found in the United States.

Assessing Cultural Competence

The nurse should take time to self-evaluate his or her progress in becoming culturally competent. The following two tools take slightly different approaches to examining cultural competence, but both help the nurse as educator reflect upon the role of culture in client care. Campinha-Bacote and Narayan state that cultural awareness is "a continual self-examination of one's own prejudices and biases toward other cultures" (2000, p. 213). Campinha-Bacote (2002) provides a mnemonic, ASKED, to help nurses assess their cultural awareness:

A is for awareness
S is for skill
K is for knowledge
E is for encounters
D is for desire

TABLE 8-1

Culhane-Pera and Colleagues' Levels of Cultural Competence

Level 1 No insight about the influence of culture on health care
Level 2 Minimal emphasis on culture in healthcare settings
Level 3 Acceptance of the role of cultural beliefs, values, and behaviors on health, disease, and treatment
Level 4 Incorporation of cultural awareness into daily healthcare practice
Level 5 Integration of attention to culture into all areas of professional life

Source: Adapted from Blue, A. (2009). The Provision of Culturally Competent Health Care. Medical University of South Carolina: Department of Family Medicine. Retrieved on May 17, 2009 at http://www.musc.edu/fm_ruralclerkship/culture.html

Nurses as educators ask themselves if they have *awareness* of biases and prejudices; if they have the *skill* to conduct a cultural assessment; if they have cultural *knowledge*; if they have experiences *encountering* people of different cultures; and if they have the *desire* to be culturally competent. This self-assessment assists the nurse when working with diverse clients.

Culhane-Pera, Reif, Egli, Bake, and Kassekert (1997) describe five levels of cultural competence with respect to health care. With this tool nurses can track their progress in becoming culturally competent as they advance through the levels (**Table 8-1**).

CULTURALLY CONGRUENT CLIENT EDUCATION

The definition of **culturally congruent client education** is drawn from the concept of culturally congruent care, initially conceptualized by Leininger, who defines culturally congruent care as "those cognitively based assistive, supportive, facilitative, or enabling acts or decisions that are tailor made to fit with individual, group, or institutional cultural values, beliefs, and lifeways in order to provide or support meaningful, beneficial, and satisfying health care to well-being services" (1991, p. 49). Schim, Doorenbos, Benkert, and Miller further explain Leininger's definition by saying that "culturally congruent care is a holistic construct, heavily influenced by negotiated experiences, meanings, mutual understandings, and respect" (2007, p. 105). We use this as a foundation to define culturally congruent client education. Culturally congruent client education involves providing meaningful and useful education for clients by incorporating diverse ways of knowing from the viewpoint of various cultural groups. It is a harmonious approach to working with clients that shows sensitivity and respect for individual cultural differences and a willingness to collaborate with them to meet their health education needs. Culturally competent nurses who are educators welcome client collaboration and cooperation. They have a foundation of knowledge about client cultures and reflect on their own personal cultural values and beliefs. This self-examination helps them understand how their beliefs influence the way they teach.

The need for culturally congruent client education is based on the fact that diverse clients respond culturally to health and illness. In the United States, healthcare disparities are a leading cause of morbidity and mortality among minorities and those of lower socioeconomic status. Because of this it is important that nurses incorporate cultural perspectives into all facets of health education delivery (Anderson, Scrimshaw, Fullilove, Fielding, & Normand, 2003). This approach addresses the need to promote equal access to quality health care and equal treatment of clients.

Later in this chapter, after we provide information about the four major cultural groups, we introduce the Stoeckel Culturally Congruent Client Education Model, which brings together culturally based actions, rationales, and health education outcomes.

CULTURALLY SPECIFIC CLIENT ASSESSMENTS AND CONCERNS

Cultural factors affect client education interactions. It is important for the nurse as educator to have an understanding of the cultural factors that shape learners from different cultural groups. Stressors and adaptive behaviors may present considerable barriers to effective client education unless nurses are sensitive to their origins and meanings and are willing to take them into account when working with clients (Falvo, 2011). By taking time to investigate a client's past experiences and cultural perceptions, the nurse takes steps to build rapport with clients, which is a basic component of effective nurse–client relationships.

Clients accept or reject the information provided by a nurse based on whether they perceive the information as truthful, in their best interest, and congruent with their beliefs. To gain a better understanding of factors related to teaching and learning with cultural groups, we have chosen to present information on four ethnic minority groups: African American, Asian American, Hispanic, and American Indian. They are the major ethnic minorities in the United States as traced by the U.S. Census Bureau. Four aspects of each group's culture that impact health education are examined: cultural norms (aspects of the culture that impact the teaching and learning process), family influence (impact and involvement of family in the teaching and learning process), beliefs about health and illness (including religious influences and folk medicine that influence clients' perception of health care), and implications for health education. Knowledge of these aspects provides insight for nurses as educators in planning and implementing teaching plans, but caution is needed to avoid stereotyping. Never assume that all clients from one ethnic group hold the same beliefs.

African American

Cultural Norms

The U.S. Census Bureau reported that the black population is expected to increase from 41.1 million to 61.8 million in 2060 (2012), which is about 14.7% of the total population.

In preparing to work with African American clients, the nurse should be aware that the initial client approach and the initial impression that you give is very important. Because interpersonal relationships are highly valued among African Americans, it is important to focus on developing a sound, trusting, and respectful relationship. This begins with consideration of the way that clients are greeted and referred to. Be aware of intracultural variations within the cultural group; for example, different generational groups may have a particular way in which they wish to be identified. Younger clients may want to be called African American; elderly clients may prefer the terms Negro or colored, and middle-aged clients may refer to themselves as black or black American (Campinha-Bacote, 2008). Most African Americans prefer to be greeted formally, with Mr., Mrs., or Miss along with their surname, because the family name is respected and indicates pride in family heritage. Unless invited, it is best to use the last name and appropriate title instead of first names. It may be necessary to clarify preferences with clients.

The attitude of healthcare professionals is one of the most significant barriers when working with African Americans. Research shows that African American clients feel they are often treated unfairly or disrespectfully because of their race (Kaiser Family Foundation, 2001). Because of this, African Americans may be suspicious of healthcare professionals and may seek out a physician or nurse only when absolutely necessary. Treating clients with respect is the foundation of the nurse–client relationship. Respect for persons has been broadly defined as the recognition that all persons have dignity and inherent worth. Expressions of respect include treatment with dignity and respect for autonomy and involvement in healthcare decisions. These expressions are associated with clients' satisfaction with care and increased adherence to treatment regimens. Beach and colleagues (2005) suggest that clients can determine when clinicians demonstrate a valuing attitude. These perceptions correlate with whether the client was treated kindly or rudely. Respectful treatment of African American clients includes acknowledging clients appropriately as described previously, shaking hands, using eye contact, listening intently, and giving physical and mental comfort.

Family Influence

Understanding African American families is an important aspect of teaching clients. Traditional family structure of husband and wife is often found, but many African American families have a matriarchal system with a single mother, aunt, or grandmother heading the household. The role of the grandmother is one of the most central roles in the African American family and is afforded great respect (Campinha-Bacote, 2008). A growing number of grandparents are functioning in the primary parental role. African American women are expected to assist family members in

FIGURE 8-1

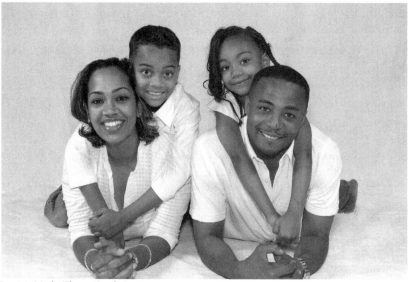

Source: © Patricia Marks/ShutterStock, Inc.

maintaining good health and determining treatment if a family member is ill. It is important for the nurse to recognize the importance of African American women in disseminating information and in assisting family members in making decisions (Cherry & Giger, 2008). If present, an African American man should also be included in the decision-making process. Some African American families have large supportive extended family networks. It is important to include involved, extended family members in planning and implementing teaching plans where appropriate because they could unknowingly sabotage the clients' progress if they are not informed.

Health Beliefs

Spiritual and religious orientation is important in some African American families, with the majority participating in Protestant denominations. Belief in God and the use of prayer and participation in formal religious service may be part of religious practices. The church community is viewed as a viable support system in developing health-promoting behaviors, and the nurse may consider a partnership with faith-based communities to support client learning.

There is evidence that African American folk medicine is practiced in all areas of the United States, but the extent of its use is not known. African American folk medicine is an offshoot of African cultural heritage in the rural South. It can involve treatment by folk practitioners who use witchcraft, voodoo, and magic. Folk medicine may be used for a variety of reasons: lack of access to traditional healthcare services, inability to afford the cost of health care, or humiliating experiences when encountering the mainstream healthcare system (Cherry & Giger, 2008).

Folk medicine perceives illness as either a natural or an unnatural occurrence. Natural illness occurs because a person is affected by natural forces without adequate protection. Unnatural illnesses are perceived as either a punishment from God or the work of the devil, which are more difficult for the nurse to address. Death is viewed as a natural part of living and is handled through strong religious beliefs (Campinha-Bacote, 2008). It is important for the nurse to assess if folk remedies are being used, and if so to assist the client in sorting out what is helpful, neutral, or harmful. This is part of the assessment information necessary to prepare the teaching plan.

Implications for Health Education

When setting up teaching sessions with African American clients, keep in mind that they may prefer a closer personal space and that extended family may accompany them. When teaching how to perform psychomotor skills, structure the learning activities in ranked order to produce maximum learning results. If timing is involved with an activity, it is important to be clear about when timing is flexible and when it is not, such as with the giving of medication. Keep in mind that a teaching plan that is congruent with the client's beliefs has a better chance of being successful. The most common health concerns for African Americans requiring health education are listed in **Table 8-2**.

Asian American

Cultural Norms

The U.S. Census Bureau projects that the Asian American population will double from 15.5 million in 2012 to 34.4 million in 2060 (2012). Its share of the total population will rise from 5.1% to 8.2% in the same period. Asians Americans emigrate from more than 20 countries and

TABLE 8-2

Most Common Disorders Requiring Health Education: African Americans

Ethnic/Racial Group	Most Common Disorders Requiring Health Education
African American	■ Heart disease
	■ Hypertension
	■ Stroke
	■ Cancer
	■ Asthma
	■ Influenza/pneumonia
	■ HIV/AIDS
	■ Homicide
	■ Obesity
	■ Sickle cell anemia

speak more than 100 languages. The Asian American population is diverse and represents people from a variety of countries and cultures. The largest subpopulations are persons of Chinese, Filipino, Japanese, Asian Indian, Korean, and Southeast Asian ancestry. Recent Asian immigrants represent the highest foreign-born percentage among all racial and ethnic groups in the United States.

Establishing rapport with Asian American clients begins with establishing trust. It is important to remember as you approach Asian American clients to be aware that their values include hard work, acceptance of what life brings, respect for nature, self-control, respect for elders, and loyalty to family. Cultural values stress politeness in verbal discourse, and if mistrust develops you may find the client reluctant to discuss lifestyle issues and behaviors. Many Asian Americans view relationships in health care as hierarchical and therefore expect the health professional to take charge (Management Sciences for Health [MSH], 2005). Clients may not want to participate in making decisions about their treatment and may appear passive in the process. Nurses as educators should acknowledge their role and use it to their advantage when working with clients. This can be particularly effective in encouraging patients to adopt healthy behaviors and adhere to teaching plans. It is important, however, that the client not feel intimidated by the nurse. Feelings of intimidation may prevent the client from telling the truth about customs, beliefs, or behaviors that may impact the success of the teaching plan. You should also be aware that some clients may silently decide not to adhere to recommended treatments (MSH, 2005).

Asian American clients view health from a variety of perspectives and often combine Eastern and Western perspectives of health. They use acupuncture, acupressure, and herbs in combination with dietary therapy, Western medicine, and supernatural healing to achieve maximum results. When beliefs contradict each other, however, some Asians will not adhere to Western medicine. It is also important to be aware that clients do not always disclose the use of complementary and alternative medicine (CAM), which can increase the chances of adverse interaction with conventional Western treatments. Clients may be reluctant to share their use of these methods, fearing disapproval from the nurse and worrying that they might appear disrespectful of Western traditions. To determine the use of CAM, you should ask clients directly and clearly what remedies they use. Nurses need to educate themselves about traditional Asian approaches to healing and encourage their clients and their healers to collaborate for the client's good. A common belief of Asian clients is that Western medicine is very potent and that it can cure illness rapidly (MSH, 2005). This belief may manifest itself by the client reducing dosages. Clients also may stop medications as soon as symptoms are relieved. These are all areas that require attention when preparing teaching plans.

When meeting Asian elders, it is a sign of disrespect to look them straight in the eyes. A limp handshake from Asian clients is a way of showing humility and respect. For many, physical contact such as a handshake or a hug between a man and a woman is interpreted as a sexual advance. For some Asian subcultures it may be appropriate for you to first address the oldest male in a group or family before greeting other members (MSH, 2005). Be aware that a lack of facial expression or a low level of verbal communication may not indicate a lack of emotion or opinion. Neither does it indicate agreement with the diagnosis or recommended treatment. Try to determine your clients' true feelings or opinions before accepting their apparent acquiescence of the treatment plan. Asian clients tend to be more comfortable with a health professional who shares their language and culture, perhaps because they believe that a person of their own culture will not dismiss their traditional Asian practices and home remedies (MSH, 2005).

Family Influence

Traditionally, the Asian family unit is strong, stable, and cohesive for all its members. The family plays a critical role in the ongoing development and support of children through adulthood.

FIGURE 8-2

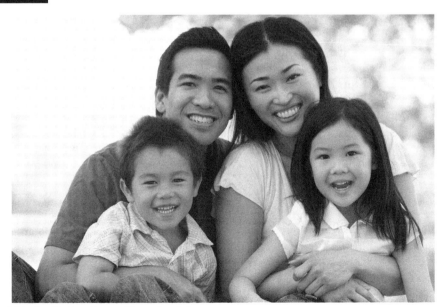

Source: © Monkey Business Images/ShutterStock, Inc.

The importance of the extended family, emphasized in Asian culture, often results in the extended family being highly involved in the client's care and medical decision making (MSH, 2005). Family members can provide valuable information regarding the client's diet, health behavior, daily activities, and types of alternative medications used. Their involvement in a treatment plan may be vital to the client's ability to adhere to the recommended teaching plan. Families may decide what the client will eat, when to take medication, whether to exercise, and when to seek medical attention. The family also exerts influence on youth to prevent antisocial and self-defeating behaviors.

Many Asian immigrants experienced stressful and painful episodes in their native countries that affect their health and influence their perception of the U.S. healthcare system. The effects of war, migration, detention camps or torture, and experiences associated with adjustment to the U.S. culture are all major factors that might result in mistrust, fear, or helplessness and prevent the client from taking an active role in their health care.

Nurses as educators need to be sensitive to the diversity and generational differences within the Asian population and decide on an individual basis whether it is culturally appropriate to involve family members. The culturally competent educator will discuss with the client the patterns of decision making in the family. Understanding and respecting complex and often delicate interactions among family members enables nurses to use the client's family as a valuable resource rather than an intrusion into the nurse–client relationship (MSH, 2005).

Health Beliefs

Asian medical tradition centers on a belief in the interconnectedness of the mind, body, and spirit and the need for balance and a holistic approach to the treatment of illness. Buddhism and other Eastern philosophies teach that art and science coexist and that healing is spiritual as well as scientific (Yee, Mokuau, & Kim, 1999). A common belief held by many Asians is that of Taoism, which originated in China. Tao, or the way, is based on the idea of balancing the natural processes and forces of yin and yang. Yin is negative female energy associated with cold and water, and Yang is positive male energy associated with heat and fire. These forces remain in balance through a combination of practices of holistic medicine, acupuncture, herbalism, and meditation. Beliefs about health and illness strongly influence clients' behavior. They may avoid the wind, be reluctant to go out after surgery, or refuse to have blood drawn (MSH, 2005). Many Asians perceive life in fatalistic terms and may feel less able to do something about their illness. Beliefs in supernatural spirits may result in reliance on religion or spiritual healing rituals in addition to Western medicine. All these factors influence your approach to teaching Asian clients.

Implications for Health Education

As an educator, you need to provide strong encouragement because Asian clients need assurance that the recommended treatment plan is the right thing to do. This may mean urging family members to encourage the client. Being an advocate also means helping to locate other supportive healthcare providers. In some communities, Asian American organizations (temples, churches, benevolent association, cultural associations, etc.) serve as focal points for social and other activities. Developing contacts with and working through these community-based

TABLE 8-3	
Most Common Disorders Requiring Health Education: Asians	
Ethnic/Racial Group	*Most Common Disorders Requiring Health Education*
Asian	▪ Cancer ▪ Heart disease ▪ Stroke ▪ Accidents ▪ Diabetes ▪ Tuberculosis ▪ Liver disease

organizations can be a useful way for you to develop an understanding of the health and social needs of clients (MSH, 2005). Be aware that Asian clients usually expect something concrete, such as prescriptions for medications, at the conclusion of a teaching session for the meeting to live up to their expectations. Without this, they might be reluctant to return for routine teaching visits or preventive care. Also be aware that Asian women may prefer to work with a female educator. The most common health concerns for Asians requiring health education are listed in **Table 8-3**.

Hispanic

Cultural Norms

The U.S. Census Bureau projects that the Hispanic population will double from 53.3 million in 2012 to 128.8 million in 2060 (2012). At the end of this period nearly one in three U.S. residents will be Hispanic, up from one in six in 2013. This will continue to make Hispanics the largest ethnic minority group in the United States. Hispanics are classified as one ethnic group, but they are actually multiple, culturally similar ethnic subgroups. The subgroups that make up the Hispanic population in the United States are Mexicans, Puerto Ricans, Cubans, Central Americans, South Americans, Dominicans, and other Hispanics and Latinos.

When working with Hispanic clients, it is important to be aware of the different terms used to refer to Hispanics. The U.S. Census Bureau (2012) uses the term *Hispanic* to describe any person, regardless of race, creed, or color, whose origins are in Mexico, Puerto Rico, Cuba, Central or South America, or some other Hispanic region. *Latino* or *Latina* refers to a person of Latin American or Spanish-speaking descent who is living in the United States. The terms *Hispanic* or *Latino* may be used interchangeably (Zoucha & Zamarripa, 2003). It is not recommended to use the terms *Chicano*, *Mexicano*, or *Xican* unless the client refers to himself or herself in these ways because these terms may be considered derogatory. The term *Tejano* is used to describe a Texan of Hispanic decent. It is important to ask clients how they would like to be referred to.

Several cultural characteristics impact the way that Hispanic clients perceive interactions with healthcare professionals. The concepts of respeto (respect), **personalismo** (personal relationships), and **confianza** (trust) are important concepts for the nurse to be aware of when interacting with Hispanic clients (Gonzalez, Owen, & Esperat, 2008). Respecto is a behavior that shows differential attention toward others based on age, sex, social position, economic status, and authority. It is important for you to show respect by addressing Hispanic clients by their surname and title in English or Spanish, such as Mrs. Rodriquez or Senora Rodriquez, and by avoiding a condescending attitude. Hispanic clients may avoid eye contact with authority figures. To be respectful, personal or private questions should be approached in an indirect way to avoid client embarrassment. Personalismo is about the nurse conveying to the client that he or she wants a personal relationship. This is demonstrated by being friendly and taking interest in the client's life. This is shown by engaging in a greeting that inquires about how they are doing and puts the client at ease. Personal contact and touch are acceptable parts of the relationship and are considered important aspects of the nurse–client relationship. Hispanic clients prefer to be close and are comfortable with the nurse giving a handshake, sitting closer, leaning forward, and giving a comforting pat on the shoulder or other gestures that indicate interest in the client. Hispanic clients demonstrate stronger attachment to the healthcare provider than to the healthcare institution and will follow the provider if they move (MSH, 2005). This emphasizes how strongly they value personal relationships. Confianza, or trust, develops over time in relation with Hispanic clients. When trust is established between the nurse and the client, it becomes more likely that the client will value the time spent with the nurse and be more likely to adhere to teaching plans.

It can be frightening for clients that cannot speak English to enter the U.S. healthcare system. Studies show that Hispanic clients view nurses who attempted to speak some Spanish as caring and respectful (Gonzalez et al., 2008). It is common for Hispanic clients to appear agreeable on the surface and to be courteous, but if they disagree they may not carry out the suggested treatment. It is uncommon for Hispanic clients to be aggressive when interacting with healthcare professionals, but their response may be silence or not adhering to the teaching plan. Joking by the nurse is considered rude, insulting, and offensive, and it may cause stress and result in a negative response (Gonzalez et al., 2008). When under stress, Hispanic clients may revert back to using their native language. Hispanic clients also may prefer educators of the same gender.

Family Influence

Family is a highly valued part of Hispanic life, and family involvement is often critical in providing health care to the client. Family matters take precedence over work and all other aspects of life. Hispanic families are large, and respect for parental authority is emphasized. Typical Hispanic families are patriarchal, with the male family members having the dominant role as head of the household. They are the decision makers. Hispanic men typically have a strong sense of machismo. This is an attitude that the man is wiser, smarter, stronger, and more knowledgeable (Zoucha & Zamarripa, 2003). Hispanic women defer to men and have subdued qualities. Mothers may influence family decisions but do not play a dominant role. Any dishonor or shame that may occur for an individual family member is considered a reflection on the entire family. Elderly Hispanics are respected and may live with married children if they are not self-sufficient. Changes in these patterns are seen in more educated clients and families with higher socioeconomic status. Overall change to a more egalitarian family structure is slow to happen.

Many clients live in multifamily arrangements that include extended family who offer social and economic support. The term **familismo** describes the Hispanic belief in family

FIGURE 8-3

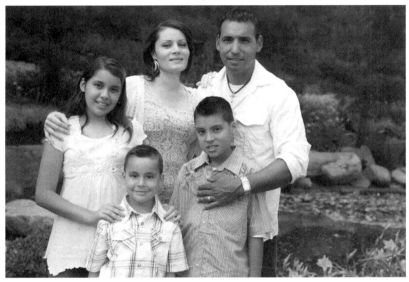

Source: © Feverpitch/ShutterStock, Inc.

interdependence that curtails exposure to outside influences, and that may be a major cause of resistance to change (Gonzalez et al., 2008). An important aspect of Hispanic families is that they are the main source of assistance before seeking out assistance from the community. By including family members, nurses as educators can build greater trust and confidence and in turn increase adherence to teaching plans.

Health Beliefs

Hispanics believe in an external locus of control, which is the belief that outside forces control their lives. For some Hispanics, health is viewed as the result of good luck or a reward from God. Some also believe in the theory of hot and cold imbalances. The basis of this belief is that illness is caused by prolonged exposure to hot or cold. Many of the illnesses are digestive in nature. To ensure good health, both hot and cold foods must be taken into the body. It is important for the nurse to be aware that the use of self-medication with alternative therapies is prevalent in Hispanic culture, and this information is seldom reported to healthcare professionals. The nurse should understand that Hispanics will have more respect for the nurse who accepts the spiritual and folk basis of their health beliefs (Gonzalez et al., 2008). If the teaching plan is incongruent with folk beliefs, the nurse as educator should attempt to find compromises or solutions to resolve the incongruence and allow clients to maintain their belief system while following the plan. Folk healers are part of **curanderismo,** which views illness from a religious and social perspective rather than the Western scientific perspective. Curanderas, santera, and espiritistas are folk healers who are sought out to treat illness and are preferred over the medical community because they are personal, less dehumanizing, know the family, and are an integral part of the Hispanic community (Gonzalez et al., 2008).

Implications for Health Education

Begin with an assessment of the Hispanic client's ability to communicate and understand English. Establishing rapport is an essential part of building a trusting relationship. There should be continuous evaluation of learning by questioning and return demonstration; problem solving should be encouraged. You need to understand the perceived causes for folk-related diseases and show respect for cultural differences, such as amulets that the client might wear to protect from the **evil eye** or evil spirits. Also be aware that some Hispanics feel that medication is always necessary, and many may not believe that their illness is being treated adequately unless medication is ordered (MSH, 2005). Your long-term goal working in the Hispanic community should be to gain an understanding of folk medicine beliefs and try to establish a relationship with the healers in the hope of eliciting acceptance and understanding of the rationale for the teaching plan. You need be aware of the client's cultural health beliefs to have an effect on the client's behavior and recovery. The most common health concerns for Hispanics requiring health education are listed in **Table 8-4**.

American Indian

Cultural Norms

The number of American Indians and Native Alaskans in the United States is 3.9 million, and it is projected to increase by more than half to 6.3 million in 2060. This will increase their share of the population from 1.3% to 1.5%. The Bureau of Indian Affairs recognizes more than 500 different Indian tribes, with the largest number being Cherokee and Navajo (Hanley, 2008). Native Alaskans are divided into five cultural and linguistic groups: Interior Indians, Aleuts, Southeast Coastal Indians, Northern Eskimos, and Southern Eskimos (Davidhizar & DeLapp, 2008). For the purposes of this discussion, American Indians and Native Alaskans are referred to as American Indians.

The first meeting with American Indian clients is considered a time for building rapport and not for carrying out essential work. American Indians may introduce themselves by stating the clan and the location of their home. They often initially appear silent and reserved; quiet voice tones are usually used when speaking. On initial greeting they may extend a hand and

TABLE 8-4

Most Common Disorders Requiring Health Education: Hispanics

Ethnic/Racial Group	*Most Common Disorders Requiring Health Education*
Hispanic	▪ Heart disease ▪ Cancer ▪ Accidents ▪ Stroke ▪ Diabetes ▪ Hypertension ▪ Obesity ▪ HIV/AIDS

FIGURE 8-4

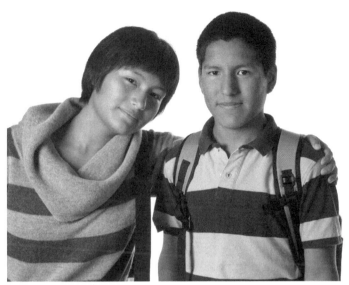

© ZanyZeus/ShutterStock, Inc.

touch the hand of the other person lightly out of respect, but touch is generally reserved for those people that the client knows well. Eye contact is to be avoided, and pointing at another person should not be done because it is considered rude.

Family Influence

Family is very important to American Indian clients and includes all members of the extended family. The primary goal of the family is the development of children and adolescents. They follow the concept of clanship, in which the nuclear family and extended family are in close relationship (Hanley, 2008). Usually a male member of the family is looked upon as the leader; however, all members of the family may be involved in healthcare decisions. A family member may travel long distances to be with an ill family member. Although men are seen as important, grandmothers and mothers are often at the center of many American Indian traditions (Zoucha & Zamarripa, 2003). Elders are a source of cultural information and can provide advice and support to the nurse. The time orientation for many American Indians is focused on the present, which affects how they perceive future events. This may result in difficulties knowing when to take medications and the importance of being on time for appointments. Many American Indians believe that the shared space of the hogan, or round open room, provides spiritual security and a sense of trust (Hanley, 2008). Some clients may not feel comfortable outside their normal surroundings.

Health Beliefs

American Indians believe that wellness is a state of harmony with one's surroundings and with families. Illness results from something that the client has done to cause disharmony. When they are ill, they may seek out the services of a medicine man to find out what is causing disharmony. The different types of medicine men and women include diagnosticians, singers, and herbalists. The use of the healing ceremony is used to return to a harmonious state. The **Blessingway ceremony** attempts to remove ill health by means of stories, songs, rituals, prayers, symbols, and sand paintings (Hanley, 2008). They have jish, or medicine bundles, containing symbolic and sacred items, such as corn pollen, feathers, stones, arrowheads, and other instruments used for healing and blessing (Hanley, 2008). Pain is considered something that must be endured, and clients may not ask for pain medication. An important cultural belief is that American Indians should not touch a dead or dying person because they believe that the spirit of the deceased may contaminate them. They also may avoid discussing the topics of death and dying. They blend traditional beliefs with Western health practices.

Implications for Health Education

It is important to remember that American Indian beliefs depend on clients' personal experiences and the degree of acculturation into U.S. society. If the client uses folk medicine, it is important for you to determine which cultural health practices are beneficial, neutral, or harmful to provide culturally congruent care. When teaching American Indians, you should be aware that they are comfortable with extended periods of silence, so allow them adequate time for information processing. You should use straightforward and easily understood language and clarify misconceptions in a direct manner. The most common health concerns for American Indians requiring health education are listed in **Table 8-5**.

CROSS-CULTURAL COMMUNICATION

Cross-cultural communication factors must be considered when nurses interact with clients and their family members from cultural backgrounds that differ from their own (Andrews, 2012). To be culturally competent, the nurse as educator needs to examine ways in which people from diversified cultural backgrounds communicate. Research has shown that communication

TABLE 8-5

Most Common Disorders Requiring Health Education: Native Americans

Ethnic/Racial Group	*Most Common Disorders Requiring Health Education*
Native American	▪ Heart disease ▪ Cancer ▪ Accidents ▪ Diabetes ▪ Stroke ▪ Alcohol abuse ▪ Hepatitis ▪ Obesity ▪ Sudden infant death syndrome (SIDS)

between healthcare professionals and clients is linked to client satisfaction, adherence to medical instructions, and health outcomes (Stewart et al., 1999). This discussion on cross-cultural communication focuses on verbal and nonverbal communication, focused communication tools, and the use of interpreters. These factors are reviewed for the four major cultural groups: African American, Asian, Hispanic, and American Indian.

Verbal Communication

Some African American clients speak in what is called African American English. This dialect, a mixture of English, Creole, and West African languages, is sometimes misinterpreted as uneducated but is actually a way to share unique cultural ideas and symbolize racial pride and identity (Campinha-Bacote, 2003). You may have to seek clarification if words are not understood. The volume of African American voices is sometimes louder than those of other cultures, but this should not be interpreted as anger or aggression.

A hallmark of Asian communication is to think before speaking and to be polite. When working with Asian clients, you may find that they respond with "yes" to a question as a way of being polite or avoiding conflict, even when they do not understand the question (Hoang & Erickson, 1985). Also, some Asian clients may feel uncomfortable about giving and receiving compliments or saying "thank you." Their communication style is based on a cultural tradition that emphasizes self-humility in social situations. An interpreter may be needed to communicate with Asian clients.

For Hispanics in the United States, an inability to speak and understand English can be a serious complication to receiving healthcare services. Most Hispanics speak some English, but many continue to speak Spanish at home with family. Communication may be complicated by the fact that Hispanics often learn a mixture of English and Spanish, which makes it difficult for you to understand. An interpreter may be required to facilitate communication. Hispanic clients expect that nurses will give direct eye contact when interacting with them, but they do not reciprocate with direct eye contact. When looking at or admiring a Hispanic child, it is important to touch the child to avoid giving the child the "evil eye" (Gonzalez et al., 2008).

Communication with American Indian clients may require you to use interpreters because many still speak native tribal languages. Another complicating factor when developing teaching plans is that many of the native languages do not have equivalent single words in the English language, which makes understanding difficult. American Indians consider silence essential to understanding and may pause after questions to carefully consider the answer.

Nonverbal Communication

African American clients are generally more comfortable with touch and a close personal space. You will see more demonstrative facial expression and use of animated gestures when talking. Using humor is acceptable with African Americans and can be a way to release feelings and reduce stress. Asian clients often will be serene and stoic, suppressing negative emotion. Asians consider the head sacred, so it is not polite to pat the head (Giger & Davidhizar, 2008). Be aware that the lack of facial expression of Asian clients or a low level of verbal communication may not indicate a lack of emotion or opinion. It is important to determine Asian clients' true feelings or opinions before deciding what they think. Hispanic clients are often tactile in their relationships and show affection for each other. They may appear agreeable on the surface to avoid confrontation, especially during health education. Dramatic body language is used when Hispanic clients describe emotional problems (Gonzalez et al., 2008). If a disagreement develops, Hispanic clients may become silent and not adhere to the teaching plan. American Indian clients prefer listening to speaking and rarely practice small talk except among close acquaintances. In social situations when they are angry or uncomfortable, American Indians may remain silent. Often they will avoid eye contact and may look at the floor while you are talking as a way of showing they are listening intently.

Focused Cultural Assessment Tools

A thorough cultural assessment helps you as the educator to develop a teaching plan that, if possible, should be done in advance of the teaching session. Specific assessment tools for an in-depth cultural assessment were described earlier in the chapter and can be selected based on client needs. Often, however, a client presents with a specific problem that needs immediate attention. In this situation it is important to first assess how the client views current health problems and what care he or she believes is needed to resolve it. Kleinman (1980) developed the following list of questions that you can use to better gain insight into the client's perception of his or her illness:

1. What do you call your problem (sickness)? What name does it have?
2. What do you think caused your sickness?
3. Why do you think it started when it did?
4. What does your sickness do to you? How does it work?
5. How severe is it? Do you think it will last a short time or a long time?
6. What do you fear most about your sickness?
7. What are the chief problems that your sickness has caused for you?
8. What kind of treatment do you think you should receive? What are the most important results you hope to receive from the treatment?

When you have an understanding of the client's perception of the health problem, there may be a need to negotiate the plan of care. The LEARN model is a framework for creating new health patterns through effective listening, education, and negotiation (Berlin & Fowkes, 1983). When using this framework for health education, you should first attempt to understand, then to be understood, and finally to negotiate a teaching plan that fits the client's cultural framework. Negotiation includes a preserve–accommodate–restructure approach (DeRosa & Kochurka, 2006). You should preserve cultural practices that help the client achieve his or her health goals and accommodate neutral cultural practices that neither help nor hinder the client. Negotiation is called for in restructuring harmful cultural practices that might risk or impair the client's health. This approach of honoring cultural values and practices helps the client feel respected and comfortable, and it is more likely that they will adhere to the treatment plan.

L: Listen with sympathy and understanding to the patient's perception of the problem.
E: Explain your perceptions of the problem.
A: Acknowledge and discuss the differences and similarities.
R: Recommend treatment.
N: Negotiate agreement.

Use of Interpreters

Interviewing non-English-speaking clients requires a bilingual interpreter for full communication. This requirement is in line with The Joint Commission standard RI.01.01.03 that states, "The hospital respects the patient's right to receive information in a manner in which he or she understands" (The Joint Commission, 2014). Even a person who has basic English skills may need the services of an interpreter when placed in teaching situations that require give and take. Whenever possible, use a bilingual team member or trained medical interpreter. The interpreter should possess a high level of fluency and a strong sense of ethics. Family members, children, or friends are not good choices for interpreting. Using them violates confidentiality, plus they are not trained to understand medical terminology. A professional interpreter has the special skills needed to fully understand what the nurse and client want to say and to make messages clear in two languages. In addition, a qualified interpreter knows the role, limitations, and responsibilities of an interpreter.

If possible, the interpreter should meet the client ahead of time to build rapport. Arrangements should be made in advance because the teaching session will take more time. Prepare ahead of time and focus on the major teaching points and prioritize information. During the session, the nurse, client, and interpreter should sit so they form the points of a triangle. The nurse should look at the client when speaking. Two different interpretive styles are possible in the teaching session: line by line and summarization. The line-by-line approach ensures accuracy but takes more time. Information needs to be presented on a concrete level because abstract conceptualizations do not readily translate and may confuse the client (Putch, 1985). The nurse must choose words carefully and use gestures sparingly. A normal tone of voice should be used, not too fast or too loud. The nurse and client should say only a sentence or two so the interpreter will have time to interpret. Simple language, without medical jargon, should be used. Summary translation is faster and works well when teaching simple procedures with which the translator is already familiar. The interpreter summarizes the points that the nurse wants to teach. The interpreter and the nurse observe the nonverbal messages throughout the teaching session. At the end it is important to ask the client to confirm understanding of what was taught.

The use of on-site medical interpreters or translators is only one way that language access services may be available to nurses. There are also telephone interpreter services, video medical interpreting services, translation software for written materials, bilingual clinical staff, and language classes for staff.

LINGUISTICALLY AND CULTURALLY APPROPRIATE TEACHING STRATEGIES AND INSTRUCTIONAL MATERIALS

Linguistic competence is the capacity of an organization and its personnel to communicate effectively and convey information in a manner that is easily understood by diverse audiences, including persons with limited English proficiency, those who are not literate or have low health literacy skills, and individuals with disabilities (Goode & Jones, 2006). To address cultural linguistic competence, the National Standards on Culturally and Linguistically Appropriate Services Standards (CLAS) were developed by the U.S. Department of Health and Human Services Office of Minority Health (2001) to ensure that all people entering the healthcare system receive equitable and effective treatment in a culturally and linguistically appropriate manner. Standard 6 mandates that healthcare organizations must provide competent language assistance from interpreters and bilingual staff to clients with limited English proficiency. The standards are intended to be inclusive of all cultures, not limited to any particular population group. They are designed to address the needs of racial, ethnic, and linguistic population groups that experience unequal access to healthcare services. These standards serve as guidelines for nurses and can be accessed online through the Office of Minority Health.

The Patient Protection and Affordable Care Act (2010), Title V, defines health literacy as "the degree to which an individual has the capacity to obtain, communicate, process, and understand basic health information and services to make appropriate health decisions" (This is similar to the definition provided by Healthy People 2010 (2009). Research shows that health literacy is the single best predictor of client health status (Campinha-Bacote, 2008). Low health literacy affects older people, immigrants, impoverished people, and minorities. It is often brought about by inadequate communication between clients and nurses. Clients frequently attempt to hide their inability to read, and the nurse cannot judge literacy level solely by a client's years of education. Clients with low reading ability and comprehension skills may not be able to express what is not understood and therefore may choose to conceal their low literacy skills (Maurer & Smith, 2004). Ways to assist clients with low health literacy include limiting the amount of medical jargon, using pictures or models to explain important health concepts, assuring understanding with demonstration techniques, and encouraging clients to ask questions. Goode, Brown, Mason, and Sockalingam (2006) identified six principles to create culturally competent health materials that should be considered when choosing, adapting, or creating health-promoting instructional aids:

1. Acknowledge the unique issues of biculturalism and bilingual status of both healthcare providers and service populations.
2. Incorporate client preferences in choosing instructional materials. Health messages should demonstrate respect for client uniqueness and cultural differences.
3. Involve members of the target population in the creation of instructional materials.
4. Use the family as the focal point of intervention when developing health messages.
5. Base health education and promotion on cultural aspects of epidemiology (concepts of causation and cure).
6. Education and promotion should exist in concert with natural and informal healthcare and support systems within the community.

Culturally appropriate teaching strategies and instructional materials are necessary when the client's culture dictates how a problem should be addressed. These teaching strategies and instructional materials include the following:

▪ Use a variety of teaching strategies and instructional materials that are specific to the culture and language. This includes written materials (posters, brochures, etc.), short films, computer-assisted instruction, group teaching, and websites.
▪ Consider clients' cultures and language skills when developing learning objectives, teaching strategies, and instructional materials.
▪ Facilitate comparable learning opportunities for clients with differing characteristics and learning styles. For example, consider learning opportunities for clients who differ in race, sex, disability, ethnicity, religion, socioeconomic status, and ability.

- Incorporate learning objectives for personal development based on cultural beliefs, and clearly communicate the learning objectives.
- Use concrete terms, choose words that do not have multiple meanings, and avoid medical jargon and slang.
- Give clients an overview of the teaching plan and tell them about the learning objectives. Relate the plan to previous learning, and summarize the main points.
- Provide frequent review of the content learned.
- Facilitate independence in thinking and action by helping clients find answers themselves.
- Promote on-task behavior by keeping clients actively involved.
- Check with clients during the teaching session to see if they have any questions about what they are doing and if they understand the content.
- Provide frequent feedback and reinforcement.

DeRosa and Kochurka (2006) developed a six-step approach to providing culturally competent care, which we have adapted for nurses to provide culturally congruent health education.

Stoeckel Culturally Congruent Client Education Model

The increasingly multicultural profile of the U.S. population requires that nurses provide culturally congruent care. Providing culturally congruent client education has the potential to improve health outcomes, increase the efficiency of healthcare professionals, and result in greater client satisfaction with services (Brach & Fraser, 2000). The Stoeckel Culturally Congruent Client Education Model brings together the concepts presented in this chapter to summarize the essential framework of what it means to provide culturally congruent client education.

BOX 8-1

Evidence-Based Nursing Practice

Collins, C.A., Decker, S.J. & Esquibel, K.A. (2006) Definitions of health: Comparison of Hispanic and African-American elders. *The Journal of Multicultural Nursing & Health, 12*(1), 14–19.

Purpose: This study described the definitions of health among Hispanic and African American elders.

Method: The study used a qualitative framework in a doctoral-level multicultural nursing course. Quasi-statistics and a semistructured interview format were used to tabulate the frequency of themes. A convenience sample of Hispanic and African American clients at senior citizen centers was used. Data were gathered throughout the class and were shared with the class, which was a limitation of this study.

Results: The participants shared some differences, but more similarities, in their definitions. Eight reoccurring themes were identified: spirituality, without pain/feeling good, positive attitude with good mentality, high priority, independent/active, health promotion/maintenance, socialization, and helping others. The findings of the study were consistent with the literature and emphasized the importance of avoiding stereotyping individuals from any cultural background.

FIGURE 8-5

The Stoeckel Culturally Congruent Client Education Model

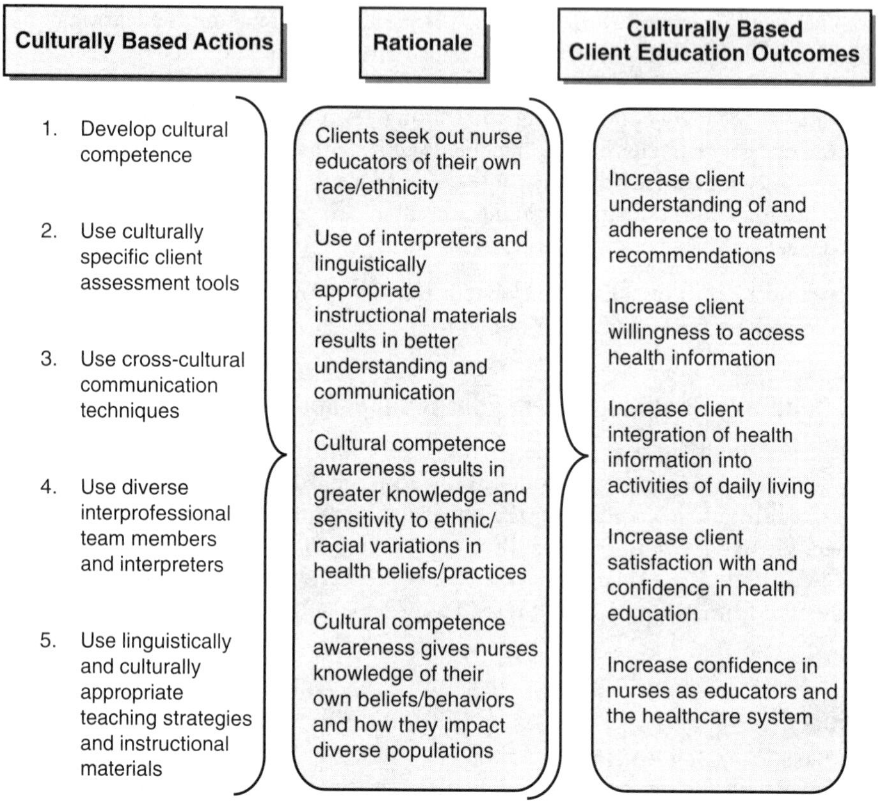

The three major components of the model are culturally based actions, rationales, and culturally based client education outcomes (**Figure 8-5**).

Culturally Based Actions

The culturally based actions in this model begin with developing cultural competence. This chapter provides Campinha-Bacote's cultural competence model that identified the steps in the process of becoming culturally competent: cultural desire, cultural awareness, cultural knowledge, cultural skill, and cultural encounters.

The second culturally based action is using culturally specific client assessment tools to develop individualized teaching plans. This chapter presented in-depth assessment tools by a variety of authors and a focused assessment option to gather client information. The nurse chooses the cultural assessment tool that is appropriate for the situation.

The third culturally based action is using knowledge of cross-cultural communication techniques to interact with clients in developing teaching plans. A preserve–accommodate–restructure approach (DeRosa & Kochurka, 2006) is taken in working with clients so that cultural practices are preserved, except for those that hinder the client's health. The LEARN technique—L: listen, E: explain, A: acknowledge, R: recommend, N: negotiate—is an example of cross-cultural communication (Berlin & Fowkes, 1983). It is a negotiation framework that supports a cross-cultural approach to client communication.

The fourth culturally based action is to use diverse interprofessional team members and interpreters that reflect the client's culture. Diverse clients are more likely to access and use healthcare services when they encounter health professionals of their own race and ethnicity (Purnell, 2013). The correct use of interpreters or bilingual team members is an important culturally based action that allows for cultural congruency. A lack of interpreter services is a significant factor associated with client dissatisfaction and poor comprehension.

The fifth culturally based action is using linguistically and culturally appropriate teaching strategies and instructional materials to enhance and support learning. This action involves providing culturally appropriate oral and written language services to clients with limited proficiency. This action increases client adherence to treatment and improves the quality of health education.

Rationales

Nurses as educators gain knowledge through developing cultural competence, which includes becoming aware of their own beliefs and behaviors as well as those of clients. The use of assessment tools facilitates gathering clients' cultural data that can be used to build individualized teaching plans. When possible, nurses of the clients' race or ethnicity should be involved in teaching clients. A goal for the future is to increase the number of culturally diverse nurses to meet this need. The use of interprofessional team members, interpreters, and linguistically appropriate instructional materials results in better understanding, adherence to treatment plans, and improved cross-cultural communication.

Culturally Based Client Education Outcomes

Culturally based actions result in meeting the needs of diverse populations. The desired culturally based client education outcomes meet the needs of diverse populations by increasing client understanding of treatment and adherence to treatment recommendations. When nurses take the recommended culturally based actions, clients are more willing to access health information. This increases their satisfaction with health education and increases their confidence in nurses as educators. These outcomes result in clients who are better able to integrate health teaching into their activities of daily living.

SUMMARY

This chapter looked at the importance of cultural competence for nurses who provide health education. Changing demographics and disparities in health care are powerful reasons that require nurses to become culturally competent. Becoming culturally competent is a developmental process and involves self-awareness and insight into the workings of other cultures. To provide meaningful health education, it is important for nurses to adapt the Stoeckel Culturally Congruent Client Education Model, which looks at culturally based actions, their rationales, and outcomes.

EXERCISES

Exercise I: Health Beliefs and Home Remedies

Purpose: Examine the health beliefs of various cultural, ethnic, and racial groups.
Directions:

1. Divide into small groups composed of individuals who are most culturally, ethnically, and racially alike.
2. Discuss how your parents and grandparents (1) defined good health and poor health, and (2) list the home remedies they used to treat individuals in poor health.
3. Share your findings with the entire class. How were your findings similar and dissimilar?
4. What did you learn about individuals who are supposedly alike?

Exercise II: Health Beliefs and Home Remedies

Purpose: Examine the health beliefs of various cultural, ethnic, and racial groups.
Directions:

1. Divide into small groups composed of individuals who are most culturally, ethnically, and racially dissimilar.
2. Compare and contrast the findings discovered in Exercise I. How were the beliefs about good health and poor health alike and different?
3. Compare and contrast the various home remedies identified in Exercise I. How were the home remedies across the cultural, ethnic, and racial groups alike and different?
4. Share your findings with the entire class.

Exercise III: Cultural Reflection

Purpose: Reflect on the health education needs of various cultural, ethnic, and racial groups.
Directions:

1. Individually reflect on the new knowledge you gained from participating in Exercises I and II. What are the implications for health education? How will this impact you in your role as an educator? Take about 15 minutes for reflection.
2. As a group, share your thoughts and conclusions with others in your class. Did others have similar thoughts and conclusions?
3. Using the Campinha-Bacote mnemonic, ASKED, described in this chapter, discuss how this exercise made you more culturally competent.

REFERENCES

American Nurses Association. (2001). *Code for nurses.* Washington, DC: Author.

Anderson, L. M., Scrimshaw, S. C., Fullilove, M. T., Fielding, J. E., & Normand, J. (2003). Task Force on Community Preventive Services. Culturally competent healthcare systems: A systematic review [Suppl. 1]. *American Journal of Preventive Medicine, 24*(3), 68–79.

Andrews, M. M. (2012). Culturally competent nursing care. In M. M. Andrews & J. S. Boyle (Eds.), *Trans-cultural concepts in nursing care* (6th ed., pp. viii–xiii). Philadelphia, PA: Wolters Kluwer/Lippincott Williams & Wilkins.

Andrews, M. M., & Boyle, J. S. (2012). Andrews/Boyle transcultural nursing assessment guide for individuals and families. In M. M. Andrews & J. S. Boyle (Eds.), *Transcultural concepts in nursing care* (6th ed., pp. 451–455). Philadelphia, PA: Wolters Kluwer/Lippincott Williams & Wilkins.

Beach, M. T., Sugarman, J., Johnson, R., Arbelaez, J. J., Duggan, P. S., & Cooper, L. A. (2005). Higher satisfaction, adherence, and receipt of preventive care? *Annals of Family Medicine, 3*(4), 331–338.

Berlin, E. A., & Fowkes, W. C., Jr. (1983). A teaching framework for cross-cultural health care. *Western Journal of Medicine, 139,* 934–938.

Blue, A. (2012). The provision of culturally competent health care. Retrieved from http://academicdepartments.musc.edu/fm_ruralclerkship/curriculum/culture.htm

Brach, C., & Fraser, I. (2000). Can cultural competency reduce racial and ethnic disparities? A review and conceptual model. *Medical Care Research and Review, 57*(1), 181–217.

Burchum, J. L. R. (2002). Cultural competence: An evolutionary perspective. *Nursing Forum, 37*(4), 5–15.

Campinha-Bacote, J. (1998). *The process of cultural competence in the delivery of healthcare services: A culturally competent model of care* (3rd ed.). Cincinnati, OH: Transcultural C.A.R.E. Associates.

Campinha-Bacote, J. (2002). The process of cultural competence in the delivery of healthcare services: A model of care. *Journal of Transcultural Nursing, 13*(3), 181–184.

Campinha-Bacote, J. (2003). Many faces: Addressing diversity in health care. *Online Journal of Issues in Nursing, 8*(1), Manuscript 2.

Campinha-Bacote, J. (2008). People of African American heritage. In L. D. Purnell & B. J. Paulanka (Eds.), *Transcultural health care* (3rd ed., pp. 56–74). Philadelphia, PA: F. A. Davis.

Campinha-Bacote, J., & Narayan, M. (2000). Culturally competent health care in the home. *Home Care Provider, 5*(6), 213–219.

Cherry, B., & Giger, J. N. (2008). African-Americans. In J. N. Giger & R. E. Davidhizar (Eds.), *Transcultural nursing: Assessment and intervention* (5th ed., pp. 190–238). St. Louis, MO: Mosby Elsevier.

Collins, C. A., Decker, S. J., & Esquibel, K. A. (2006). Definitions of health: Comparison of Hispanic and African-American elders. *The Journal of Multicultural Nursing & Health, 12*(1), 14–19.

Cross, T., Bazron, B., Dennis, K., & Isaacs, M. (1989). *Towards a culturally competent system of care: A monograph on effective services for minority children who are severely emotionally disturbed: Volume I.* Washington, DC: Georgetown University Child Development Center.

Culhane-Pera, K. A., Reif, C., Egli, E., Bake, N. J., & Kassekert, R. (1997). A curriculum for multicultural education in family medicine. *Family Medicine, 29*(10), 719–723.

Davidhizar, R. E., & DeLapp, T. D. (2008). American Eskimos: The Yup'ik and Inupiat. In J. N. Giger & R. E. Davidhizar (Eds.), *Transcultural nursing: Assessment and intervention* (5th ed., pp. 323–356). St. Louis, MO: Mosby Elsevier.

DeRosa, N., & Kochurka, K. (2006). Implement culturally competent healthcare in your workplace. *Nursing Management, 37*(10), 18–26.

Falvo, D. R. (2011). *Effective patient education: A guide to increased adherence* (4th ed.). Sudbury, MA: Jones & Bartlett Learning.

Flowers, D. L. (2009). Culturally competent nursing care a challenge for the 21st century. *Critical Care Nurse, 24*(4), 48–52.

Giger, J. N., & Davidhizar, R. E. (2008). *Transcultural nursing: Assessment and intervention* (4th ed.). St. Louis, MO: Mosby Elsevier.

Gonzalez, E. W., Owen, D. C., & Esperat, C. R. (2008). Mexican Americans. In J. N. Giger & R. E. Davidhizar (Eds.), *Transcultural nursing: Assessment and intervention* (5th ed., pp. 239–275). St. Louis, MO: Mosby Elsevier.

Goode, T., Brown, M., Mason, J., & Sockalingam, S. (2006). A guide for using the cultural and linguistic competence policy assessment instrument. Washington, DC: National Center for Cultural Competence, Georgetown University Center for Child and HumanDevelopment. Retrieved from http://www.clcpa.info

Goode, T., & Jones, W. (2006). *Definition of linguistic competence.* Washington, DC: National Center for Cultural Competence, Georgetown University Center for Child and Human Development.Hanley, C. E. (2008). Navajos. In J. N. Giger & R. E. Davidhizar (Eds.), *Transcultural nursing: Assessment and intervention* (5th ed., pp. 276–299). St. Louis, MO: Mosby Elsevier.

Harvard Medical School. (2009). Culturally competent care online resource center. Retrieved from http://medweb.med.harvard.edu/cccec/about/index.htm

Healthy People 2010. (2009). Health communications. (Definition of health literacy.) Retrieved from http://www.healthypeople.gov/document/html/volume1/11healthcom.htm#_Toc490471359

Hoang, G. N., & Erickson, R. V. (1985). Cultural barriers to effective medical care among Indochinese patients. *Annual Review of Medicine, 36*(2), 229–239.

Institute of Medicine. (2002). *Unequal treatment: Confronting racial and ethnic disparities in health care.* Washington, DC: National Academies Press.

Kaiser Family Foundation. (2001). Generation Rx.com: How young people use the Internet for health information. Retrieved from www.kff.org/entmedia/20011211a-index.cfm

Kleinman, A. (1980). *Patients and healers in the context of culture.* Berkeley, CA: University of California Press.

Leininger, M. (1991). *Culture care diversity and universality: A theory of nursing.* New York, NY: National League for Nursing.

Management Sciences for Health. (2005). Introduction to cultural competence. Retrieved from http://erc.msh.org/aapi/cc1.html

Maurer, F., & Smith, C. (2004). *Community/public health nursing practice: Health for families and populations.* St. Louis, MO: Elsevier Health Sciences.

Patient Protection and Affordable Care Act. (2010). Retrieved from http://www.gpo.gov/fdsys/pkg/BILLS-111hr3590enr/pdf/BILLS-111hr3590enr.pdf

Purnell, L. D. (2013). *Transcultural health care: A culturally competent approach* (4th ed.). Philadelphia, PA: F. A. Davis.

Putch, R. W. (1985). Cross-cultural communication: The special case of interpreters in health care. *Journal of the American Medical Association, 254*(23), 3344–3348.

Schim, S. M., Doorenbos, A., Benkert, R., & Miller, J. (2007). Culturally congruent care: Putting the puzzle together. *Journal of Transcultural Nursing, 18*(2), 103–110.

Smith, W. R., Betancourt, J. R., Wynia, M. K., Bussey-Jones, J., Stone, V. E., Phillips, C. O., . . . Bowles, J. (2007). Position paper: Recommendations for teaching about racial and ethnic disparities in health and health care. *Annals of Internal Medicine, 147*(9), 654–665.

Stewart, M., Brown, J. B., Boon, H., Galajda, J., Meredith, L., & Sangster, M. (1999). Evidence on patient–doctor communication. *Cancer Prevention and Control, 3*(1), 25–30.

The Joint Commission. (2014). Hospitals (CAMH). Retrieved from http://www.jointcommission.org/standards_information/hap_requirements.aspx

U.S. Census Bureau. (2012). U.S. Census Bureau projections show a slower growing, older, more diverse nation a half century from now. Retrieved from http://www.census.gov/newsroom/releases/archives/population/cb12-243.html

U.S. Department of Health and Human Services. (2010). *Healthy People 2020.* Washington, DC: Author

U.S. Department of Health and Human Services, Office of Minority Health. (2001).

Yee, B., Mokuau, N., & Kim, S. (Eds.). (1999). *Developing cultural competence in Asian and Pacific Islander communities: Opportunities in primary health care and substance abuse prevention* (Publication No. SMA 98-3193). Washington, DC: U.S. Department of Health and Human Services.

Zoucha, R., & Zamarripa, C. A. (2003). People of Mexican heritage. In L. D. Purnell & B. J. Paulanka (Eds.), *Transcultural health care* (3rd ed., pp. 309–324). Philadelphia, PA: F. A. Davis.

IV

Planning and Implementing Health Education

9

Learning Objectives

INTRODUCTION

In this chapter we illustrate the steps of developing a teaching plan and show its progression in subsequent chapters. Developing a teaching plan helps you see the totality of the approach to client education and keeps you on track in carrying out the plan. The teaching plan has four sections: (1) learning objectives, (2) teaching content, (3) teaching strategies and instructional materials, and (4) evaluation. To optimize learning as you move through the chapter, we suggest you identify a client for whom you wish to provide health education and begin to develop a teaching plan that is appropriate for that client. In this chapter we address the first step of the teaching plan, which is to write learning objectives.

LEARNING OBJECTIVES DEFINED

Objectives provide direction and indicate the desired end point of an effort or activity (Webster's, 2013). In health education, objectives for learning are essential to providing a framework around which the nurse as educator builds the teaching plan. Objectives clarify what you intend to teach and what the client is to learn.

The words *goal* and *objective* are often used interchangeably, but *goal* has a broader meaning than *objective*. **Goals** are statements that refer to the overarching learning outcomes to be achieved over a period of time. They are the general intentions or aims for what is to be learned. Objectives are included under goals and are more focused, yet they are consistent with the goals. They address specific behaviors to be learned. Objectives are precise, measurable, and obtainable statements describing what will be learned and who will do what, when, and how.

Objectives must be met before the goal can be achieved (Bastable & Doody, 2008). An example of a goal for an obese client is to learn weight management, whereas objectives would focus on specific behaviors to bring about that goal. Three examples of **learning objectives** related to weight management include the following:

- The client will demonstrate how to correctly weigh herself at the conclusion of the teaching session without assistance from the nurse.
- After completing the learning module, the client will correctly identify three healthy foods from a list of foods provided by the nurse.
- Upon completion of the course, the client will make the association between physical activity and weight control from memory in a personal written reflection.

Clearly stated goals and learning objectives give direction to both the learner and the nurse as educator. They keep the teaching and learning process on track to achieve the desired learning outcomes. The main purpose for establishing learning objectives is to focus the instruction and guide the planning, implementation, and evaluation of the desired learning. Evaluating learning objectives reveals client learning and the educator's effectiveness in the teaching and learning process. **Figure 9-1** illustrates the critical role of clearly stated learning objectives in developing the teaching plan.

In the education literature objectives are referred to as behavioral objectives, instructional objectives, and learning objectives. We prefer *learning objectives* and use that term in this chapter to develop the teaching plan.

FIGURE 9-1

Learning Objectives as the Basis for the Teaching Plan

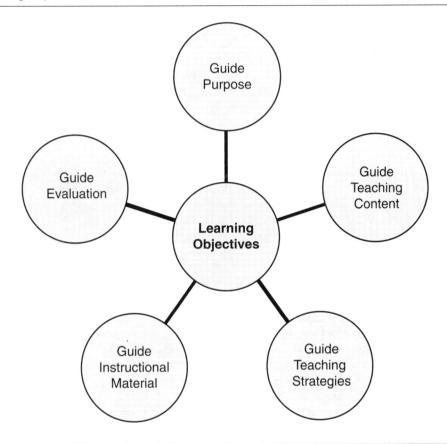

FACTORS TO CONSIDER BEFORE WRITING LEARNING OBJECTIVES

Before writing learning objectives you need to take into account five factors that affect your approach. The first factor is to consider your educational philosophy, the educational philosophy of the client's healthcare provider, and beliefs about education held by the institution at which you work. Recall that hospitals are required by The Joint Commission to provide health education. Clinics may also have educational protocols to follow. Questions to ask include the following: What does the client's healthcare provider believe about the role and purpose of health education? What and how much does the client's provider want you to teach and the client to know? Does the healthcare institution have a statement of philosophy and policies regarding health education? Does it have health education guidelines from accrediting bodies? Is there an established curriculum? What are your beliefs about the type and extent of information that clients should receive about their diagnoses, treatment regimens, and alternative therapies? Knowing who determines what clients should be taught and knowing the institution's health education policies are important when you work in a team to meet the client's needs.

A second factor is to identify what clients want to learn. Ask the client what his or her expectations are and plan to collaborate in writing the learning objectives. Find out the client's learning goals so the objectives will be relevant. Engaging the learner helps the client to be motivated and attentive.

A third factor is to assess what you think clients need to learn. It is important to assess clients' level of knowledge so that new learning relates to what they already know. If you are teaching to health team members, gather information from the literature and from other sources that can inform you of learning needs. Part of your assessment should include consideration of the client's developmental, emotional, and experiential readiness because these factors influence one's ability to grasp information. An example of using these factors in writing objectives is that clients who are in denial are less likely to benefit from teaching than those who are willing to face their health challenges. Another example is if a client cannot read, you will need to choose learning objectives that do not depend on reading ability. The objectives should be appropriate to the abilities of the learner. For example, young clients should not be expected to acquire knowledge or perform skills that are beyond their developmental level. A client paralyzed from a cerebral vascular accident (stroke) should not be expected to engage in tasks requiring muscular control that he or she is incapable of performing.

A fourth factor when establishing learning objectives is the time available for teaching and learning. Nurses and clients are busy, so you need to identify time constraints and make the best use of the time available. This may involve collaborating with colleagues who could teach at other times or after discharge. It may also mean that you consider a different method of delivering your message, such as in online format. Some health information takes time to learn, which may mean establishing priorities, selecting intermediate objectives, and making arrangements to provide for continuity of teaching. This includes communicating clearly to colleagues how far the client has progressed in learning and what remains to be taught and learned.

A fifth and final factor affecting the establishment of learning objectives is the environment in which the learning will take place. This includes the physical environment and the psychological atmosphere. The nurse as educator should take into consideration that some students may be in a virtual environment and others may be in a face-to-face environment. Before you write learning objectives, consider the environment:

▪ What is the physical environment like? Is it conducive to learning?
▪ Is functional audiovisual equipment and Internet connectivity available?
▪ Are instructional materials available and functioning appropriately?
▪ Is the learning atmosphere unhurried and structured properly for learning?
▪ Is there sufficient space? Is the space comfortable? Is the online environment well designed and user friendly?
▪ Is there a nonthreatening atmosphere in which clients feel free to learn?

WRITING LEARNING OBJECTIVES

After you identify what you wish clients to learn, the next step is drafting text that clearly and specifically tells them what they can expect to learn. Learning objectives are composed of four parts adapted from Mager (1997), who is credited as being the first person to focus the educational community on learning objectives. The parts are distinguished as the ABCD approach to writing learning objectives:

- *Audience* (who the learner is)
- *Behavior* (what the learner is to do)
- *Conditions* (the conditions under which the learner is to perform)
- *Degree* (how well the learner is to perform)

A summary of the parts of the ABCD approach to writing learning objectives is shown in **Table 9-1**. The bold text indicates the addition of each part of the learning objective writing process.

Before we explain the ABCD approach to writing learning objectives, there are two general guidelines to be aware of (Mager, 1997):

- Objectives should be written from the perspective of the learner, not the teacher.
  - *Correct*: Describe how a pacemaker affects the heart rate.
  - *Incorrect*: Teach how a pacemaker affects the heart rate.
- Objectives should focus on a learning outcome, not the process for achieving the outcome.
  - *Correct*: Count the pulse rate for 1 minute.
  - *Incorrect*: Learn how to obtain the pulse rate for 1 minute.

Audience

The first step in the ABCD approach to writing learning objectives is to identify the *Audience* or the person to whom the objective is directed. This part of the learning objective describes who

TABLE 9-1

The ABCD Approach to Writing Learning Objectives

Objective part	Description	Example
Audience	To whom is the objective applied?	**The client will**
Behavior	What will the client do? What is the action verb? What learning domain is addressed?	The client will **create a time line of the main events that occur with hypoglycemia.**
Conditions	How will the action be accomplished? What specifics about the situation must be met?	The client will create a time line of the main events that occur with hypoglycemia **by drawing a diagram of the process using a list of items provided by the teacher.**
Degree	Describe the minimum criteria for acceptable student performance. ■ How often? ■ How well? ■ How many? ■ How much? Define expectations regarding accuracy, quality, and speed.	The client will create a time line of the main events that occur with hypoglycemia by drawing a diagram of the process using a list of items provided by the teacher **showing the order that the events normally occur.**

the learner is. For example, the audience may be a student, a learner, or a diabetic patient. In our case, the learner is a client, so the objective begins with "The client will."

Behavior

The second step in writing learning objectives is to clearly state the *Behavior* that the client will do and how he or she will demonstrate the knowledge, attitude, or skill you are attempting to teach. Behavior is about the activity in which the client is to engage. The activity can be visible (such as writing or doing) or invisible (such as adding or solving); however, the results are visible or audible.

Behavior is best described through action verbs that have few interpretations. Avoid using ambiguous verbs such as *learn* or *know*, and avoid verbs that express the nurse's view, such as *inform* or *teach*. Appropriate action verbs convey the learner's perspective and state precisely what the client will do following instruction. Examples of poorly and clearly stated objectives are shown in **Table 9-2**.

Table 9-3 provides a sample list of verbs that have few interpretations and vague verbs that have many interpretations (Gronlund & Brookhart, 2009).

Domains of Learning

Verbs are categorized by the domains of learning and hierarchies within the domains. Bloom, Englehart, Furst, Hill, and Krathwohl (1956) were pioneers in categorizing the domains and levels. They classified various academic achievements according to educational outcomes and called the classification system the Taxonomy of Learning Objectives (Anderson et al., 2001). The domains of learning help make clear what is expected of different levels of intellectual behavior. By writing learning objectives, nurses as educators take an active role in health education. As health education becomes an increasingly large part of health and illness care, nurses must be knowledgeable about how to structure, write, and evaluate learning objectives. Learning objectives may be written in all three domains. The three domains of learning are as follows:

TABLE 9-2

Poorly and Clearly Stated Objectives

Poorly Stated Objectives	*Clearly Stated Objectives*
The client will *know* the symptoms of diabetes.	The client will *verbally state* the three signs and symptoms of hyperglycemia and state why they occur to the nurse.
The client will *understand* the distinction between hypoglycemia and hyperglycemia.	The client will *correctly identify the signs and symptoms* of hypoglycemia from a list on a written exam.
The client will *know how* to test his or her blood sugar.	The client will *demonstrate the proper use of* a glucometer to test his or her blood sugar to the nurse during a home visit.

TABLE 9-3

Verbs with Few and Many Interpretations

Verbs with Few Interpretations	Verbs with Many Interpretations
Apply	Appreciate
Compare	Be familiar with
Construct	Be interested in
Contrast	Believe
Define	Enjoy
Demonstrate	Feel
Describe	Grasp the significance of
Explain	Have faith in
Identify	Internalize
List	Know
Order	Learn
Recall	*Really* understand
Recite	Think
Recognize	Understand
Select	
Solve	
State	
Verbalize	
Write	

- ▪ **Cognitive** domain, which emphasizes thinking
- ▪ **Affective** domain, which emphasizes attitudes and feelings
- ▪ **Psychomotor** domain, which emphasizes doing and performing skills

It is important to choose the correct verb to illustrate the domain for which you are writing objectives. In writing learning objectives, you will soon realize that many behaviors do not fall exclusively in one of the three domains. Learners learn as an integrated whole; however, you must isolate the particular behavior of concern. For example, irrigating a colostomy is not only a psychomotor activity; it also requires cognition and an affective response. Thus, learning objectives may involve more than one domain.

Cognitive Domain

We now examine the domains of learning by looking first at the cognitive domain. The cognitive domain is concerned with knowledge, beliefs, and reasoning. Bloom initially divided the cognitive domain into six levels or hierarchies: knowledge, comprehension, application, analysis, synthesis, and evaluation. During the 1990s the **taxonomy** was updated. The changes

FIGURE 9-2

Hierarchy of the Cognitive Domain

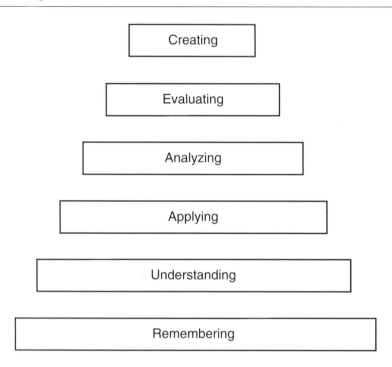

included renaming the six categories, changing the categories from noun to verb form, and rearranging the categories. This new taxonomy reflects a more active form of thinking that is evident in 21st century learning. The new cognitive levels are remembering, understanding, applying, analyzing, evaluating, and creating (Anderson et al., 2001) (**Figure 9-2**).

The six categories are examined in further detail in **Table 9-4**, which gives the category description, verbs, and sample objectives. **Table 9-9** includes a detailed list of verbs that can be used to write cognitive objectives.

Affective Domain

The next classification of objectives is the affective domain, which is related to the client's attitudes, interests, attention, awareness, and values. The cognitive domain was previously listed in increasing order of complexity, but the affective domain is listed in increasing order of depth into the client's emotions and value system. Affective objectives are more difficult to isolate and express accurately; consequently, they are difficult to evaluate through measurement. The levels of the affective domain are receiving, responding, valuing, and organization, and they are characterized by values (Krathwohl, Bloom, & Masia, 1964). **Table 9-5** illustrates descriptions, verbs, and sample objectives of the five levels of the affective domain. **Table 9-10** reviews verbs in depth used for affective objectives.

TABLE 9-4

Cognitive Categories with Sample Objectives

Cognitive Category	Description	Verb	Sample Objective
Remembering	Client recalls information	Define	The client will define the terms *hypoglycemia* and *hyperglycemia*.
Understanding	Client explains ideas and concepts	Describe	The client will describe the signs and symptoms of insulin shock.
Applying	Client grasps ideas and concepts	Interpret	The client will interpret his or her blood sugar level to determine if more insulin is needed.
Analyzing	Client distinguishes among different parts	Compare, contrast	The client will compare and contrast the signs and symptoms of hypoglycemia and hyperglycemia.
Evaluating	Client justifies a stand or takes a position	Support	The client will support the need to keep blood sugar within normal limits.
Creating	Client creates a new product or point of view	Design	The client will design a calendar to keep track of daily blood sugar levels.

TABLE 9-5

Affective Categories and Sample Objectives

Affective Category	Description	Verbs	Sample Objective
Receiving	Client is aware of or attending to something in the environment	Listen to	The client will listen to a presentation on colostomy care and share the information with family members.
Responding	Client shows new behaviors as a result of experience	Choose	The client will choose to discuss his or her feelings about caring for the colostomy in a support group.
Valuing	Client shows involvement or commitment	Express	The client will express agreement with the guidelines for maintaining sterile technique in wound care.
Organization	Client integrates a new value, ranking it among priorities	Select	The client will select foods that meet the requirements of a diabetic diet.
Characterization by value	Client acts consistently with the new value	Display	By taking medication, the client will demonstrate acceptance that he or she has a chronic illness.

Psychomotor Domain

In contrast to affective learning, psychomotor skills are concerned with physical movement and coordination, which are easier to identify and measure because they are readily observable. Learning a physical skill—such as walking with crutches, manipulating a syringe, or doing a procedure—usually involves substantial psychomotor learning. More than one level of learning exists in the psychomotor domain. For example, hand washing is less complex than cleaning a wound. In these psychomotor activities, the level of skill is readily observable.

Several systems for defining psychomotor learning are available in the literature (Harrow, 1972; Simpson, 1972). We have chosen to adapt and abbreviate the system developed by Simpson (1972) because it appears to have the most relevance for client education. **Table 9-6** reviews the

TABLE 9-6

Psychomotor Categories and Sample Objectives

Psychomotor Category	*Description*	*Verb*	*Sample Objective*
Perception	Client attains sensory awareness of clues associated with the task to be performed	Watches	The client watches the nurse perform a colostomy irrigation.
Set	Client exhibits readiness to take action through verbal expressions or body language	Expresses	The client expresses willingness to try to do part of the colostomy irrigation.
Guided response	Client exerts efforts to imitate observed behavior; attempts to comply with directions and coaching	Performs	The client will perform colostomy irrigation with assistance.
Mechanism	Client achieves the ability to perform the skill, which is becoming a habit	Demonstrates	The client will demonstrate how to irrigate a colostomy without assistance.
Complex overt response	Client performs the skill easily and independently in sequence with attention to details	Coordinates	The client coordinates complete colostomy care and makes adjustments as needed in the process.
Adaption	Client achieves the ability to alter the skill to suit conditions and performs the skill automatically as needed	Adapts	The client adapts skill knowledge and performs colostomy care while on a camping trip.

Source: Adapted from Gronlund and Brookhart, 2009; and Gronlund 2004.

descriptions and provides sample objectives in the psychomotor domain. **Table 9-11** reviews verbs for writing objectives in the psychomotor domain.

Conditions

The third step in the ABCD process of writing learning objectives is to define the **conditions** under which the client will perform the desired task. This includes specifying situations and restraints during which the objective must be met, or describing important conditions under which the **performance** is expected to occur. The statement of conditions is not always necessary to a clear statement of objectives, but it should be included when pertinent. As demonstrated in **Table 9-7**, conditions might be stated with the following phrases:

- Given a list of …
- when provided with …
- without using …
- by the end of this lesson …
- the learner will be denied …
- under special conditions of …
- within 15 minutes. . . . .
- as measured against a checklist

Degree

Degree refers to the quality or level of performance that is considered acceptable and should be specified or implied when writing objectives. The degree may be based on practice standards, which the nurse should be aware of. The degree defines what level the client must perform at so you can determine if learning is successful. The **criteria** might include concepts such as amount, quality, and speed. For instance, clients may be considered successful if they are able to slow their pulse by five beats per minute during relaxation training or identify 2 out of 3 causes of hypertension. Accuracy is an important criterion when a client is preparing an insulin injection. The degree might specify without error or correctly. Other criteria might be without any verbal guidance or from memory. **Table 9-8** summarizes how the parts of the ABCD method of writing learning objectives come together to give a complete picture of client expectations.

TABLE 9-7

Audience, Behavior, and Condition

Audience	Behavior	Condition
The client will	perform a colostomy irrigation	given a syringe and a basin
The client will	verbally tell the pulse rate	when asked by the nurse

TABLE 9-8

Audience, Behavior, Condition, Degree

Audience	Behavior	Condition	Degree
The client will	perform a colostomy irrigation	given a syringe and a basin	without any verbal guidance from the nurse
The client will	verbally tell the pulse rate under which she should not take digoxin	when asked by the nurse	correctly before discharge from the hospital

TABLE 9-9

Sample Verbs for Cognitive Objectives

Remembering	Defines	Lists	Recalls	Reproduces	Tells
	Identifies	Matches	Records	Selects	Underlines
	Indicates	Names	Repeats	Shows	
	Labels	Points	Reports	States	
Understanding	Describes	Explains	Identifies	Paraphrases	Rewrites
	Discusses	Expresses	Increases	Reiterates	Summarizes
	Draws	Generalizes	Locates	Restates	Translates
	Estimates	Gives example	Outlines	Reviews	
Applying	Applies	Draws	Investigates	Predicts	Selects
	Calculates	Eliminates	Manipulates	Prepares	Shops
	Changes	Formulates	Measures	Produces	Shows
	Computes	Illustrates	Modifies	Proposes	Solves
	Demonstrates	Implements	Negotiates	Relates	Uses
	Designs	Infers	Operates	Revises	
	Develops	Interprets	Orders	Schedules	
Analyzing	Analyzes	Calculates	Criticizes	Distinguishes	Relates
	Appraises	Categorizes	Debates	Identifies	Selects
	Arranges	Classifies	Diagrams	Illustrates	Separates
	Assigns	Compares	Differentiates	Infers	Subdivides
	Breaks down	Contrasts	Discriminates	Outlines	Tests
Evaluating	Appraises	Contrasts	Distinguishes	Interprets	Selects
	Assesses	Criticizes	Estimates	Judges	Summarizes
	Calibrates	Debates	Evaluates	Justifies	Supports
	Compares	Defends	Explains	Measures	Values
	Computes	Describes		Relates	
	Concludes	Discriminates		Revises	
Creating	Arranges	Compiles	Devises	Orders	Reorganizes
	Assembles	Composes	Estimates	Organizes	Revises
	Blends	Constructs	Formulates	Paraphrases	Rewrites
	Categorizes	Contrasts	Generates	Plans	Simplifies
	Classifies	Correlates	Integrates	Prepares	Summarizes
	Collects	Creates	Manages	Rearranges	Teaches
	Combines	Defends	Mixes	Reconstructs	Writes
	Compares	Designs	Modifies	Relates	

Source: Adapted from Gronlund and Brookhart, 2009; and Gronlund 2004.

TABLE 9-10			

Sample Verbs for Affective Objectives

Receiving	Accepts	Focuses	Names
	Admits	Follows	Observes
	Allows	Heeds	Pays attention
	Asks	Identifies	Replies
	Attends	Listens	Stays
	Describes	Looks	Uses
Responding	Agrees	Discusses	Replies
	Answers	Explains	Reports
	Assists	Labels	Selects
	Attempts	Participates	Shows
	Chooses	Performs	States willingness
	Complies	Practices	Tries
	Conforms	Reacts	Verbalizes
Valuing	Asks	Differentiates	Justifies
	Asserts	Disagrees	Proposes
	Assists	Explains	Reports
	Attempts	Follows	Selects
	Chooses	Gives	Volunteers
	Completes	Helps	Works
	Defends	Initiates	
	Describes	Joins	
Organization	Adheres	Completes	Modifies
	Alters	Defends	Orders
	Arranges	Explains	Organizes
	Chooses	Expresses	Relates
	Combines	Generalizes	Resolves
	Compares	Integrates	Synthesizes
Internalizing values (characterization)	Acts	Describes	Performs
	Adheres	Discriminates	Practices
	Asserts	Displays	Revises
	Assists	Endures	Solves
	Commits	Explains	Uses
	Defends	Influences	

Source: Adapted from Gronlund and Brookhart, 2009; and Gronlund 2004.

Reordering of ABCD Components

The order of the ABCD components can be changed to make the most comprehensive and clear statement of the objective. **A**udience + **B**ehavior + **C**ondition + **D**egree can be altered to **C** + **A** + **B** + **D**. An example is as follows: Given a syringe and a basin, the client will perform a colostomy irrigation without verbal guidance from the nurse. **A** + **B** + **D** + **C** can also be used: The

TABLE 9-11

Sample Verbs for Psychomotor Objectives

Perception	Attends	Contrasts	Distinguishes	Looks	Selects
	Chooses	Describes	Focuses on	Observes	Separates
	Compares	Detects	Identifies	Perceives	
	Concentrates	Differentiates	Isolates	Relates	
Set	Aims	Begins	Gets ready	Reacts	Starts
	Aligns	Copies	Positions	Responds	Tries
	Asks	Displays	Prepares	Shows	Volunteers
	Attempts	Expresses	Proceeds	Stands up	
Guided response	Aligns	Combs	Holds	Presses	Solves
	Applies	Compiles	Inserts	Produces	Splints
	Arises	Connects	Joins	Pulls	Spreads
	Arranges	Constructs	Leans	Pushes	Squeezes
	Assembles	Cools	Lifts	Raises	Stands
	Attaches	Coordinates	Locates	Reassembles	Starts
	Attempts	Counts	Lowers	Reclines	Sticks
Mechanism	Auscultates	Covers	Makes	Removes	Stimulates
	Avoids	Crawls	Manipulates	Repairs	Stoops
	Balances	Cuts	Mends	Replaces	Stops
	Bathes	Demonstrates	Molds	Restores	Synchronizes
	Boils	Disconnects	Navigates	Rubs	Tears
	Breathes	Discriminates	Opens	Runs	Tests
Complex overt response	Brushes	Dissects	Operates	Scrubs	Ties
	Builds	Examines	Palpates	Secures	Transfers
	Calibrates	Fastens	Parts	Separates	Turns
	Catheterizes	Finds	Picks up	Sews	Types
	Changes	Folds	Pinches	Shakes	Ventilates
	Chooses	Grasps	Pivots	Sharpens	Walks
	Cleans	Guides	Places	Shortens	Washes
	Cleanses	Heats	Pours	Simulates	Weighs
	Closes	Hops	Practices	Slides	Wipes
Adaptation	Adapts	Creates	Modifies	Reverses	Substitutes
	Alters	Designs	Rearranges	Revises	Swaps
	Changes	Diverts	Reformulates	Rotates	Switches
	Composes	Exchanges	Remodels	Shifts	Varies
	Converts		Reorganizes		
	Corrects		Replaces		

Source: Adapted from Gronlund and Brookhart, 2009; and Gronlund 2004.

client will perform a colostomy irrigation without verbal guidance from the nurse when given a syringe and a basin. The order of the components should be carefully thought through to help the learner understand the learning expectations.

SELECTION OF CONTENT

The time has come for you to select appropriate **content** to develop a teaching plan. Based on a client or clients that you have identified, assessment data you have collected, and the learning objectives you have written, you must now select appropriate content for teaching. To clarify and illustrate the process of developing a teaching plan, we created a case example. The format we have chosen is widely applicable and shows the pertinent information that should be included in the teaching plan.

CASE EXAMPLE: MRS. ROSA LOPEZ

Our client is Mrs. Rosa Lopez, a 40-year-old woman of mixed race with African American and Mexican heritage. She is a single mother who is supporting and raising two teenage children, a son and a daughter, who live at home. She is a teacher's aid at a public school and has stress at work. She is also busy volunteering at her church. She was recently diagnosed with hypertension. The doctor prescribed an antihypertensive medication and recommended she limit her sodium intake to 2,000 mg per day.

Mrs. Lopez has a family history of hypertension, but she is reluctant to take medication to treat it. She stated that the hypertension is not bothering her, and she does not understand why it is necessary to take medication for it. Her behavior emphasizes the fact that hypertension is an invisible disease with multiple factors contributing to its etiology and treatment, including medications, nutrition, weight management, and stress reduction. We determined that she has educational needs in the three domains of learning: cognitive, affective, and psychomotor. Although there are many things our client needs to learn about hypertension, for the purposes of illustrating a teaching plan we will provide an example of one learning objective in each of the domains. Recall that the learning domains are not isolated entities; rather, learning in the domains overlaps. For example, psychomotor and affective objectives have cognitive components.

Our teaching plan has four columns (**Table 9-12**). The first contains the learning objectives, the second identifies the content in an outline form, the third lists the teaching strategies and instructional materials, and the fourth lists the evaluation methods. We have included only four columns because we want the teaching plan to be serviceable, a plan from which you can actually teach (it is practical to include only four columns on one page).

SUMMARY

This chapter defined learning objectives as precise, measurable, and attainable statements that describe what will be learned and who will do what, when, and how. Five factors were

TABLE 9-12

Sample Teaching Plan for Mrs. Rosa Lopez

Learning Objectives	Content Outline	Strategies and Materials	Evaluation
1. The client will correctly verbally explain how excessive salt intake affects blood pressure to the nurse by memory (cognitive).	Greeting and introductions Hypertension Definition Fluid retention Excess sodium intake Role in fluid retention Sodium and salt relationship Sodium is 40% of table salt (sodium chloride) Fluid retention and C-V system		Verbal questions Paper and pencil test
2. The client will choose to limit sodium intake by working with the nurse to prepare a dietary plan for one week (affective).	Four components of dietary plan: 1. Remove salt shaker from table. 2. Use no salt in cooking. 3. Avoid canned or processed foods that are high in sodium. 4. Use low-sodium seasonings, such as herbs and spices.		Short term: Attitude scale Long term: Implementation of dietary changes
3. The client will demonstrate how to accurately obtain her own blood pressure reading using home digital equipment without any verbal guidance from the nurse (psychomotor).	Techniques for obtaining blood pressure: 1. Read equipment directions. 2. Locate brachial artery. 3. Place arm in cuff. 4. Inflate cuff. 5. Release air in cuff. 6. Record findings.		Checklist to obtain blood pressure Record of blood pressure readings

discussed that should be considered before writing learning objectives. A four-part process for writing objectives was presented: Audience, Behavior, Conditions, and Degree (ABCD). The process emphasized writing clear and specific learning objectives. Examples of objectives were given using the ABCD method in each of the learning domains: cognitive, affective, and psychomotor. The correct choice of verbs for each domain was emphasized. The chapter concluded with the introduction of the case example of Mrs. Rosa Lopez and a format for a teaching plan.

EXERCISES

Exercise I: Writing Objectives in Each Learning Domain

Purposes:

- Differentiate among cognitive, affective, and psychomotor learning domains.
- Write clear statements to describe client learning outcomes in each domain.

Directions: Review the incorrectly written learning objectives and complete the following tasks:

1. State the learning domain or domains and **level of complexity** inferred by each objective.
2. Correct the objectives using the ABCD method of Audience, Behavior, Conditions, and Degree.
3. You may write more than one correct objective for each incorrect objective.
4. Use verbs with few meanings (listed in this chapter).

The incorrectly written learning objectives are as follows:

- Client will be integrating the mastery and competency of passive exercises to support attitudes of adequacy and self-esteem.
- Client will be able to perform at some level a return demonstration of the presented passive exercises despite his or her physical limitations.
- To teach the client to cough and deep breathe preoperatively.
- To demonstrate to the client the use of the circle bed traction and abduction splint preoperatively.
- Client will understand the importance of food groups that comprise a healthy diet.

Exercise II: Writing Learning Objectives for Clients

Purpose: Write learning objectives using the ABCD method of Audience, Behavior, Conditions, and Degree.
Directions: Divide into small working groups and (1) identify appropriate teaching content, (2) state the rationale for the content you have selected, and (3) write at least one learning objective using the ABCD method in each of the three domains that are appropriate to each client situation.

1. John Martinez is a 50-year-old farm worker who was admitted to the coronary care unit 4 days ago. This is his first myocardial infarction, and he states that he has never been ill a day in his life. He lives with his wife and their four teenaged children. He speaks very little English.
2. Suzie Scofield is a blind 6-year-old African American girl who has been admitted to the pediatric unit in preparation for a tonsillectomy tomorrow. Suzie lives with her mother, one older brother, and one younger sister. Her mother is a licensed practical nurse at the hospital.
3. Delores Johnson is a 30-year-old woman with a stormy 10-year history of ulcerative colitis. She has been hospitalized again for medical treatment. The doctors are trying to persuade Ms. Johnson to accept surgery, an ileostomy. She is a buyer for a large department store and

travels in her work. She is married and has no children, but she would like to become pregnant some time in the near future.

Exercise III: Writing Learning Objectives for Health Team Members

Purposes:

■ Apply theory to teaching health team members.
■ Write learning objectives using the ABCD method of Audience, Behavior, Conditions, and Degree.

Directions:
1. Develop a teaching plan for teaching health team members.
2. Think about possible learning deficits and potentials among the team members you plan to teach.
3. Write one learning objective in each learning domain: cognitive, affective, and psychomotor.
4. After you are satisfied with each objective, refer back to the information in this chapter. Determine the level of depth or complexity at which you have written the objective and consider if it is too high or too low; then rework it as necessary.
5. After you are satisfied that the objective is at the level you believe is appropriate, write the level beside that objective.
6. Work in small groups and consult with each other.

Exercise IV: Sample Nursing Diagnosis and Related Health Education

Purpose: Illustrate a sample nursing diagnosis and related health education.
Directions: Discuss the following situation and the implications for health education.

Situation: Acute Care/Home Care for Todd Smith

Todd is a 10-year-old white boy who has been diagnosed with osteomyelitis. He is in the hospital to receive aggressive intravenous antibiotic treatment. Your job is to prepare him and his mother for self-care of a central venous catheter at home, administration of antibiotics, maintenance of a clean insertion site, clamping off the catheter, administration of medications by learning to remove air before injection, and maintenance of a patent catheter.

Nursing Diagnosis

■ Todd is at high risk for skin integrity impairment related to central venous catheter placement as evidenced by possible redness and swelling at the site.
■ Todd and his mother's fear and anxiety are related to insufficient knowledge of catheter care, as evidenced by their questions.

Expected Outcomes/Learning Objectives

1. The client describes to the nurse the correct route of the catheter in the body.
2. The client expresses confidence in his ability to assist his mother with catheter care within 1 week of insertion.
3. The client assists his mother with catheter care without contamination while following the established protocol.
4. The client assists his mother with the established protocol for IV antibiotic administration twice daily without contamination.
5. The client keeps the catheter securely bandaged between IV treatments according to the protocol.
6. The client keeps the catheter clean and dry during bathing according to the protocol.
7. The client verbalizes to the nurse signs and symptoms of incipient infection, side effects of antibiotics, and allergic reactions immediately upon observing them.

Health Education Interventions

1. Assess the client's previous experiences with changing dressings, administering medication by syringe, and incision care.
2. Explain the anatomy and physiology components of the procedure.
3. Demonstrate full protocols for catheter care, IV antibiotic administration, and incision care.
4. Invite and reinforce step-by-step participation by the mother and the client in the procedures.
5. Explain the signs and symptoms of incipient infection, side effects of antibiotics, and allergic reactions.

Discussion

This situation is a good example of the value of audiovisual aids, objects and models, reinforcement, and demonstration/return demonstration. Using the real equipment as well as pictures and charts will facilitate teaching the mother and client the necessary skills. You should watch their facial expressions for signs of comprehension, overload, or both. Choose activities that are likely to promote immediate success. Encourage the mother and the client to participate at their own pace. Build gradually by giving the mother and the client things to hold before giving them things to do. For example, have them handle the bandage and then apply it. Assure them that they do not have to do the entire procedure until they are ready.

Explain your collaborative relationship with the home health nurse who will pick up where you have left off. Assure the client and the mother that the home health nurse will be with them the first time any of the protocols are performed at home. Send home a videotape of the procedure that they have already watched in the hospital.

REFERENCES

Anderson, L. W., Krathwohl, D. R., Airasian, P. W., Cruikshank, K. A., Mayer, R. E., Pintrich, P. R., . . . Wittrock, M. C. (Eds.). (2001). *A taxonomy for learning, teaching, and assessing: A revision of Bloom's taxonomy of educational objectives.* New York, NY: Longman.

Bastable, S. B., & Doody, J. A. (2008). Behavioral objectives. In S. B. Bastable (Ed.), *Nurse as educator: Principles of teaching and learning for nursing practice* (3rd ed., pp. 383–427). Sudbury, MA: Jones and Bartlett.

Bloom, B. S., Englehart, M. D., Furst, E. J., Hill, W. H., & Krathwohl, D. R. (1956). *Taxonomy of educational objectives: The classification of educational goals. Handbook I: Cognitive domain.* New York, NY: David McKay.

Gronlund, N. E. (2004). *Writing instructional objectives for teaching and assessment* (7th ed.). Upper Saddle River, NJ: Pearson Education.

Gronlund, N. E., & Brookhart, S. M. (2009). *Gronlund's writing instructional objectives* (8th ed.). Upper Saddle River, NJ: Pearson Education.

Harrow, A. J. (1972). *A taxonomy of the psychomotor domain: A guide for developing behavioral objectives.* New York, NY: David McKay.

Krathwohl, D. R., Bloom, B. S., & Masia, B. B. (1964). *Taxonomy of educational objectives: The classification of educational goals. Handbook II: Affective domain.* New York, NY: David McKay.

Mager, R. F. (1997). *Preparing instructional objectives* (3rd ed.). Atlanta, GA: CEP Press.

Simpson, E. J. (1972). *The psychomotor domain* (Vol. 3). Washington, DC: Gryphon House.

Webster's All-In-One Dictionary and Thesaurus (2nd ed.). (2013). Springfield, MA: Federal Street Press.

10

Teaching Strategies

OBJECTIVES

Upon completion of this chapter, you will be able to do the following:

- Define the term *teaching strategy*.
- Compare and contrast teacher-directed, teacher-facilitated, and learner-directed teaching strategies according to their advantages and disadvantages.
- Describe a teachable moment.
- Contrast formal and informal teaching.
- State at least two examples of teaching strategies for achieving learning objectives in each of the following domains: cognitive, affective, and psychomotor.
- Identify three factors that affect the choice of teaching strategies.
- Demonstrate selected teaching strategies when implementing a teaching plan.

KEY TERMS

demonstration
games
guest lecture
group activities and
    teaching
learner-directed strategy
lecture
lecture with discussion

levels of prevention
one-to-one instruction
peer counseling
programmed instruction
return demonstration
role-play
simulation
teacher-directed strategy

teacher-facilitated
    strategy
teaching strategy
team teaching
technology-assisted
    learning

INTRODUCTION

Teaching is an active process in which information is shared with others to provide them with the information needed to make behavioral changes. Learning is the process of assimilating information with a resultant change in behavior. The purposes of client teaching are to promote, retain, and restore health. Learning needs related to health education include three **levels of prevention:** primary prevention (health maintenance), secondary prevention (diagnosis and treatment), and tertiary prevention (follow-up). Health teaching in these areas is used to prevent disease and provide nurses with starting points in making effective, positive changes in the health status of clients. The challenge for nurses as educators is to choose teaching strategies that nurture health-promoting habits, values, and attitudes.

This chapter looks at the use of teaching strategies when preparing teaching plans for health education. A **teaching strategy** is defined as an instructional method that presents content in a way that is designed to bring about specific changes in learners. Teaching strategies include activities that are done by learners as well as teachers. They are a part of the teaching and learning process, which is a planned interaction that promotes a behavioral change. An important distinction in the current nurse's role as educator includes facilitating learning rather than being a source of all knowledge. The nurse helps learners construct their own knowledge rather than telling them things they are expected to memorize. The client as learner is the center of all teaching, and as a result no one single teaching strategy is effective all the time for all learners (Killen, 2000).

TYPES OF TEACHING STRATEGIES

Different teaching strategies are simply different ways of helping clients achieve learning objectives. The choices range from a totally teacher-dominated approach in which clients are passive recipients of information, to totally independent learning in which the teacher plays no active role. In between these extremes there are several major strategies and numerous variations of each strategy. No single teaching strategy is better than another in all circumstances. Your choice of teaching strategy is influenced by the outcome you want for the client. Different types of learning can be facilitated by different strategies. There is an array of teaching strategies from which to choose. This chapter discusses different teaching strategies and factors to consider in selecting them. We discuss teaching strategies under three broad headings: teacher-directed strategies, teacher-facilitated strategies, and learner-directed strategies.

TEACHER-DIRECTED STRATEGIES

Teacher-directed strategies are those in which the teacher presents information in a highly structured format and directs the activities of learners. These strategies include one-to-one individualized instruction, lecture format, **lecture with discussion** and questions and answers, **demonstration** and **return demonstration**, and team teaching. These strategies are described, the necessary preparation is identified, and the advantages and disadvantages are discussed.

One-to-One Individual Instruction

One-to-one individual instruction is either formal or informal and includes clients alone or clients and family members as appropriate. Formal one-to-one individual instruction occurs when nurses meet individually with clients at a planned time for the purpose of providing health education. A common clinical example is preoperative teaching. The nurse selects the meeting location and time, and the content to be covered based on the client's schedule for surgery. Meeting face to face allows the nurse to give clients personalized attention. This is a good initial format to provide basic knowledge in an atmosphere that gives the client an opportunity to ask questions and get immediate feedback. Individual teaching allows clients to share confidential information and problems. This format is adaptable to the needs of clients with low health literacy skills, physical impairments, or emotional difficulties (Rankin, Stallings, & London, 2005).

Plan formal one-to-one individual instruction ahead of time. Planning involves creating an outline of the content that sequences learning and choosing supplemental materials specific to the client's background and experiences. When sequencing information, teach basic concepts first and then variations and adjustments. Clients are more interested in learning what is meaningful to them, so it is helpful to begin with what clients have identified as a need or concern. To assess teaching effectiveness, ask the client to restate the information in his or her own words.

The most frequent type of teaching is informal one-to-one individual instruction that occurs at the bedside while interacting with clients for other reasons. These interactions turn into teachable moments, those unplanned moments when nurses recognize a client's readiness to learn, and capture the opportunity to facilitate learning. Romano states that "the reality of the complex environment we practice in requires us to do much of our teaching on the fly, which can be effective if done right and done often" (2009, p. 141). Watch for teachable moments during your interactions with clients and use clinical judgment to determine when teaching is appropriate. Opportune times to teach are before procedures, after a doctor's visit, while transporting a client, or when you are waiting for test results. Other opportune times to teach include the following circumstances:

- The client asks questions and shows a facial expression of curiosity or puzzlement.
- The client voices concerns about specific issues.
- The client makes innocent comments that indicate misunderstanding.
- The client shows nonverbal signs of confusion, frustration, or discouragement.
- The family voices concerns.

During teachable moments, constantly assess the clients' knowledge by listening and developing what Lowenstein and Reeder identify as "meta-cognitive empathy" (2009). In other words, be aware of what the client does and does not understand by evaluating his or her responses to pointed questions. Ask what he or she knows about the illness, what he or she considers positive lifestyle behaviors, and what lifestyle changes are needed to improve health. Avoid starting your conversation by telling clients what you think they need to know. Listen carefully to identify thoughts that may need strengthening or reinforcing. This also includes correcting misunderstandings, adding knowledge, or referring the client to appropriate resources (Lowenstein & Reeder, 2009). Information that you glean from informal conversations helps you construct a mini–teaching plan with appropriate teaching strategies on the spot to address client concerns.

Although informal client education takes place spontaneously, you still need to present information in a clear, organized manner based on the client's level of need (Falvo, 2011). Present information to clients when they are ready to receive it and in amounts they are able to comprehend. Use the teach-back method to evaluate your teaching by asking the client to restate in his or her own words what you have taught. Using this strategy, you can assess how well the client comprehended your message (Tamura-Lis, 2013).

Another form of one-to-one individual instruction is telehealth, which is the use of electronic and telecommunication technologies to support long-distance clinical health care. This strategy is used for client care and health-related education. It uses video conferencing to connect the nurse and the client. Some of the technologies used in telehealth include videoconferencing, Internet access, streaming media, and wireless communications. These approaches hold great potential for health education for homebound clients and clients in remote areas. There continues to be, however, significant barriers in making this a part of daily health practices. One barrier is the mindset of health professionals who continue to focus on face-to-face care based on tradition and fragmented delivery systems. Clients want care based in their communities, but providers today wrestle with financial, regulatory, and operational challenges. The slow adoption of electronic health records (EHR) and information sharing is another barrier. In addition, reimbursement models need to be modified with less focus on fee-for-service and face-to-face visits so clinicians and healthcare organizations get paid for the care that is delivered via telehealth. It is anticipated that the adoption of telehealth will accelerate as an understanding of cultural changes develops (Rogove, McArthur, Demaerschalk, & Vespa, 2012).

The advantages of one-to-one individual instruction are the personal approach to the client, the active learner role in a give-and-take relationship with the nurse, and the flexible format in an informal atmosphere. Individualized teaching also is done through phone calls, email, and telehealth. The disadvantages include lack of sharing with, and support from, other clients and their families. This strategy exacts a high cost in terms of staff time for instruction (Rankin et al., 2005).

Lecture

A **lecture** is an oral presentation of a given subject delivered before an audience or class for the purpose of instruction. Lectures are given in person or are televised, and they can be delivered as audio recordings such as podcasts. The nurse presents information on a topic that is divided into three major segments: introduction (5 minutes), body, and conclusion (5 minutes) (Woodring & Woodring, 2007). Usually in health education the lecture is short, lasting from 15 to 20 minutes. The introduction is your opportunity to gain the attention of the audience and state what clients should gain from the lecture. The body of the lecture should explain the main concepts and convey the critical information clients need to know. The conclusion summarizes the information that was presented and makes a link between what was taught and what the clients will be able to practically use. The lecture format is an efficient, versatile, and economical teaching strategy than can be used when time is limited or when a group of clients and family members can benefit from core factual information (Bucher & Kotecki, 2014).

Preparation for giving a lecture requires planning ahead and includes knowing the learners, clarifying learning objectives, knowing the topic, and organizing and sequencing the content. Visual reinforcement, such as a PowerPoint presentation or handouts, is used to emphasize the key points. Keep in mind that an individual's optimal attention span is approximately 1 minute per year of age up to 45 years. For example, a 5-year-old has a 5-minute attention span, whereas a 21-year-old has a 21-minute attention span (Woodring & Woodring, 2007). This illustrates the importance of varying the presentation pace and including other supplemental strategies to add interest. The effectiveness of the lecture strategy depends on the skill of the speaker. **Table 10-1** offers suggestions for how to successfully prepare a lecture and avoid pitfalls.

The advantage of a lecture is that you can address a large numbers of clients in one setting. It is also useful for poor readers, it allows auditory learners to receive succinct information quickly, and it allows you to make facts more interesting and understandable by clarifying confusing points. Disadvantages of lectures are that clients are in a passive learner role and they provide few feedback opportunities for clients. Eighty percent of lecture information is forgotten within 1 day (Woodring & Woodring, 2007). A modification of the lecture strategy that addresses the disadvantages is the interactive lecture, in which the nurse gives clients something to do during the lecture. This strategy includes segments of lecture combined with segments in which clients are interacting with each other and the teacher. An example is a lecture followed by clients answering questions using clickers or clients interacting in pairs or small groups to answer questions.

Guest Lecture

Guest lecturers are a good choice for teacher-directed learning because they provide role models with whom clients can identify. An example of an appropriate guest speaker is to invite a person who has quit smoking to talk with a group of clients who are trying to stop smoking. The testimony of a guest lecturer can have a powerful effect on clients and be a source of motivation. It should be noted that guest lecturers can be invited into online environments as well. Some important aspects of the guest lecturer strategy are as follows:

- The guest lecturer should be chosen carefully and be fully informed of the learning objectives he or she is expected to cover.
- If possible, attend a presentation, or talk with someone who has attended a presentation, by the guest lecturer to determine if the presentation is appropriate.
- Provide the guest lecturer with exact information about time, place, and location, including the URL for online sessions. Plan to have someone meet or call the guest lecturer to orient the person to the learning format or venue.
- Check with the guest lecturer to identify what equipment, special tools, and web links will be needed.

Lecture with Discussion and Questions and Answers

A lecture is most effective when used with a discussion that involves clients. Discussion is a two-way verbal interaction that involves talking, listening, asking questions, and answering questions. The discussion strategy is sometimes referred to as *teach back* when it encourages the client to verbalize what was learned. The use of discussion or an exchange of points of view helps clients become active participants in the learning process. This strategy is a good choice when clients have previous experience with a subject and have information to share. It promotes understanding and application of knowledge. It also fosters the development of desirable attitudes (Bucher & Kotecki, 2014; Rankin et al., 2005).

TABLE 10-1

Suggestions for the Lecturer

Stage of Lecture Preparation	*Suggestions*	*Avoid*
Preparation stage (weeks in advance)	■ Specify the date, time, and location of the lecture. ■ Visit the lecture venue if possible. ■ Clarify the purpose and objectives of the lecture. ■ Cover only three to five main points. ■ Gather evidence-based research on the topic. ■ Analyze the audience. Consider age, culture, socioeconomic factors, and language. ■ Make sure your tone and examples are appropriate to the audience. ■ Prepare an outline and notes for the presentation. ■ Practice giving the lecture. ■ Choose appropriate attire. ■ Check to be sure technology is working and accessible. ■ Prepare handouts in advance. ■ Prepare in advance for questions.	■ Procrastinating ■ Lack of preparation ■ Trying to wing it at the last minute
Giving the presentation (introduction)	■ Introduce yourself. ■ State the purpose and objectives of the lecture. ■ Get the attention of the audience. ■ Remain calm and cope with anxiety. ■ Place a glass of water on the podium for dry throat. ■ Gain learner attention by showing enthusiasm and self-confidence. ■ Smile and look at the audience frequently. ■ Speak clearly, strongly, and loudly; use a microphone if needed. ■ Use a conversational pace when speaking. ■ Use natural gestures. ■ Use language and expressions appropriate to the audience. ■ Provide handouts with an outline of the presentation if appropriate.	■ Distracting mannerisms or gestures, such as pacing, clearing the throat ■ Saying you are nervous ■ Apologizing ■ Looking down at your notes

(continues)

TABLE 10-1

Suggestions for the Lecturer (Continued)

Stage of Lecture Preparation	Suggestions	Avoid
Giving the presentation (body of the lecture)	■ Define the main concepts and principles. ■ Provide smooth transitions between topics. ■ Do not try to provide every detail pertaining to your topic. ■ Talk from notes, do not read from notes. ■ Use humor, stories, analogies, or metaphors to make a point. ■ If appropriate, move from behind the podium to engage the audience. ■ Use appropriate audiovisuals. ■ Provide a change of pace in longer presentations; combine strategies. ■ Provide 15-minute breaks if the lecture is longer than 20 minutes.	■ Repeating phrases or expressions such as "umm" or "you know" ■ Turning your back on the audience ■ Reading from notes ■ Talking down to the audience
Giving the presentation (conclusion)	■ Stay within the allotted time. ■ Review the key points and emphasize practical learning aspects. ■ Provide the opportunity for learners to ask questions if time allows. ■ Admit when you do not know an answer. ■ Thank the audience for their attention.	■ Stopping abruptly and leaving the podium ■ Speaking longer than the specified time

There are several different types of discussions. Open discussions occur when clients determine the topic, and the role of the nurse is to ask questions that lead learners to consider various ideas. With this format, the nurse needs to define terms and encourage different points of view. Planned discussion occurs when the nurse determines the content of the discussion, plans questions in advance, and guides clients toward a predetermined goal or conclusion. Formal debate is a type of discussion in which clients present opposing viewpoints, usually in a structured format.

Nurses play a big part in the discussion strategy by choosing the type of discussion and forming focus questions that guide clients toward the learning outcomes that are the focus of the lesson. Questions serve many purposes in the teaching and learning process. Questions help to assess what clients already know, stimulate interest in a new topic, discern whether or not clients grasped the main points, explore ideas, and promote higher levels of thinking. It is important to prepare questions ahead of time and modify them as needed.

As the teacher, you shape the discussion by the manner in which contributions are treated. If clients feel that their contributions are valued and used, they experience freedom to express themselves. Do not dominate the discussion; use the time to identify and correct inaccurate information and guide the discussion. Encourage participation by all clients; do not let the conversation be dominated by a few group members. It is important to maintain a nonthreatening environment that encourages informal sharing. A disadvantage is that this strategy takes more time, depending on the topic and the number of participants.

An important skill is the ability to manage the discussion and facilitate learning. This requires thought and preparation. The first task in leading a discussion is to get the discussion started. It is often helpful to begin by reviewing the objectives of the session with the group. Another approach is to summarize past information and then ask group members their opinions. Sometimes a skilled teacher will make a controversial statement to stimulate the group's participation. After the discussion is in progress, there are several ways to keep it on track by focusing, refocusing, changing the focus, and recapping what has been said (deTornyay & Thompson, 1982).

Focusing is keeping the group discussion centered on the learning objectives. One way to focus the group is to ask questions that specifically direct the group's attention to the point or points you wish to make. This can be done by asking open-ended questions, such as "What do you find is the most interesting part of …"

Refocusing is getting the group discussion back on the topic when it has strayed from the original topic. Sometimes groups bring interesting but irrelevant information into the discussion. You can refocus the group by saying something such as, "Let's get back to our topic." There may be times the group has deviated from the topic and you must choose whether or not to refocus the discussion. This is a judgment call because the new topic may be important to discuss. Group members may need to deal with the new topic before they can focus on anything else. When a group has discussed a topic sufficiently and no new information or ideas are forthcoming, then it is time to change the focus of the discussion. You might say, "Now that we've discussed the … let us examine another aspect of … ". Recapping is summarizing the discussion to help clients see relationships and draw conclusions.

Using Questions as a Teaching Strategy

Questioning is a useful teaching strategy to stimulate thinking. Types of questions that are useful in client education are remembering/factual, understanding/describing, clarifying, and higher order. Remembering/factual questions begin with words such as who, what, where, or when. For example, "What is the normal range for blood pressure?" Understanding/describing questions require clients to organize their thoughts in a logical relationship and respond with a longer answer. For example, "Describe the signs and symptoms of insulin shock." Clarifying questions help clients clarify an idea that is based on their own statements and go beyond a superficial response. For example, "I don't quite understand what you mean; please tell me more."

Higher-order questions help clients think critically and require considerable thought. They have a place in health education in group discussions and when working individually with clients who are confronted with complex health decisions. Higher-order questions help clients compare and contrast (find similarities and differences), analyze (examine the parts and elements), and evaluate (determine the value of) information. Examples of these types of questions are provided in **Table 10-2**.

Questions also prompt clients to examine their assumptions (a fact or statement taken for granted) and make inferences (drawing conclusions and deducing) (Webster's, 2013). A sample question to identify assumptions is, "Why must a surgery consent form be signed before your operation?" A sample question to make inferences is, "After reading this pamphlet about the risk of heart attacks in people with high cholesterol, what would you infer about the foods you usually eat?"

TABLE 10-2

Examples of Types of Questions

Sample Question	Type of Question
What is your . . . ?	Remembering/factual
Who is your . . . ?	Remembering/factual
Describe the signs of . . .	Understanding/describing
Describe how you do this at home . . .	Understanding/describing
Tell me what you mean when . . .	Clarifying
Describe how you . . .	Clarifying
How does . . . compare with . . . ?	Comparing/contrasting
How are . . . and . . . alike and different?	Comparing/contrasting
Give me an example of . . .	Applying
How will you manage . . . at home?	Applying
How would . . . work for you?	Analyzing
What can you infer from . . . ?	Analyzing
How does . . . relate to . . . ?	Synthesizing
How has your past experience . . . ?	Synthesizing
Which . . . will work best for you and why?	Evaluating
What are the pros and cons of . . . ?	Evaluating
How will you design . . . ?	Creating
How would you create . . . ?	Creating

Clients often find themselves in situations where there are few right and wrong answers. They simply must make the best decision in difficult circumstances. There is a danger of not thinking critically about the consequences of these decisions (Browne & Keeley, 2007). Clients often hear contradictory opinions when they are under the care of specialists, and sorting through this information requires thought. As educators, encourage clients and their families to think through all aspects of a situation. For example, "Your family doctor and the surgeon told you different opinions about treatment. What are the pros and cons of each? What are the long-range results of having open-heart surgery or taking medication and changing your lifestyle?" Table 10-2 can help you use questioning as a teaching strategy.

Problems with the Discussion Strategy

A disadvantage of the discussion strategy is that it requires additional time, depending on the topic and the number of participants. When using this strategy, you give up some control because you allow clients to share some of the leadership. At times this means that clients diverge on a topic that is very different from what you had in mind and you need to decide whether or not to refocus the group.

Another problem with the discussion strategy occurs if the participants lose interest. This is evident when they start side conversations, yawn, become restless, and look glassy eyed. At this point you should consider changing your strategy. For instance, you could conduct a group activity and have the participants move their chairs into a new arrangement that is more appropriate for the activity. Or you could have everyone stand up and stretch or perhaps call for a 15-minute break. Another option is to change the topic of the discussion.

Other problems with the discussion strategy are nonparticipants, overparticipants, and rude participants. When the participants know each other and are comfortable being together, most clients will participate. If you have a very quiet nonparticipant in the group, you can encourage that person to speak up. For example, after some participants have commented, you can say, "What do some of the rest of you think about this?" It rarely helps to call on a specific participant unless the learning objective is to learn to be verbally assertive. Keep the environment welcoming, and usually quiet people will eventually share their thoughts.

Handling an overly talkative participant can be a challenge. This is a client who is outgoing, has lots of ideas, and likes to talk. There are several ways to handle this situation. For example, you can say to the overparticipant, "That is a great idea. Now, what do some of the rest of you think?" or "Do you all agree with …?" or "Does … speak for all of you?" It helps when you look away from the overparticipant and look at other members of the group. If the overparticipant continues to talk, you can say, "Now I'd like to hear from some others in the group." If the person persists, you may need to have a private conversation with the person away from the group. This is also true for a rude participant.

Demonstration and Return Demonstration

Demonstration is performing a practical activity to teach skills. It is also called the show-back method, which asks clients to verbalize and demonstrate what they learned from the nurse educator. This strategy requires that clients have an adequate sense of sight and manual dexterity. Demonstration is useful for cognitive and psychomotor learning (Bucher & Kotecki, 2014; Rankin et al., 2005). An example of the demonstration strategy is teaching child care skills to parents of an ill child. Demonstration can be done in person or by video. It involves a single client or small or large groups.

Begin by informing the clients about the learning objectives and the purpose of the demonstration. It is important for you to understand the procedure before attempting to perform it for others. Gather the essential equipment at the beginning of the demonstration to avoid fumbling and false starts when your clients are present. Be sure that all clients are positioned so they can see the demonstration and hear your comments. Provide a running commentary throughout the demonstration to focus the attention of clients on the relevant components. If possible, hold the demonstration in the actual place where clients will carry out the procedure. Clarify and repeat your demonstration as needed; then have each client return the demonstration. Be sure to define unfamiliar terms and have a discussion period after the demonstration to answer questions. The entire process should last no more than 15 to 20 minutes. If clients are learning motor skills, provide time for clients to practice as soon as possible after the demonstration. **Table 10-3** reviews the steps to follow when performing a demonstration.

TABLE 10-3

Demonstration Guidelines

Phase	Guidelines
Predemonstration phase	▪ Assess client needs. ▪ Identify learning objectives. ▪ Become familiar with the procedure. ▪ Choose the location. ▪ Gather essential equipment and supplies.
Demonstration phase	▪ Inform clients of objectives and purpose. ▪ Define unfamiliar terms. ▪ Be sure clients can see and hear. ▪ Give commentary about the procedure. ▪ Clarify and repeat as needed.
Postdemonstration phase	▪ Provide time for discussion and questions. ▪ Limit time to 20 minutes. ▪ Provide time for practice as soon as possible.

Team Teaching

Team teaching occurs when two or more teachers with different preparation, abilities, and skills cooperate and share with one another the responsibilities for planning, teaching, and evaluating client learning. In team teaching, teachers combine their strengths to make the presentation stronger. Refer to the guidelines for effective team teaching found in **Box 10-1**.

TEACHER-FACILITATED STRATEGIES

Teacher-facilitated strategies are a bridge between teacher-directed strategies and learner-directed strategies. The teacher takes the role of facilitator rather than directing the process of

BOX 10-1

Guidelines for Effective Team Teaching

1. All team members participate in formulation of the objectives.
2. All team members contribute to the specific planning of each member's presentation.
3. All team members should be conversant with the specific plans of the other team members.
4. All team members should carry on teaching functions in the presence of others whose roles might be to assist, observe client reactions, and offer constructive criticism in subsequent discussion.
5. All team members participate in periodic evaluation of the class.
6. Conflicts should be viewed as opportunities for growth. They should be addressed before the team encounters the clients.

learning. The strategies in this group include **group activities and teaching**, role-play, simulation, and web-based delivery of health education.

Group Activities and Teaching

Teaching in groups occurs when two or more clients work together on an activity. All approaches to group work have the distinguishing feature that clients are working together without direct intervention by the teacher at least some of the time (Killen, 2000). The principal reason to use this teaching strategy is to offer greater active learning opportunities. Cognitive and affective learning objectives are addressed through group activities. Community-based group interventions offer a cost-effective approach to developing a network of social support based on principles of social learning theory to affect change (Todd et al., 2010). Some examples of situations in which group work might be an appropriate teaching strategy are as follows (Killen, 2000):

- When you want to increase clients' depth of understanding of the course content by having them explore it and discuss their understanding with other learners
- When you want clients to exchange ideas and learn from one another by exploring issues from many perspectives, such as with parent education interventions
- When you want to enhance clients' motivation and increase their active participation in learning

You facilitate the group process by making the learning objectives clear and explaining the directions for the group activities. You should also develop guidelines to help clients participate productively in the group process. Some disadvantages of group activities and teaching are that clients who are accustomed to teacher-directed strategies may have difficulty changing their expectations. Some clients may find the activities a waste of time. Also, you may find it difficult to assess individual clients fairly when they have worked within a group. Group work requires preparation and an adequate room arrangement to accommodate the planned activities. High-ability learners may lose their incentive to learn when placed in mixed-ability groups (Curry, as cited in Killen, 2000).

Role-Play

In **role-play** clients act out their own situation or that of another person. Role-playing requires maturity, confidence, and flexibility on the part of clients. This strategy is effective in meeting cognitive, affective, and psychomotor learning objectives. It is most often used when clients need to examine their attitudes and behaviors, when they need to understand the viewpoints and attitudes of others, and when they need to practice carrying out ideas or decisions. For example, a parent may want to rehearse how he or she will talk to a son or daughter about drug use (Bucher & Kotecki, 2014).

Assertiveness training is an example of a situation in which role-playing works well. Your role is that of facilitator; you give instructions and provide time for feedback and evaluation. It is important to remember that this strategy takes extra time, and some clients may feel uncomfortable and inhibited with this method.

Simulation

Patient **simulation** is a frequently used teaching strategy in the health professions that allows learners to gain new knowledge and apply previously acquired knowledge using technology as a tool to complete the teaching and learning process. We present this strategy because it shows promise as a tool for client education. A patient simulator is a highly sophisticated, technologically advanced mannequin in adult, child, or infant size. These mannequins fully integrate with computer software and support the development of preplanned scenarios that mimic a wide variety of patient situations (Beyea & Kobokovich, 2004). Currently simulation has three categories of complexity: low, medium, and high fidelity. Static mannequins represent low-fidelity simulation and are used to learn skills that are performed as tasks that do not necessarily require complex thinking. Medium-fidelity mannequins provide a more realistic experience and allow the assessment of vital signs and heart and lung sounds. High-fidelity simulators incorporate vocal interaction to imitate actual clinical situations through realistic patient responses (Diener & Hobbs, 2012). A benefit of using simulation is that learning can occur without fear of harming a real person (Beyea & Kobokovich, 2004). Learners may be less likely to apply knowledge that led to failure in a similar situation, and they may be more likely to repeat behavior that was successful. An important part of the simulation experience requires the educator to create the simulation scenario and be familiar with the technology. The educator must also be knowledgeable about conducting the simulation and have a debriefing session afterward to integrate learning. Immediate feedback following a simulation experience is a key component for client learning (Diener & Hobbs, 2012). Competency can be evaluated using a rubric grading system.

Educators have just begun to explore the usefulness of patient simulation in health care. It is being used to develop, maintain, and evaluate nursing competencies so it is useful for teaching team members. Patient simulation provides a way to help health team members make transitions to actual patient care. This strategy enhances client safety while helping team members to develop clinical skills that reduce the potential for errors (Beyea & Kobokovich, 2004). The nurse as educator should recognize the potential of using multiple learning preferences to promote a positive learning environment. It is likely that this technology will eventually be used in client education to address specific learning needs. Your role as educator is to create the learning scenario, facilitate the learning experience, and conduct the debriefing. The disadvantages of this strategy are the costs of the mannequins, software, and support technology.

Simulated experiences do not always require high-fidelity equipment to be effective. It is possible to create lifelike virtual environments to help clients learn to maneuver safely and use trial and error to learn how to handle real-life situations. An example is rehabilitation programs that use mock city streets and avatars to help disabled clients learn to be independent (Steward-Gelinas & Romano, 2009).

Web-Based Delivery of Health Education

Technology is changing the way health education is provided to clients because 81% of American adults now use the Internet (Fox, 2013). Web-based delivery of health education is a cooperative activity between the teacher and clients. The teacher is responsible for preparing the health education materials, facilitating periodic interaction with clients, and measuring learning outcomes. Clients engage with the health education materials at their own pace, interact

BOX 10-2

Evidence-Based Nursing Practice

Moussa, M., Sherrod, D., & Choi, J. (2013). An e-health intervention for increasing diabetes knowledge in African Americans. *International Journal of Nursing Practice, 19*(Suppl. 3), 36-43.

Purpose: To determine if the eCare We Care e-health intervention program for diabetes improves diabetes knowledge among diabetic African American with low diabetes literacy.

Method: An equivalent comparison group with pre- and posttest design was used. Forty-six African American patients with type 1 or type 2 diabetes were randomly assigned to receive either the e-health intervention, eCare We Care or the paper-based, text-only diabetes tutorials. Four weekly sessions included: introduction to diabetes, eye complications, foot care, and meal planning.

Results: Significantly greater improvements in scores on the diabetes knowledge survey were demonstrated by the e-health intervention group than the comparison group except in week 1, introduction to diabetes. The e-health intervention group showed significant improvement in scores on diabetes knowledge for all 4 weeks.

with the teacher periodically, and participate in evaluation of their learning. Nurse educators are developing web-based health education programs such as those shown in **Box 10-2**. Other educators have found web-based education effective for parent training (Breitenstein & Gross, 2013) and nutrition education (Neuenschwander, Abbott, & Mobley, 2013). Web-based health education programs are flexible, convenient, easy for clients to use, and more efficient in terms of cost and time for nurse educators.

LEARNER-DIRECTED STRATEGIES

Learner-directed strategies focus on clients as the initiators and designers of the learning process. These strategies include the use of e-health interactive tutorials, games, self-directed instruction (**technology-assisted** strategies and program instruction), and peer counseling groups.

E-health Interactive Tutorials

Many websites are available for clients to learn about health. Last year 56% of American adults reported searching the Internet for health information (Fox, 2013). Many were looking for specific information for themselves or a family member. Excellent health tutorials can be found on MedlinePlus, a service of the U.S. National Library of Medicine, and the Mayo Clinic website. The abundance of web-based health information facilitates self-education for large segments of the population.

Many clients are health conscious and track health parameters and monitor their progress in achieving health-related goals. For example, 60% of adults track their weight, diet, or exercise routines, and 33% of adults track their blood pressure, blood sugar, headaches, or sleep patterns. To track this information, 21% use some form of technology, such as a spreadsheet, a website, a device, or an app (Fox & Duggan, 2013). Teaching clients to track their health parameters helps motivate them by monitoring their progress in achieving their health goals.

In addition, 91% of adults report owning some kind of cell phone, 56% report their phone operates on a smartphone platform (Smith, 2013), and 60% access the Internet on their phone (Duggan, 2013). Multiple health apps are available for the iOS and Android platforms. For example, apps are offered by health organizations (such as Kaiser Permanente and Aetna); the Centers for Disease Control and Prevention; and commercial vendors (such as Lose It! and Weight Watchers for weight loss, and Strava and Fitbit for activity and calorie tracking). In addition to smartphones, tablet ownership has increased. According to Zickuhr (2013), 34% of adults now own a tablet computer such as an iPad, Samsung Galaxy Tab, Google Nexus, or Kindle Fire, all with Internet access to health information.

Games

A **game** is an organized, active competition or contest engaged in by players who act individually or collectively as a team. The objective of a game is winning. Rules define the method of play and the criteria for winning. Instructional games use a body of knowledge or set of skills that must be drawn on as resources. Games provide a pleasurable structure for providing information, testing the level and application of skills and knowledge, and offering practice in simulated situations. They are often used with pediatric patients for preoperative teaching that introduces them to hospital procedures, the environment, and the staff before surgery (Rankin et al., 2005). During a game clients take a course of action and view the consequences in a nonthreatening way. Problem solving can be incorporated into the game. Clients should succeed, yet be challenged in the exercise. Gaming has become increasingly sophisticated. Players can adopt avatars that allow them to live in and interact with the virtual or game-based environment. Bauman (2012) believes that gaming can be used to enhance patient education. He describes a learning environment that has been specifically engineered to replicate actual existing environments that allow for "suspension of disbelief." This encourages clients to learn within a social context. Today's learners have an advanced degree of technical and digital literacy with expectations of how information should be disseminated, presented, and transferred. To engage these learners, consider virtual environments as a learning tool. Games may use flash cards, pictures, or computer applications. They may be modifications of popular games such as Bingo, Scrabble, or crossword puzzles. A benefit is that games can be inexpensive to purchase or make. Before introducing a game, evaluate its appropriateness for each specific client. An important aspect of games is that they should be entertaining because there is a clear relationship between learning and fun (Baranich & Currie, 2004).

Self-Directed Learning (Technology-Assisted Strategies and Programmed Instruction)

Self-directed learning is the process of clients engaging in learning activities that they, rather than the teacher, define (Schmidt, 2000). Clients who use this strategy identify their learning needs, formulate goals, identify resources, select and implement learning strategies, and evaluate learning outcomes. Clients demonstrate the initiative and consciously accept responsibility for their own learning. This involves searching out information and resources. Clients focus on information gathering. When used effectively, this strategy has many advantages over teaching-directed strategies. Some of the advantages of this strategy are as follows (Killen, 2000):

- It encourages clients to ask questions and investigate, discover, and create answers for themselves, rather than waiting for someone to provide answers for them.
- It enables clients to develop a deeper level of understanding of the subject than would be possible if other teaching strategies, such as lectures, were used.
- It shows clients that their existing knowledge is valuable and can form the basis for future learning.

Clients use this strategy when they access the Internet and resource centers in libraries and hospitals to find information about health and illness. Personal computer competency is a necessary skill for clients who want to search online. They need to be taught how to identify reliable and accurate information. Encourage them to use websites from the government, universities, or reputable medical or health associations.

Programmed instruction is another self-directed learning strategy that comes prepackaged from a book or computer software company. All the steps necessary to systematically learn the information are presented sequentially. The information is broken into small steps called frames. Clients are required to make frequent responses as they work through the information. Immediate feedback is given about the correctness or accuracy of responses. Programmed instruction is particularly useful for clients who are independent learners and who learn better when they have no time constraints.

Peer Counseling

Peer counseling is a self-help activity that is learner directed. The members of a peer counseling group provide support for one another by giving information, sharing experiences, and accepting and understanding each other. Peer counseling also provides useful suggestions about a problem or concern. Support groups help clients improve their coping skills, provide motivation to get further help, or take a more active role in their treatment. Participation gives clients hope and the knowledge that they are not alone. Peer counseling groups exist for clients with virtually all health-related problems, such as cancer, diabetes, and disabilities. You can refer clients or family members to a peer counseling group to help with follow-up care after initial treatment. Research indicates that attending support groups is beneficial. Studies indicate that clients who participate in support groups, in addition to their medical treatments, report less anxiety and depression and live longer than those who did not attend (Campbell, Phaneuf, & Deane, 2004). It is speculated that having the social support of others in the group boosts the immune system by reducing anxiety and psychological stress. Support groups take place in person, on the Internet, or by phone. Peer counseling helps clients connect with others who share the same problem. It helps people improve their coping skills, motivates them to get further help, or encourages them to take a more active role in treatment. Support groups give hope.

SELECTING THE RIGHT TEACHING STRATEGY

We now review important factors to take into consideration when selecting teaching strategies to implement the teaching plan. There are many factors to consider, but the most important is to choose a strategy based on what you want clients to be able to do as a result of your teaching.

To help you select appropriate teaching strategies, the following factors are briefly reviewed: the client's educational needs and learning objectives, characteristics of the client and the teacher, the learning context, and the content to be taught. **Figure 10-1** illustrates these factors.

The first factor to consider in selecting teaching strategies is to determine the client's educational needs and learning objectives. Carefully listen to what clients want to know and determine what they need to know. Determine their current health knowledge and if they have misinformation or a history of health problems. Consider readiness to learn, ability to learn, motivation to learn, and barriers to learning. Each of these impacts how you state the learning objectives and your choice of teaching strategies. Most teaching plans have learning objectives in each of the three domains: cognitive, affective, and psychomotor. When you are clear about the client's expected learning objectives, appropriate teaching strategies can be considered. When choosing teaching strategies, it is important to consider whether the client has the necessary abilities, including intellectual, emotional, and physical, to learn the skill (Onega & Devers, 2008). Keep in mind that the client's age, developmental stage, sensory impairments, educational background, nature of the illness, and culture should be taken into consideration. Teaching strategies should match the client's strengths and needs and help them reach the level

FIGURE 10-1

Selecting Teaching Strategies

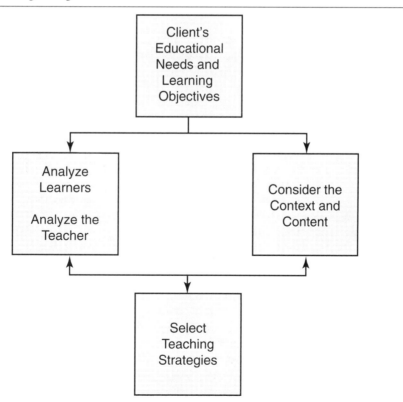

of mastery you set for them. For example, a client with hearing problems does not respond well to a lecture format. A client with poor vision does not learn through the use of demonstration. Also consider the time frame available for teaching. Choose a strategy that allows you to achieve the objectives within the available time frame. If you need to present information as quickly as possible to a group, a lecture is the best choice.

The second factor to consider in selecting teaching strategies is the characteristics of the client and the teacher. Knowing clients' learning styles is particularly important when selecting teaching strategies. Learning styles are characteristic ways that clients perceive, interact with, and respond to their environment. They are the clients' preferred mode of gaining knowledge. Styles are auditory (through hearing), visual (through seeing), kinesthetic (through the whole body), or a combination of these. As the teacher, you should also be aware of your preferred teaching and learning styles. Your clients will achieve learning objectives more quickly if your teaching style is compatible with their learning style. Based on this information about styles, choose from the teacher-directed, teacher-facilitated, or learner-directed approaches. Selecting among these approaches is more complex than just choosing one. A variety of teaching strategies helps to maintain clients' attention and increases achievement. For example, supplement the lecture with a group activity (Kindsvatter, Wilen, & Ishler, 1988).

The third factor to consider in selecting teaching strategies is the learning context. Learning context refers to the circumstances surrounding teaching and learning and includes both the physical and psychological environment. The physical environment may be the hospital, long-term care or assisted living facility, private home, school, worksite, or community. Consider the need for privacy and how much space is needed. Ensuring privacy and minimizing extraneous noises and interruptions are important.

If you are teaching a group of clients using the lecture strategy, assess the physical environment. Arrive at the location ahead of time to confirm that the environment is adequate and the seating is sufficient, comfortable, and arranged to support learning. Environmental factors are important and affect client learning (Dunn, 1983).

The psychological context is important and must support the teaching strategies. Be actively involved in creating the psychological context. The psychological environment should be relaxed, nonthreatening, and inviting to clients. Maintain a respectful, warm, and enthusiastic attitude.

The fourth factor to consider in selecting teaching strategies is the content to be learned. Content is the basic information you want to teach. You should choose teaching strategies to facilitate the efficient and successful accomplishment of learning objectives. Your task is to structure learning experiences that encourage clients to think in particular ways about the things you want them to learn (Killen, 2000). Choose the simplest, clearest, and most succinct manner of presentation (Onega & Devers, 2008). Focus first on must-know content and save nice-to-know information if time allows. Be aware of and take into consideration the client's current knowledge and previous experiences related to the content. Emphasize the relevance of the content to the client's age and lifestyle. You will find that certain content lends itself to specific strategies. For example, children will respond well to teaching strategies that permit them to participate actively. Would a lecture be an appropriate strategy to teach hand washing to a class of 6-year-olds? Probably not. A hands-on demonstration better meets the needs of this group.

Schedule and pace learning according to the clients' needs and abilities. When giving information, use simple but accurate words. Avoid using medical jargon and periodically check for understanding and interpretation of the information. Avoid information overload; repetition helps to emphasize important points. Using more than one teaching strategy enhances learning.

Written materials clarify information and give clients something to refer to at home. Verbal and written communication should complement each other (Falvo, 2011). Finally, remember that interactive teaching strategies are more effective than those that are not (Killen, 2000).

In **Table 10-4** we summarize the various teaching strategies, learning domains, and a description of the strategy.

Table 10-5 summarizes this information to help you choose strategies that fit the learning needs and objectives.

TABLE 10-4

Teaching Strategy, Learning Domain, and Description

Teaching Strategy	Learning Domain	Description
Teacher Directed		
Lecture	Cognitive	▪ Teacher-directed content and pace ▪ Feedback determined by teacher ▪ Use with individuals or groups ▪ Encourages retention of facts
One-on-one discussion	Affective Cognitive	▪ Teacher-directed content and pace ▪ Encourages participation by clients ▪ Permits reinforcement and repetition at client's level ▪ Supports introduction of sensitive subjects
Guest lecturer	Cognitive Affective	▪ Teacher-directed content and pace ▪ Modeling by an expert
Team teaching	Cognitive	▪ Teacher-directed content and pace ▪ Use with groups ▪ Encourages retention of facts ▪ Offers varied viewpoints ▪ Members present based on their teaching strengths
Lecture with discussion and questions and answers	Cognitive Affective	▪ Teacher controls most content and pace ▪ Teacher must know the content and be prepared to answer questions ▪ Use with individuals and groups ▪ Teacher confirms understanding by asking questions
Demonstration	Cognitive Psychomotor	▪ Teacher-directed content and pace ▪ Modeling of skills and behaviors by teacher ▪ Gives commentary with demonstration ▪ Use with individuals and groups ▪ Does not include hands-on experience
Demonstration, return demonstration, practice	Cognitive	▪ Teacher-facilitated content and pace ▪ Allows repetition and immediate feedback ▪ Includes hands-on experience

(continues)

TABLE 10-4

Teaching Strategy, Learning Domain, and Description (Continued)

Teaching Strategy	Learning Domain	Description
Teacher facilitated		
Group activities and discussion	Affective Cognitive	■ Teacher-facilitated content and pace ■ Clients obtain assistance from supportive group ■ Group members learn from one another
Role-playing	Affective Cognitive	■ Teacher-facilitated content and pace ■ Encourages expression of values, attitudes, and emotions ■ Assists in the development of communication skills ■ Involves active participation by client
Simulation	Cognitive Affective Psychomotor	■ Teacher facilitated ■ Use with individuals and groups ■ Group members learn from one another ■ Encourages expression of values, attitudes, and emotions
Learner directed		
Peer group	Affective Cognitive	■ Client directed ■ Support and modeling from clients with similar issues ■ Encourages expression of values, attitudes, and emotions
Games	Cognitive	■ Client directed ■ Permits reinforcement and repetition at client's level ■ Offers practice and application of skills ■ Fun, competitive ■ Individual or with a partner
Technology-assisted instruction	Cognitive	■ Client directed ■ Promotes individual initiative and responsibility for learning ■ Stimulates information gathering and questioning

TABLE 10-5

Teaching Strategies: Advantages and Disadvantages

Teaching Strategy	Advantages	Disadvantages
Lecture	■ Easy to organize ■ Predictable ■ Efficient ■ Good for large group ■ Allows teacher control	■ Lacks client feedback ■ Lacks client participation ■ Can create information overload

(continues)

TABLE 10-5

Teaching Strategies: Advantages and Disadvantages (Continued)

Teaching Strategy	Advantages	Disadvantages
One-on-one individual instruction	▪ Personalized attention ▪ Provides basic knowledge ▪ Immediate feedback ▪ Clients can share confidential information ▪ Adaptable to clients with low health literacy skills, physical impairments, or emotional difficulties ▪ Flexible and informal	▪ Lack of sharing with and support from other clients and family ▪ High cost in terms of staff time
Guest lecturer	▪ Source of motivation ▪ Role-modeling	▪ May not follow learning objectives ▪ May deviate from topic ▪ May exceed the allotted time
Lecture with discussion and questions and answers	▪ Continual feedback ▪ Attitude development and modification ▪ Picks up confusion and helps resolve difficulties ▪ Vehicle for clients to network with each other ▪ Active learning process ▪ Assess client's knowledge	▪ Teacher can dominate the discussion ▪ Takes more time ▪ Nonparticipant ▪ Overparticipant
Demonstration and return demonstration	▪ Activates many senses ▪ Clarifies the whys of principles ▪ Correlates theory with practice ▪ Commands interest	▪ Takes a lot of time ▪ Does not cover all aspects of cognitive learning ▪ Must have adequate sight and manual dexterity ▪ Practice is needed
Team teaching	▪ Enhances teaching by using competencies of more than one teacher ▪ Allows teachers to learn from each other ▪ Accentuates divergent points of view	▪ Lacks continuity and internal consistency ▪ Requires more planning time ▪ Makes group processing slower ▪ Forces teachers to give up autonomy

(continues)

TABLE 10-5

Teaching Strategies: Advantages and Disadvantages (Continued)

Teaching Strategy	Advantages	Disadvantages
Group activities and teaching	<ul><li>Increases depth of client understanding</li><li>Encourages clients to exchange ideas</li><li>Clients learn from one another</li><li>Increases active participation and learning</li></ul>	<ul><li>Clients may find activities a waste of time</li><li>Clients may have difficulties changing their expectations</li><li>Requires increased preparation time</li><li>Adequate room accommodations are needed</li><li>Some learners lose interest in mixed-ability groups</li></ul>
Role-play	<ul><li>Helps examine attitudes and behaviors</li><li>Helps examine viewpoints of others</li><li>A way to practice carrying out ideas or decisions</li></ul>	<ul><li>Requires maturity, confidence, and flexibility from clients</li><li>May embarrass clients</li><li>Requires some self-disclosure</li></ul>
Simulation	<ul><li>Mimics clinical situations</li><li>Requires hands-on participation</li><li>Learning without fear of harming a real person</li><li>Beneficial in evaluating competencies</li><li>Promotes the greatest transfer of learning</li></ul>	<ul><li>The cost of mannequins and support technology</li><li>Scenarios have to be developed and carried out</li><li>Time consuming</li><li>Requires teachers who are familiar with the technology and process</li></ul>
Games	<ul><li>Fun</li><li>Challenging</li><li>Competitive</li><li>Active learning</li><li>Encourages problem solving</li><li>Relatively inexpensive</li><li>Application of knowledge</li></ul>	<ul><li>Makes achievement of outcomes difficult to assess</li><li>Some clients may not like them</li><li>Cost and development of games</li><li>Not effective for presenting information</li></ul>
Computer-assisted learning and programmed instruction	<ul><li>Allows clients to go at their own pace</li><li>Repeat a section at will</li><li>Breaks material down into manageable increments</li><li>Saves teacher time</li></ul>	<ul><li>Depends on motivation of learner</li><li>Does not account for unplanned feedback, which can distract clients</li></ul>
Peer counseling	<ul><li>Clients provide support for each other</li><li>Useful suggestions about a problem or concern</li><li>Helps clients improve coping skills</li><li>Provides motivation</li><li>Gives hope</li></ul>	<ul><li>Challenge is for clients to stay in contact with the group</li><li>Information may be incorrect</li><li>May not be suitable for all clients</li></ul>

CASE EXAMPLE: MRS. ROSA LOPEZ

In this case example we are working on a teaching plan for Mrs. Rosa Lopez. We are ready to include teaching strategies. Refer to Table 10-5 to see how to include teaching strategies in the teaching plan. The cognitive objective, to have the client correctly verbally explain how excessive salt intake affects blood pressure to the nurse by memory, is to increase knowledge. Because our example is an individual client, we would use the strategy of one-to-one discussion to increase her knowledge about the relationship between excessive sodium intake and hypertension. Discussion is a useful strategy for assessing what the client already knows and building on that knowledge. We identify specific questions to ask her during the discussion in addition to answering her questions.

The affective objective seeks to have the client choose to limit the intake of sodium by working with the nurse to prepare a dietary plan for one week. We note that Mrs. Lopez is at the valuing level, so we would have her think through the steps of how she will prepare a dietary plan and put it into effect. This is important because she is not only cooking for herself, but also for her two children. We would have her identify any barriers she sees to preparing a dietary plan and explore how she can work around those barriers.

The psychomotor objective seeks to have the client demonstrate how to accurately obtain her own blood pressure reading and record it without any verbal guidance. We would use the strategy of demonstration and return demonstration to achieve this. We would have Mrs. Lopez read the directions as we demonstrate how to take the blood pressure using the client's own digital equipment. Mrs. Lopez would then perform a return demonstration using the equipment and record the findings using the procedural guidelines (**Table 10-6**).

Before instructing Mrs. Lopez, we would arrange a room to facilitate learning. The room should be quiet and have comfortable seating with a table nearby for the digital blood pressure equipment. The room should have a clearly visible place to hang the chart explaining hypertension and its relationship to excess sodium. The room should have the pamphlets and handouts we will give to Mrs. Lopez. It would be desirable to have a computer available with Internet access to demonstrate how to search online for information about low sodium diets that are

TABLE 10-6

Sample Teaching Plan for Mrs. Rosa Lopez

Learning Objectives	Content Outline	Strategies and Materials	Evaluation
1. The client will correctly verbally explain how excessive salt intake affects blood pressure to the nurse by memory (cognitive).	Greeting and Introduction Hypertension Definition Fluid retention Excess sodium intake Role in fluid retention Sodium and salt relationship Sodium is 40% of table salt (sodium chloride) Fluid retention and C-V system	Talking and discussion Answer questions Discussion question: What is the relationship between sodium intake and hypertension?	Verbal questions Paper and pencil test

(continues)

TABLE 10-6

Sample Teaching Plan for Mrs. Rosa Lopez (Continued)

Learning Objectives	Content Outline	Strategies and Materials	Evaluation
2. The client will choose to limit sodium intake by working with the nurse to prepare a dietary plan for one week (affective).	Four components of dietary plan: 1. Remove salt shaker from table. 2. Use no salt in cooking. 3. Avoid canned or processed foods that are high in sodium. 4. Use low-sodium seasonings, such as herbs and spices.	Talking and discussion Answer questions Read sample labels for sodium content Discussion question: How can you incorporate these changes into your meal planning and usual diet?	Short term: Attitude scale Long term: Implementation of dietary changes
3. The client will demonstrate how to accurately obtain her own blood pressure reading using home digital equipment without any verbal guidance (psychomotor).	Techniques for obtaining blood pressure: 1. Read equipment directions. 2. Locate brachial artery. 3. Place arm in cuff. 4. Inflate cuff. 5. Release air in cuff. 6. Record findings.	Talking and discussion Demonstrate procedure Have client demonstrate procedure, answer questions, develop record-keeping system	Blood pressure Checklist to obtain blood pressure Record of blood pressure readings

culturally appropriate. If a computer is not available and Mrs. Lopez is Internet savvy, we would walk her through the requisite search steps and suggest websites for her to investigate at home.

The digital blood pressure equipment would be placed on the table and be ready for use. Mrs. Lopez would read the directions as we demonstrate how to use the equipment. Then she would perform a return demonstration using the procedure checklist and record the findings. Mrs. Lopez would be given an opportunity to evaluate her own performance based on the guidelines in the checklist. When the procedure is performed correctly, we would compliment her and reinforce her newly acquired skills.

SUMMARY

Teaching strategies involve much more than transmitting information. It is the process of collaborating with clients to achieve learning objectives. This chapter emphasized the importance of engaging clients in the teaching and learning process so they can benefit from their experiences. The desired learning objectives, characteristics of the client, the learning context, and the content must guide the choice of teaching strategies. When selecting teaching strategies, there are teacher-directed, teacher-facilitated, and learner-directed strategies from which to choose. Base your choice on the learning objectives and desired outcomes for the teaching content. After you choose an overall strategy, select instructional materials to complement your teaching strategies. It is important to vary your approach to instruction, keeping in mind that clients have different needs, abilities, and learning preferences.

EXERCISES

Exercise I: Choosing Learning Strategies

Purpose: Distinguish among teacher-directed, teacher-facilitated, and learner-directed teaching strategies.
Directions:

1. Make a list of various topics that require client health education.
2. Review the list and describe whether each topic should be addressed through teacher-directed, teacher-facilitated, or learner-directed teaching strategies.
3. Identify the specific type of teacher-directed, teacher-facilitated, or learner-directed teaching strategy that you would use.
4. Discuss how each group member made his or her decision and why.

Exercise II: Develop and Implement a Teaching Plan

Purpose: Select appropriate strategies to teach a self-selected topic.
Directions:

1. Divide into groups of five or six members.
2. Identify topics about which each member wants to know more.
3. Each member should choose a topic and then independently do the following:
   a. Prepare two learning objectives using the ABCD method of writing objectives.
   b. Prepare a teaching plan that includes an outline of the content.
   c. Select suitable teaching strategies.
4. Have each member give a 15-minute presentation of his or her teaching plan.
5. Share and reflect on the experience of presenting your teaching plan.

REFERENCES

Baranich, K. L., & Currie, C. C. (2004, September/October). Using games to teach motivate and engage. *The Games Journal*, 6–9.

Bauman, E. B. (2012). *Game-based teaching and simulation in nursing and healthcare*. New York, NY: Springer.

Beyea, S., & Kobokovich, L. (2004). Human patient simulation: A teaching strategy. *AORN Journal, 8*(4), 738–742.

Breitenstein, S. M., & Gross, D. (2013). Web-based delivery of a preventive parent training intervention: A feasibility study. *Journal of Child and Adolescent Psychiatric Nursing, 26*, 149–157.

Browne, M. N., & Keeley, S. M. (2007). *Asking the right questions: A guide to critical thinking* (8th ed.). Upper Saddle River, NJ: Pearson Prentice Hall.

Bucher, L., & Kotecki, C. N. (2014). Patient and caregiver teaching. In S. L. Lewis, S. R. Dirksen, M. M. Heitkemper, & L. Bucher (Eds.), *Medical-surgical nursing: Assessment and management of clinical problems* (9th ed., pp. 47–60). St. Louis, MO: Elsevier Mosby.

Campbell, H. S., Phaneuf, M. R., & Deane, K. (2004). Cancer peer support programs: Do they work? *Patient Education and Counseling, 55*(1), 3–15.

deTornyay, R., & Thompson, M. A. (1982). Strategies for teaching nursing. New York, NY: John Wiley and Sons.

Diener, E., & Hobbs, N. (2012). Simulated care: Technology-mediated learning in twenty-first century nursing education. *Nursing Forum, 46*(1), 34–38.

Duggan, M. (2013). Cell phone activities 2013. Retrieved from http://www.pewinternet.org/Reports/2013/Cell-Activities.aspx

Dunn, R. (1983). Can students identify their own learning styles? *Educational Leadership*, *40*(5), 60–62.

Falvo, D. R. (2011). *Effective patient education: A guide to increased adherence* (4th ed.). Sudbury, MA: Jones & Bartlett Learning.

Fox, S. (2013). Health online 2013. Retrieved from http://www.pewinternet.org/Reports/2013/Health-online.aspx

Fox, S., & Duggan, M. (2013). Tracking for health. Retrieved from http://www.pewinternet.org/Reports/2013/Tracking-for-Health.aspx

Killen, R. (2000). *Effective teaching strategies: Lessons from research and practice* (4th ed.). Lansdowne, South Africa: Juta.

Kindsvatter, R., Wilen, W., & Ishler, M. (1988). *Dynamics of effective teaching*. New York, NY: Longman.

Lowenstein, A., & Reeder, J. A. (2009). Making learning stick. In A. Lowenstein, L. Foord-May, & J. C. Romano (Eds.), *Teaching strategies for health education and health promotion: Working with patients, families, and communities* (pp. 151–177). Sudbury, MA: Jones and Bartlett.

Moussa, M., Sherrod, D., & Choi, J. (2013). An e-health intervention for increasing diabetes knowledge in African Americans [Suppl. 3]. *International Journal of Nursing Practice*, *19*, 36–43.

Neuenschwander, L. M., Abbott, A., & Mobley, A. R. (2013). Comparison of a web-based vs in-person nutrition education program for low-income adults. *Journal of the Academy of Nutrition and Dietetics*, *113*(1), 120–126.

Onega, L. L., & Devers, E. (2008). Health education and group process. In M. Stanhope & J. Lancaster (Eds.), *Public health nursing: Population-centered health care in the community* (2nd ed., pp. 290–315). St. Louis, MO: Mosby Elsevier.

Rankin, S. H., Stallings, K. D., & London, F. (2005). *Patient education in health and illness* (5th ed.). Philadelphia, PA: Lippincott Williams & Wilkins.

Rogove, H. J., McArthur, D., Demaerschalk, B. M, & Vespa, P. M. (2012). Barriers to telemedicine: Survey of current users in acute care units. *Telemedicine and e-Health*, *18*(1), 48–53.

Romano, J. C. (2009). Teaching on the fly. In A. F. Lowenstein, L. Foord-May, & J. C. Romano (Eds.), *Teaching strategies for health education and health promotion: Working with patients, families, and communities* (pp. 139–150). Sudbury, MA: Jones and Bartlett.

Schmidt, H. G. (2000). Assumptions underlying self directed learning may be false. *Medical Education*, *34*(4), 243–245.

Smith, A. (2013). Smartphone ownership 2013. Retrieved from http://www.pewinternet.org/Reports/2013/Smartphone-Ownership-2013.aspx

Steward-Gelinas, D., & Romano, J. (2009). Individualized instruction. In A. Lowenstein, L. Foord-May, & J. C. Romano (Eds.), *Teaching strategies for health education and health promotion: Working with patients, families, and communities* (pp. 117–128). Sudbury, MA: Jones and Bartlett.

Tamura-Lis, W. (2013). Teach-back for quality education and patient safety. *Urologic Nursing*, *33*(6), 267–271.

Todd, S., Bromely, J., Ioannou, K., Harrison, J., Mellor, C., Taylor, E., & Crabtree, E. (2010). Using group-based parent training interventions with parents of children with disabilities: A description of process, content and outcomes in clinical practice. *Child and Adolescent Mental Health*, *15*(3), 171–175.

Webster's All-in-One Dictionary & Thesaurus (2nd ed.). (2013). Springfield, MA: Federal Street Press.

Woodring, B. C., & Woodring, R. C. (2007). Lecture is not a four-letter word. In M. J. Bradshaw & A. J. Lowenstein (Eds.), *Innovative teaching strategies in nursing and related health professions* (4th ed., pp. 109–130). Sudbury, MA: Jones and Bartlett.

Zickuhr, K. (2013). Tablet ownership 2013. Retrieved from http://www.pewinternet.org/Reports/2013/Tablet-Ownership-2013.aspx

11

Instructional Materials

OBJECTIVES

Upon completion of this chapter, you will be able to do the following:

- State at least two purposes of instructional materials.
- Describe the importance of health literacy in evaluating instructional materials.
- Evaluate the readability and appropriateness of selected health education materials.
- Identify reliable sources for obtaining health-related pamphlets and brochures.
- List five criteria for evaluating the accuracy and reliability of websites.
- Critique the advantages and disadvantages of at least 10 types of media.

KEY TERMS

35 mm slides	education pathways	posters
analogy	email	PowerPoint slides
appropriateness	flip charts	readability
audiocassettes	health literacy	replica
brochures	instructional handouts	storyboard
bulletin boards	Internet	symbol
computer-assisted	LCD projector	transparencies
instruction	objects and models	videotapes
digital camera	overhead projector	whiteboards/chalkboards
DVD audio	pamphlets	World Wide Web
DVD video	photographs	

INTRODUCTION

In this chapter we examine a number of instructional materials that help you supplement the teaching strategies to achieve the learning objectives.

Instructional materials are the actual matter or substance physically manipulated with the aim of promoting client learning. These materials are used by the teacher and the client. Instructional materials provide ways to use all senses to enhance learning. Some materials allow for the physical contact that kinesthetic learners need, whereas others enhance and reinforce cognitive knowledge. Still other materials invite emotional involvement, which is crucial for changing attitudes.

Instructional materials serve several purposes (Pohl, 1981). These purposes include extending the client's sensory experience, introducing variety into the teaching and learning process, giving meaning to abstractions, and making otherwise complicated explanations understandable. Pohl identified a number of factors to consider when determining which instructional materials to use. These factors include assessment of the topic being presented, the clients who are being addressed, and the available materials.

It is important to emphasize that instructional materials do not take the place of an effective teacher. Instructional materials enrich the learning experience of clients if they are appropriate to the learning objectives. Instructional materials must be carefully examined, evaluated, and selected on the basis of how they supplement the learning objectives to achieve the educational outcomes. The clinical judgment of nurses as educators is essential in this process.

Although instructional materials are available from a number of different sources, they may not be more effective than materials you develop yourself. By tapping into your creativity, you can develop materials that are specific to the health concerns of clients who are served by your employer or healthcare institution.

In this chapter we discuss health literacy and examples of instructional materials such as print media, multimedia, and the Internet and the World Wide Web (Web). There are a variety of instructional materials available, and each has advantages and disadvantages for any specific teaching and learning situation. We discuss these advantages and disadvantages of selected materials along with their purposes and helpful hints for using them.

HEALTH LITERACY

Health literacy is receiving increased attention by health professionals, and it has particular importance for nurses as educators. It is an important consideration in selecting instructional materials, especially printed materials given to clients in the form of pamphlets and handouts, and information downloaded from the Internet. To benefit from instructional materials, clients must be health literate, and nurse educators must be capable of assessing literacy and suitability of materials.

Literacy is defined as the ability to read and write (Webster's, 2013). Health literacy expands that definition by its focus on the client's abilities in the healthcare environment. The Patient Protection and Affordable Care Act (PPACA), Title V, defines health literacy as the degree to which an individual has the capacity to obtain, communicate, process, and understand basic health information and services to make appropriate health decisions (2010). The health literacy goal (HC/HIT-1) of Healthy People 2020 is to "improve the health literacy of the population." One of its subgoals (HC/HIT-1-1) is to "increase the proportion of persons who report their health care provider always gave them easy-to-understand instructions about what to do to take care of their illness or health condition" (HealthyPeople.gov, 2014).

A quick and accurate assessment tool called the Newest Vital Sign can determine a client's ability to read and apply information from a nutrition label. According to the National Assessment of Adult Literacy, in the United States in 2003, approximately 22% (47 million) of the population had basic health literacy skills and 14% (30 million) had below basic skills (National Center for Education Statistics [NCES], 2003). Combined, these groups represent 36% (77 million) of the population. Individuals in these groups have difficulty processing and understanding basic health information and services and making appropriate health decisions. According to Clancy (2008), those with basic or below basic health literacy skills have now increased to almost 90 million. This latter figure is important and indicates a substantial health literacy problem that affects you in preparing teaching plans.

Health literacy is required to understand how to take medications, follow a treatment regimen, follow directions to prepare for diagnostic examinations, and respond to radio and television public warnings about recalls of unhealthful products, equipment, and drugs. Health literacy is required for communicating with healthcare providers, describing symptoms, and understanding treatment recommendations. It is also required to critically evaluate newspaper and magazine advertisements and determine the credibility of information found on the Internet. It involves being able to fill out complex forms, understand insurance coverage, and navigate the healthcare system. It is fundamental to making informed decisions about promoting, retaining, and restoring health.

Low health literacy is observed across the demographic spectrum. However, it is more often seen in clients aged 65 years and older, clients with limited English-speaking skills, racial and ethnic minorities, low-income groups, and clients who have not attended or completed high school (Mooney & Prins, 2013; NCES, 2003). It is easy to assume that clients who appear to be middle class, well groomed, and articulate are also health literate, but this is not always the case (Doak, Doak, & Root, 1996). Even clients who are well educated can have difficulty understanding health-related information. Consider a diabetic client who does not understand how to use food exchanges or a client on a fat-restricted diet who thinks pork is a white meat and is therefore low in fat.

Low health literacy has a financial impact. Clients with low literacy skills have poorer health outcomes and adhere less to medical recommendations than those with higher literacy skills. They have higher rates of hospitalization and use emergency services more, perhaps attributed to using fewer preventive and treatment services (Levy & Royne, 2009). The ramifications of low health literacy are particularly important in the treatment of clients with chronic illnesses, who must manage their own health and implement lifestyle changes for success (Seligman et al., 2007).

TYPES OF INSTRUCTIONAL MATERIALS

We are fortunate today to have an abundance of instructional materials to facilitate learning that appeal to all learning styles: visual, auditory, and kinesthetic. However, it is important to remember that they cannot substitute for good teaching. Instructional materials enrich and supplement the teaching and learning process. They do not replace the teacher. They help clients understand concepts and retain information when teachers use a variety of materials. Illustrations quickly bring to life concepts that may take many words to describe. A teacher is essential to assess client needs, develop the teaching plan, provide guidance, answer questions, and evaluate teaching effectiveness. Take-home handouts remind clients about your teaching.

In selecting instructional materials, you are constrained by what is available where you are employed. Make use of what your employer has available and, if possible, recommend the purchase of new materials and equipment. Be sure the materials are current. Clients may be turned off by visual images of out-of-date clothing, hairstyles, and equipment, and they may consider the information irrelevant to their situation (Falvo, 2011). If what you need is not available, we encourage you to adapt and be creative. Is there some way to improvise or create illustrations? Healthcare institutions are cost conscious, and your employer may appreciate your creativity. In this section we discuss printed materials, multimedia, and the Internet and World Wide Web.

PRINTED MATERIALS

Printed material is the most widely used source of information given to clients. Examples of common printed materials include pamphlets, brochures, instructional handouts, and booklets. It is common for clients participating in health education classes to expect handouts and to leave with reading material that supplements and enhances their learning. Falvo (2011) recommends having a good supply of written materials on hand for the common health problems seen in clients who are served by your employer or healthcare institution.

There are multiple sources of printed material. Every voluntary healthcare organization, such as the American Cancer Society, is more than happy to supply you with printed materials. This is also true for local, state, and federal governments, depending on the type of information you request. Pharmaceutical firms and commercial sources also have printed materials that you can distribute to clients. When you cannot find exactly what you want from these sources, consider preparing your own materials.

All printed materials are not equal. They need to be evaluated carefully to determine which ones best meet your purposes. You may want to have a committee help you evaluate the printed materials distributed to clients. Things to consider include the philosophy of your department, healthcare institution, or physicians; the clients and their needs; the availability of appropriate materials; and cost.

If you decide to prepare your own materials, consider the amount of time and cost it requires. You need to conceptualize and write the copy, then arrange for artistic design, layout, printing, and duplicating the material. This process can be lengthy and costly, and the effort needs to be worthwhile (Falvo, 2011). It may be not as cost effective to prepare your own materials as it may first seem.

Selecting Printed Materials

As the educator, you are responsible for providing clients with understandable health information (Wood, Kettinger, & Lessick, 2007). Clients vary greatly in their ability to read and translate symbols on a piece of paper into information that is meaningful to them. You may be tempted to depend on printed materials to convey information to clients. This is especially true when you feel pressed for time and depend on reading materials to enhance the client's knowledge regarding the topic at hand. Brochures, written instructions, and consent forms are often sources of information. Many of them are written above the reading level of the average adult client, which is eighth-grade level (Winslow, 2001).

The essential issues in evaluating written materials are readability and appropriateness (Hasselkus, 2009). It is your responsibility to review all written materials before sharing them with clients. Select materials that are at a suitable reading level for clients and are appropriate to the learning objectives.

Readability

Readability of written materials refers to the language level (expressed in terms of grade level), layout, and design (Hasselkus, 2009). Readability involves examining the number of syllables in each word and the number of words in each sentence. Words with many syllables require a higher level of reading skill than words with fewer syllables. Short sentences are easier to read than long sentences.

In selecting written materials, consider the client's background and the purpose of the materials. The client's background and educational level provide clues to reading ability; however, most clients read at three to five grade levels below their educational attainment (Doak et al., 1996). Observe the reading materials in the client's room. If none are available, ask the client what his or her favorite reading materials are. Listen to the vocabulary clients use. How simple or complex are the individual words? If the client is employed, try to determine how much reading is required on the job. Answering these questions provides a quick overview of reading ability.

Next consider the purpose of the written materials. What information does the client need that the material is expected to provide? What must the material communicate? Is the purpose to supplement your teaching, fill in gaps that you did not have time to explain, or expand on a topic of interest? Is the material a set of instructions on how to do a procedure? Is the material designed to encourage or inspire?

Online software programs can quickly calculate readability. Word processing software evaluates a selected passage according to the formula chosen by the manufacturer. The SMOG Readability Formula and WordsCount Analytics are two such services. The SMOG Calculator estimates the years of education needed to understand a piece of writing (McLaughlin, 1969). WordsCount Analytics provides similar information plus additional readability services. The readability level of any written material can be determined by submitting a representative passage on either website and having it evaluated. The following are websites that will help you evaluate the readability of written materials. The Suitability Assessment of Materials (SAM) site assesses not only readability, but also usability and suitability elements:

- Iowa Department of Public Health Fry Readability Graph: http://www.idph.state.ia.us/search/search.aspx?as_q=readability&searchtype=advanced
- Harry McLaughlin SMOG Calculator: http://www.harrymclaughlin.com/SMOG.htm
- WordsCount: http://www.wordscount.info/
- SAM (Suitability Assessment of Materials): http://www.beginningsguides.com/upload/sam-for-beginnings.pdf

When the written material is beyond the reading ability of the client, comprehension is decreased and recall is sketchy and inaccurate. The client also may interpret the information differently than what was intended. As a result, the client's motivation to seek further instruction from written sources may be reduced. One way to assess a client's ability to make use of a pamphlet is to have him or her look it over and ask questions about the content. For example, you could say, "I want to give you a pamphlet that explains things clearly. Will you look at this and tell me if it appeals to you?"

Another way is to ask the client to read a pamphlet and report its comprehensibility. For example, you could say, "Tell me what this pamphlet says to you. Is it boring? Confusing?"

Look carefully at the client while he or she is reading. Does the client show signs of tension? Watch the client's eyes. Do his or her eyes move across and down the page in a systematic manner? These answers provide clues to both readability and appropriateness.

Appropriateness

The **appropriateness** of written materials focuses on the information itself. Is it suitable given the client's health problem and circumstances? Does the physician want the client to have this information? Is the information appropriate to the client's ethnic and cultural values and beliefs (Hasselkus, 2009)? Written materials should be age, gender, and culturally appropriate and respectful (Zarcadoolas, Pleasant, & Greer, 2006). Whatever written materials are provided, it is important to assess the client's ability to understand and use the information to improve health and well-being.

Generational differences may influence the type of printed material you give to clients. Something that a young person finds captivating may be insulting to an older client. Whatever the case, you do not want to offend clients by distributing materials that they consider beneath their intelligence.

In the acute care setting, many clients who need instruction are affected by medications they are receiving. It is not unusual for certain drug-induced states and other postsurgical or disease conditions to blur vision and slow intellectual processing. Visual acuity may be a problem, and it may be affected by mundane problems, such as the need to put on eyeglasses. Fear and anxiety can reduce reading ability or even make it impossible for the client to grasp the meaning of printed words. Selecting an appropriate time to discuss and share written materials is as important as selecting appropriate materials. Avoid meal times and visiting hours.

Pamphlets and Brochures

Pamphlets and **brochures** are attractive, readily available, and often free. You can use them before, during, or after a presentation. Clients can hold them and use them to study and learn at their own pace so they can exercise more control over the learning experience. Voluntary health organizations are a rich source of printed materials, and many are provided in both English and Spanish. Examples include the American Cancer Society, the American Heart Association, and the American Lung Association. Virtually every disease that affects a specific population is served by an organization that provides public education and written materials.

Some websites offer print-on-demand health information that is current and cost effective. For example, health information is available from The Joint Commission through the Speak

Up initiative (The Joint Commission, 2009). These brochures can be downloaded and used as needed. Their brochures are not copyrighted; however, The Joint Commission requires that it be credited as the source of the material. The topics are varied; examples include medication safety, preventing infection, pain management, and preventing medical mistakes.

It is important to give careful consideration to the timing of pamphlet distribution if you are using them in a class. If the pamphlets contain the actual information you wish to discuss, use them as advance organizers and a substitute for note taking. If you decide they are distracting, keep them out of sight until the presentation is completed.

Instructional Handouts and Patient Education Pathways

Instructional handouts refer to information specifically prepared for a client or group of clients served by a specific physician or healthcare institution or agency. They typically cover preparation for diagnostic procedures, following treatment regimens, and follow-up care after a treatment or a procedure. If you are preparing these handouts, you need to have a final draft approved by the physician or your employer. Follow the guidelines for writing instructional materials. Place this information on video or audio media for clients who have low health literacy (Roberts, 2008).

Patient **education pathways** are instructional tools that facilitate client education. They inform clients about what to expect in their course of treatment and their role in recovery and restoration of health, which are both major goals of the pathways. When they are shared with clients, pathways are personal educational tools that encourage participation in self-care routines and symptom management. Pathways assume that clients who are well informed and knowledgeable about their treatment are more likely to adhere to the treatment plan. The information provided in the pathways is comprehensive, consistent, and specific to the treatment a client is undergoing. It covers every aspect in the course of treatment; for example, diet, tests, treatments, medications, activities, education, and discharge planning. Patient education pathways are similar to the multidisciplinary critical pathway tools used to manage a client's hospital stay (Clarke, 2002).

Bulletin Boards

Bulletin boards supplement health education. Depending on clients' needs and health topics of interest, bulletin boards can display a variety of information. For example, they can highlight accident prevention, advertise national health awareness months, and announce health fairs. Specific health-related topics are often of interest, such as the nature of heart disease, cancer, and diabetes. Information can be related to the season of the year, such as preventing the common cold and flu during the fall months and healthful eating during holidays. Not only do bulletin boards supplement health education, but they also reinforce information you have taught. The display reminds clients of the important points of your presentation.

Bulletin boards are a type of informal learning that allows clients to learn at their own pace. Place them in conspicuous spots that are suitable for browsing. Keep in mind that pausing and glancing are the usual activities of browsers. Information that is deep or wordy will languish unread or may disappear if someone wishes to really delve into it. High-traffic areas are good places for bulletin boards, such as waiting rooms (hospital, clinic, and office), hallways, and cafeterias. If the bulletin board is to be read by children or clients in wheelchairs, lower the height of the board from the normal erect adult's eye-level position.

Bulletin boards display pictures, photographs, tables, graphs, and cartoons as well as text information. The content, text, and graphics should be simple, clear, and at a reading level appropriate for the target population. Determine the central message for the bulletin board and then organize the content to support that message. Organizers, such as headings, should be clearly marked and easy to differentiate from the body of the text.

The font used for headings should be larger than the font for text. The lines of the text should be short enough to scan with sufficient space to separate distinct messages. Paragraph and sentence length should be short and easy to read. Block style fonts, such as Times New Roman, Gothic, and Verdana, are easier to read than script fonts or italics, which resemble handwriting. Use both upper- and lowercase lettering. Avoid using all capital letters because they are difficult to read (Thomas, 2007). They are also perceived as shouting.

Avoid cluttering the board with too much text or graphs and tables. Too much information, and information that is too complex, are difficult for clients to quickly grasp. Display just the essential information and avoid extraneous information that detracts from your message. The display and text should be current and updated as necessary.

Although bright, primary colors attract children, these colors are difficult for older adults to read. Age-related changes in the eyes make it difficult for older adults to discriminate shades of blue, green, and violet. The warm colors of red, orange, and yellow are easier for older adults to see (Linton, 2007). Make the background of the bulletin board a light color to avoid the glare that occurs with white backgrounds. Dark-colored text on a light-colored background is easier for older adults and others to read (Thomas, 2007).

If you have handouts or pamphlets to distribute that reinforce the message on the bulletin board, place them in a folder attached to a lower corner of the board. If the handouts or pamphlets are too bulky or heavy, consider placing a small table next to the bulletin board.

Posters

Many of the suggestions pertaining to bulletin boards also apply to the preparation of posters. **Posters** are another effective way to communicate health information. They can accompany a presentation or be located in conspicuous places for viewing. Posters are easy to make and also commercially available. They are especially useful for limited periods of time to communicate a specific message such as a health month, a workshop announcement, or safety precautions. If posters remain in place too long or are overused, they lose their ability to attract attention and can lead to boredom (Pittman, 2009). Posters are low cost, portable, and allow for self-paced learning.

Posters should use only key words to communicate a message, rather than complete sentences. Use bullets or list the essential information by numbers for brevity. If you use a picture, figure, or cartoon, it should be clear and large enough to be understood immediately. Illustrations should appeal to the age, gender, socioeconomic status, and cultural characteristics of clients. Sensitivity and delicacy are important, especially if you inject humor.

As with bulletin boards, use appropriate colors and block-style fonts rather than script fonts for ease of reading. If your clients are older, use large, bold fonts. If you are using a poster with a presentation, remember the 6-W formula. It means that the last row of the audience should be no farther from the poster than six times the width of the poster. For example, if the poster is 2 feet wide, the last row of viewers should be no farther than 12 feet from the poster. For a larger audience, transform the poster into a transparency, slide, or PowerPoint slide.

Flip Charts

A **flip chart** is versatile because it is portable and is used like a whiteboard or chalkboard. Creative uses of flip charts include composing instantaneous posters, gathering and preserving audience contributions, and having clients write out their thoughts. A flip chart combines the advantages of posters and whiteboards or chalkboards. You can plan ahead and prepare your charts, or you can have the blank pages available while teaching for spontaneous use.

If you prepare the flip chart ahead of time, take the time you need to prepare exactly what you want: written information, pictures, cartoons, or a combination thereof. A flip chart also is used as an advance organizer because it allows you to write your outline and have the clients follow along as you move through the presentation.

If you plan to use a flip chart spontaneously as you teach, have a good supply of colorful pens on hand. Spontaneous use is appropriate when you want to elicit responses from the audience or when you want your clients to work in small groups and write their contributions down to be shared later with a larger group. If you use this method, hang the finished charts around the room. When you do this, clients feel like valued contributors to the teaching and learning process. Your flip charts also can be saved for future use. The material you have collected can be transcribed and sent to all the participants. The major disadvantage to using a flip chart is you must have at least some artistic talent to be effective. Also your audience must be small enough so everyone can see the flip chart.

Whiteboards or Chalkboards

A **whiteboard** or **chalkboard** is available in most classroom settings. It is valuable for making a spontaneous drawing, diagram, or illustration. You can add to or take away from the drawing while using it to explain the meaning or purpose of the topic under discussion. A whiteboard or chalkboard is an excellent device for involving clients. To promote contributions, ask a question and then write down the responses from the clients. Most individuals find it reinforcing to see their words written on the board. The best questions to ask first are those to which everyone can respond, such as questions about personal experience. For example you can ask, "How can you tell when you are stressed out? What do you do, or what have you seen others do, when they are stressed out?"

The whiteboard or chalkboard also helps with organizing information. You can link ideas in a circle or list problems on one side and solutions on the other. The board also allows you to compare and contrast various points of view or to organize contributions from the audience into whatever schema you choose. Whenever possible, transfer complicated ideas to a handout that clients can refer to during your presentation.

When using the whiteboard or chalkboard, determine if your cursive writing is more legible than your printing, and use the more readable style. Write a brief notation on the board; then step aside and face the audience. This allows you to maintain contact with your clients and receive their feedback on the clarity of your point. By stepping aside you also allow clients to copy the message, which means they can integrate both visual and auditory stimuli. Stepping aside also keeps you from becoming so involved with your creation on the board that you start talking to the board instead of the clients.

Preparing Your Own Written Materials

Consider preparing your own written materials if nothing suitable is available. When preparing your own, it is important to write at the sixth-grade reading level or lower to benefit clients (Winslow, 2001). Do this by shortening words with multiple syllables, eliminating extraneous words, and simplifying sentence structure. Use everyday, plain language consistent with the client's vocabulary; avoid using medical jargon that clouds the health message.

Plain Language is a U.S. government initiative emphasized by President Clinton in 1998 when he issued an executive memo requiring federal agencies to write in plain language. It requires written materials to be understandable the first time a person reads or hears it so they can (1) find what they need, (2) understand what they find, and (3) use what they find to meet their needs. Plain language is grammatically correct with accurate word usage and complete sentence structure. It is clear writing that tells clients exactly what they need to know without using unnecessary words. Plain language makes information more informative and easier for clients to understand.

Begin preparing your own teaching materials by assessing the clients carefully. Know who you are writing for and what their needs are. Consider involving selected members of your target audience as a focus group. Also involve selected healthcare providers who plan to use the material. There may be a difference between what the healthcare providers think is most important for clients to know and what the clients actually want to know.

After you identify the content to communicate, focus on the two to three most important points. Begin developing the most important point first, and then develop the others one at a time. Do not overload clients with too much information; decide what is essential and focus on that. If you must use technical terms such as the names of diagnostic procedures, be sure to define exactly what you mean. Keep the message and examples concrete because they are easier for clients to understand. Abstract messages may be difficult to grasp for those with low health literacy (Seligman et al., 2007; Zarcadoolas et al., 2006). It is important that your information is accurate and updated as necessary. As your focus groups (clients and providers) review your material, make changes based on their feedback.

The layout and presentation of your material are important (Pittman, 2009). Consider the general appearance of the text and margins. The text should be limited so the material does not appear crowded, and the margins should be ample. The material should have a clear title that indicates its purpose. Use headings, subheadings, and bullets to present the information in a logical and organized format. Using different fonts, bold fonts, highlighting, bullets, and numbers make the text more readable. Add pictures, illustrations, and diagrams to illustrate important points. They often communicate health messages more effectively than text (Bryan, 2008). Be sure the material is appropriate for the age, gender, and culture of your target audience. Color always livens up a message if it is cost effective to add it. The goal in preparing your own written material is to simplify the message while communicating essential health information. **Box 11-1** lists guidelines for writing your own instructional materials.

BOX 11-1

Guidelines for Writing Instructional Materials

Planning:
- Identify the purpose of the materials.
- Identify the most important points to communicate (two or three).
- Assess the characteristics and needs of the target audience.
- Involve selected members of your target audience as a focus group.
- Involve selected healthcare providers who will use the materials.

Organizing:
- Group like information together.
- Develop each point or group one at a time.
- Keep paragraphs brief.

Writing:
- Use short, simple sentences that express only one idea.
- Use plain language and familiar words with only one or two syllables.
- Be consistent in how you define and use words.
- Avoid medical jargon, technical terms, abbreviations, and acronyms.
- Write at the fourth- to sixth-grade reading level.
- Use conversational style with an active voice.
- Use concrete, not abstract, examples.
- Avoid extraneous words.
- Update the material as necessary to maintain currency and relevance.

Appearance and layout:
- Add pictures, illustrations, and colors that support the message.
- Use pictures and illustrations that are appropriate to the age, gender, and culture of the clients.
- Use attractive spacing and layout with generous white space.
- Use 12-point type for text.
- Use larger type, bold, or underlines to separate headings and subheadings.
- Use bold fonts; avoid script fonts and italics.
- Use highlighting, bullets, and numbers as appropriate.
- Use upper- and lowercase lettering; avoid all caps.

Evaluating Printed Materials

Printed information must be accurate and from a reliable source. This is important for all printed materials, whether in the form of pamphlets, brochures, or instructional handouts. If the purpose of the printed material is to assist clients with treatment choices about a health problem, you can use the DISCERN, an online tool to evaluate the quality of the printed health care information. It was a project funded from 1996-97 by the British Library and the NHS Executive Research and Development Programme and is available to health professionals. Nurses as educators can use the tool to evaluate written materials they develop or to evaluate printed materials already available. The tool rates, from 1 to 5, printed material in three areas: the reliability of the material, the specific details of the information about treatment choices, and an overall quality rating of the printed material.

Always consider the source of the printed materials. Many health and disease-related brochures that healthcare institutions or agencies use are prepared by voluntary healthcare organizations. Examples of reputable voluntary healthcare organizations are the March of Dimes and the American Heart Association. These are accurate and reliable sources of information.

Instructional handouts are usually prepared by a committee in the healthcare institution or by a physician who has approved the content. These are also accurate and reliable sources. In contrast, newspaper and magazine advertisements are less reliable, although they are not necessarily inaccurate. Each source must be evaluated on its own merits.

MULTIMEDIA

Video Media

Videotapes and **DVDs** are excellent instructional tools. Both show action images with sound; however, DVDs are replacing videotapes in popularity and usage. Regardless of format, video is the closest substitute to the actual experience because it stimulates both hearing and sight. Videos evoke imagery and intense emotion because they invite clients to experience the scenes along with the actors. Visual images are more likely to be remembered than information clients read or hear (Doak et al., 1996).

Videos allow clients to observe action without being direct participants, which is consistent with Bandura's social cognitive theory (1986, 2001) of how people learn. The actor models the desirable behavior; for example, child-rearing practices or performing a procedure. Videos are also excellent for generating an affective response in the audience and for promoting discussion. Videos can be stopped to discuss a particular action or generate problem-solving options from the audience. They help clients anticipate experiences for which they must prepare, such as childbirth. Visual images are also effective with non-English-speaking clients.

Videos are easy to store and transport. If you are making a presentation at another location, most facilities have a videocassette recorder (VCR) or DVD player and television monitor. You need to confirm this in case you need to bring your own equipment. Many health departments and community health organizations will lend videotapes and DVDs for presentations. Contact the appropriate agency to determine what is available and reserve the materials.

Consider making your own video recordings; they are relatively easy to make if you have access to the requisite equipment. If you are dissatisfied with the results, you can easily remake it. Using a video camera to record a client's performance, such as a team member performing a procedure, is an excellent teaching tool. Clients can then watch the performance and receive immediate and accurate feedback as they attempt to learn a particular procedure. If you make a video recording, keep it to 8 minutes or less because clients tend to lose interest if it is longer. If the video needs to be longer, stop it periodically and discuss it to keep the clients' attention. Videos that tell captivating stories or have multiple scene changes hold clients' interest for longer periods (Doak et al., 1996).

As with any learning experience, videos are most valuable if they are prefaced by advance organizers. An introduction includes a title, the length of the video, a synopsis of the message or story, and what you expect clients to gain from the viewing. It is helpful to tell clients specifically what they should notice and what they are expected to do with the experience afterward, such as discuss the plot or perform the procedures. If unfamiliar words are used, introduce them beforehand. Put the words on a transparency, handout, or a whiteboard or chalkboard before the video is shown.

Audio Media

Audiocassettes, DVDs, and CDs are formats for recording sound. These formats are widely available, as are their respective players. Audio messages are also supported by other portable media players, such as the iPod and other MP3 players. Audio media are especially useful when clients must learn an auditory skill, such as teaching the parents of an asthmatic child to recognize various breath sounds. By listening to different types of breathing, parents can learn which types of breathing require an emergency response and which types can be improved with routine treatment.

Audio media are useful for hearing directions when the client cannot look at the speaker. Consider a client who is lying prone while following directions for exercise or relaxation. Many people find it easier to concentrate when their eyes are closed or when they listen to soothing music or directions for creating healing images. Clients can make an audiocassette tape of their favorite therapeutic music or download therapeutic music onto an iPod or other MP3 player (Pittman, 2009).

In these days of early discharge, clients often leave the hospital before they or their families are confident of the procedures they must perform at home. Audio recording of health instructions for use after discharge reminds clients of the information they were taught. For example, by recording your voice during the client's final teaching session, you can talk the client through a procedure with a minimum of extra time and effort. First review with the client the necessary equipment and record this information at the beginning of the tape. Then, as the client performs the procedure, record each step, pausing when the client needs more time. You should offer words of reinforcement and encouragement during this session. When the client and family go home, they will hear your reassuring words, which are comforting to those who must now handle the procedure on their own. In addition to being a reassuring experience that lowers tension, the familiarity of your voice recreates a mindset that more closely approximates the last teaching session. This promotes more accurate recall. You need the proper audio equipment for recording a tape or DVD. Most healthcare institutions have the equipment, and most families have playback equipment at home.

When you are in community health settings and clients live far away, such as in rural settings, consider depending on the telephone between home visits. Or an audiotape, DVD, or CD containing reminders, complicated instructions, and so forth could be left with the family.

Audio media have many advantages. They are used with individuals or groups. They are inexpensive, readily available, and can be tailor-made, erased, or remade in the client's language. Also, they help clients develop listening skills. Audio media capture nuances of speech that are impossible to convey in written communication. However, audio media have some drawbacks as well. Listeners find it difficult to listen for more than 15 minutes without other stimuli because they get bored. Remember that tapes, DVDs, and CDs are somewhat fragile and need protection from moisture and temperature extremes.

Computer-Assisted Instruction

Many health maintenance organizations and healthcare institutions or agencies have special areas where clients can access interactive software to supplement health education. **Computer-assisted instruction** (CAI) is an excellent resource for self-paced learning. It does not become impatient; its pace can be controlled by the client, and it gives immediate, objective, and consistent feedback. The software allows clients to repeat all or part of a lesson and progress at their own rate. Clients acquire information in private, and no one else has to know what they think or how long they take to obtain the expected knowledge. CAI is useful for clients of any age, especially if they can control the pace at which they progress. For younger clients, CAI may evoke the fun and excitement of an arcade game. Self-paced learning takes initiative on the part of clients. The CAI may lead you to expect too much independent learning from clients. If CAI is provided in a healthcare setting, be available to answer questions from clients and assist them with the software as the need arises.

Many interactive websites are available on the Internet. For example, the website MedlinePlus is a service of the National Library of Medicine (NLM) and National Institutes of Health (NIH). The site offers Easy to Read instructional materials that are available in more than 40 languages and interactive health tutorials on topics in the following categories: diseases and conditions, tests and diagnostic procedures, surgery and treatment procedures, and prevention and wellness (U.S. National Library of Medicine and National Institutes of Health, 2012). These sites can be accessed from a client's home.

Interactive bulletin boards serve as a continuing education resource for updating health team members (Flournoy, Turner, & Combs, 2000). Short, succinct lessons, messages, and updates can be created for health team members. It is self-paced learning that health team members use when they have the time and interest.

Digital Camera and Photographs

Digital cameras have largely replaced their older counterpart, the 35 mm camera. A digital camera takes video or still **photographs** by recording images on an electronic imaging sensor. Images are displayed immediately after they are recorded and can be stored or deleted as desired. Images can be printed on photo printers or taken to any commercial print service.

Digital photos can be displayed with an **LCD projector**, which is suitable for large groups. Everyone in your audience sees the same photo at the same time. Single photographs are best used on an individual basis or in a small group. When they are passed around, however, they may be distracting to the audience.

Slides

Film **35 mm slides** may still be available for health education purposes in some healthcare institutions or agencies. The slides are placed in a carousel and require a slide projector to view them. They can also be inserted into a PowerPoint presentation. A slide presentation is excellent for visual learners and helps to clarify your comments. The order of slides can be replaced or rearranged in the carousel if you change the nature of your presentation. You need to prepare a script to accompany the slide presentation. Slides are easy to store and transport. Because 35 mm film is no longer common, it is wise to learn to use a digital camera.

Objects and Models

Objects should be used for demonstration when possible. For example, use a real syringe when you teach self-injections, and use a real dressing when you teach how to change a dressing. **Models** are used when the real object, such as a heart, is not available or not feasible to use. Three types of models are replicas, analogies, and symbols.

Replica

A **replica** is a model that resembles a real object. It is a scaled construction that magnifies the features of the original object. The increased size of the features makes demonstration easier. This type of model can be picked up and manipulated and helps convey the concept of dimensions. Replicas are useful for kinesthetic clients who learn better with hands-on opportunities. For example, clients can take a model of a kidney apart and put it back together again, thus getting a better idea of how the kidney works. By handling the replica, clients can control the pace of learning.

A replica can be used to help clients develop a skill. Learning to clean a central line or to examine breasts for lumps are challenging procedures that are best learned on something other than a human being. Replicas exist for practicing these skills, but they are expensive, fragile, and require storage space.

Replicas best serve only a few clients at a time. Compensate for this by using team teaching and placing different replicas at different stations. Such an arrangement divides the larger group into several smaller ones and allows each station to become an area of concentrated focus with fewer competing stimuli.

Analogy

An **analogy** is something that has features similar and a likeness to something else (Webster's, 2013); it compares the familiar with the unfamiliar for explanatory purposes (Ruhl, 2009). Analogies build on clients' existing knowledge to communicate complex medical concepts. They emphasize a shared quality that helps make something unfamiliar become more understandable. A good analogy is familiar, short, clear, and visual.

When you create an analogy, the unfamiliar concept is the target, and the familiar concept you use for comparison is the analog. The target and the analog are connected with the words *like* or *as*. For example, you could explain that the action of the heart is like a pump that moves water. Ruhl (2009) identifies five things to remember when using analogies:

1. Determine the need for the analogy. Use an analogy when you are trying to explain something that is hard to understand.
2. Confirm that the client understands the analogy. You could say, "Tell me how you understand what I said"; then have the client state in his or her own words what you explained.
3. Follow up with a full explanation and use other instructional materials to augment your explanation.
4. Point out the limitations of the analogy. For instance, it is true that the brain is like a computer, but there are differences that the client should be aware of.
5. Make the client aware that the analogy is just a starting point. After he or she understands the concepts, use that understanding to move forward.

Ruhl encourages health educators to be creative and spontaneous, adapt analogies to the client's style of language, and build on common references that clients use.

Analogies demand conceptual sophistication and an ability to understand how things are alike and different. Because not everyone perceives the same way, practice using the analogy on others to find out if they understand the point and if it fits the message you intend to convey.

Symbol

A **symbol** stands for something else that it represents by association or resemblance. Often a printed or written sign is used to represent an operation, element, quantity, quality, relation, or something invisible (Webster's, 2013). The treble clef sign and notes on lines are examples of musical symbols. Words are examples of symbols. They are combinations of circles and lines arranged in special patterns to convey a certain meaning. The meaning varies according to the language familiar to the speaker, writer, listener, and reader.

Words are symbolic models that you use to convey a concept or idea to clients. Words are such familiar symbols that you no longer perceive the circles and lines with which words are drawn unless you are dyslexic. If fact, unless you have a photographic mind, you could not even report the exact words on this page. You would probably report the ideas, general concepts, and meanings you attached to what you read.

You may draw diagrams, signs, or cartoons, all of which are attempts to convey meaning through the use of symbols. International traffic signs are examples of such symbols. The picture conveys the meaning. Circles have many meanings. If they are arranged on top of each other and colored red, yellow, and green, they would be perceived in the United States as parts of a traffic light. Smiley faces are recognized by most people in this culture as conveying happiness or approval.

The practice of representing something by symbols is so widespread in this culture that it is difficult to describe by example. The symbol + means plus, and the symbol = means equal to. Stick figures can be used by a teacher to symbolize people regardless of artistic talent. The figure can help you focus a client's attention on the desired point. Distinct symbols are used in health care to distinguish between male and female people.

Symbols are gaining widespread application in areas that cater to multilingual groups and international travel. Examples include airports, roadway traffic signs, lodging and food, and handicapped parking symbols. You should avoid using abbreviations that are common among healthcare personnel but are not common to clients. These abbreviations include NPO, PO, and PRN. Although these abbreviations convey meaning to certain groups, they might add confusion to other groups. **Figure 11-1** illustrates some common symbols.

Transparencies

Transparencies remain a popular choice for illustrating a presentation and are used as backup to other media, such as PowerPoint presentations. They can be seen with the room lights on. They are useful to highlight important points in a verbal presentation. The highlights can be in the form of brief, well-spaced outlines, pictures, simple drawings, or cartoons. You can prepare transparencies in advance or on the spot in response to interaction with the clients.

FIGURE 11-1

Common Symbols

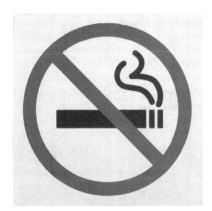 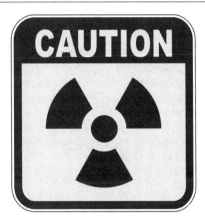

© AbleStock (left), © WilleeCole/ShutterStock, Inc. (right)

You can prepare permanent or nonpermanent transparencies in several ways. To create permanent transparencies, construct a drawing or write text on paper, copy the material in a copy machine, then run the copy together with a blank transparency through a thermal fax machine. The thermal fax and carbon on the copy interact to make the transparency in the presence of heat. The same process is used to create picture transparencies. To create nonpermanent transparencies, use nonpermanent, washable color marking pens. This works well for illustrating as you are presenting. The transparency is reusable because the ink will wash off. Transparencies are relatively inexpensive to purchase and can be stored flat in pocket envelopes that fit a standard note binder.

Transparencies are projected onto a screen via an **overhead projector,** and they are useful for any size audience. A projector is bulky and has a long arm with a mirror and lens that focus and redirect light forward onto a screen. When a transparency is placed on the projector, the image is directed onto the screen. The projector has a very bright halogen lamp, a fan to cool the machine, and a storage place for additional lamps.

An overhead projector needs to be adjusted before the presentation to ensure a good projected image on the screen. This means adjusting the size of the screen and the distance from the projector to the screen. We recommend that you stand to one side of the projector and look at the audience when giving a presentation. Place the projector so you can face the audience. The audience looks at the screen while you look at the transparency on the projector to see what the audience sees.

PowerPoint Slides

Microsoft **PowerPoint** is a presentation software program widely used by educators. It is useful for large audiences and requires an LCD projector to display the images onto a screen for viewing. The presentation can be accessed from the computer, a disc, or a flash drive. The room may need to be darkened for best viewing.

BOX 11-2

Guidelines for Creating and Using PowerPoint Slides

- Choose a format that best illustrates your points with headings and subheadings.
- Choose a plain background to limit the distractions on the slides.
- Choose a soft background color that contrasts with the lettering.
- Use bullets or numbers to separate the information.
- Use upper- and lowercase lettering; avoid all capitalized lettering.
- List as few words as possible to communicate the message.
- Limit the amount of information on each slide; avoid overcrowding.
- Limit the number of slides so the audience focuses on your comments.
- Advance the slides to match your comments.
- Be sure the hardware and software are operating properly before your presentation.
- Give a copy of the slides to the audience to reinforce learning.

Identify what you want to illustrate through PowerPoint slides. You can input text, graphics, movies, or other objects on the slides and arrange and rearrange them as you wish. The software provides a template with a variety of formats and backgrounds to create the slides. You can navigate through the slides as you make your presentation. The slides can be printed, or you can display the presentation live on a computer. The software is easy to use but requires the proper equipment. See **Box 11-2** for help in preparing your presentation.

Storyboards

A **storyboard** is a visual presentation of text or graphic information. Storyboards tell a story or explain sequential information (Pittman, 2009). Microsoft PowerPoint software is commonly used for creating storyboards. The software provides many options for layout, text, and graphics.

Storyboards are easy to develop, edit, and distribute for client education purposes. They are low cost and provide consistent, current information to clients. The development of storyboards begins by selecting a health-related topic followed by identifying the essential information to include. A committee can help determine the topic, content, and accuracy. After they are developed, storyboards can be distributed via email, they can be printed, or they can be made into posters with the correct type of printer (Kisak & Conrad, 2004).

Cartoons

Cartoons can be transferred to a transparency or PowerPoint slide and projected for large groups; or cartoons may be circulated among members of a small group or shared with an individual. Humorous cartoons provide comic relief and make a point much more clearly than many words. Before you decide to use humor, test it out on people similar to your intended audience. Drawings that are intended to be humorous also can evoke unexpected reactions among clients who may perceive the material differently than you do. Cartoons are not necessarily cross-cultural, so you should show prospective cartoons to someone from the target culture and have them critique it for you. As with photographs, cartoons can be placed in clear plastic covers for protection.

Mobile Devices

The ownership and use of mobile devices has increasingly become how we communicate and access information both within the United States and around the world. They are rapidly replacing landline telephones with their powerful computing and battery capabilities and expanding wireless broadband networks. A goal of Healthy People 2020 is to "use health communication strategies and health information technology (IT) to improve population health outcomes and health care quality, and to achieve health equity" (HealthyPeople.gov, 2014, para. 1). Mobile devices are useful tools for educating clients, promoting the use of preventive services, managing chronic conditions, and improving overall health.

In addition to the web-based delivery of health education and e-health interactive tutorials, mobile devices can also serve as an interface between clients and healthcare providers by the real-time transmission of information about vital body functions. For example, iPhones were used to monitor adolescents with type 1 diabetes. One group kept a food diary, whereas another used the cell phone camera to record their dietary intake. The photographs were downloaded and analyzed, along with the food diaries. Although there was no significant difference between the two groups, it demonstrates a novel use of the cell phone to monitor clients (Donald, Franklin, & Greene, 2009). Text messaging was effective in improving self-efficacy and adherence in adolescents with type 1 diabetes (Franklin, Waller, Pagliari, & Greene, 2006), and mobile devices were effective in monitoring client vital signs (Mark, 2013). Many healthcare institutions and agencies provide telephone numbers for clients who have concerns. Health advice lines are also available. Telephones are used to follow up with clients to offer encouragement and help with any problems they have in adhering to a treatment regimen.

INTERNET AND WORLD WIDE WEB

The **Internet** is a huge global network that connects computers for the purpose of transferring information from one computer to another. It connects millions of private, public, academic, business, and government computers. The Internet is the infrastructure that supports the Web. The **Web** is a network of hypertext documents called webpages that are accessed via the Internet. Webpages may contain text, images, videos, audio, and other multimedia. Users can easily navigate these pages with the click of a mouse. The Web was created to display information, whereas the Internet was created to exchange information. The Internet and the Web are not synonymous terms, although they are often used as if they were (Sopczyk, 2008; Wikipedia, 2014).

To access the Web, clients must have a computer, or have access to one, with a telecommunication link and special software to connect to an Internet service provider (ISP). Clients navigate the Web through a browser such as Microsoft Internet Explorer. When a person is on the Internet, search engines (Google) and directories (Yahoo!) allow users to search for specific information and websites (Sopczyk, 2008).

The technology and supporting software are developing rapidly and changing daily. By the time that you read this, today's technology will have advanced and the number of health-related websites will have greatly expanded. Nurses who work with this technology need to keep abreast of these changes to assist clients who need health education.

Wikipedia (2014), an online encyclopedia, estimates that by 2009 one-fourth of the world's population will use services on the Internet. The Pew Internet/California HealthCare Foundation survey found that 74% of U.S. adults go online, and 61% of them look online for health information (Fox & Jones, 2009). A nurse who works as an educator must be computer and information literate to use this medium to assist clients (Sopczyk, 2008).

Because so many clients access the Internet, you should ask them if they are looking at health-related websites. If so, ask which ones they find useful and evaluate if they are accessing reliable sources of information. By listening to what clients have learned about health issues, you have the opportunity to evaluate that knowledge. You can refer clients to reliable websites if that is indicated. Clients may have questions about what they are learning, or they may be overwhelmed with the amount of information they are finding. Urge clients to use online health information to supplement that given by their healthcare provider, not as a substitute. Many clients misunderstand or misinterpret health information and require clarifying explanations.

E-health Websites

The Web is the newest source for interactive health information, often referred to as e-health. Electronically available health information includes access to personal health records online, health education libraries, professional health journals, and self-assessment tools. When health information is so widely available and accessible, it has the potential to improve the quality of health if used by clients. It also has the potential to create problems for clients and providers if the health information is inaccurate and influences their decision making and healthcare practices.

The Internet is advantageous for clients because it is accessed in private in their own homes. Information is read at clients' speed and convenience. Taking advantage of this technology is more effective for clients with adequate health literacy skills. Those at low health literacy levels may find accessing and understanding health information on websites more challenging.

Clients without a personal computer have free access through public libraries, community centers, or senior centers. Clients who are enrolled in health maintenance organizations, such as Kaiser Permanente, have access to onsite interactive health education software. Electronic sources of health information are available from The Joint Commission through the Speak Up initiative (The Joint Commission, 2009) and Medline Plus, both described earlier in this chapter.

The Web has become a source of information and an educational tool for clients with a variety of health issues (Hawn, 2009; Jacobi et al., 2007; Scharer, 2005; Schultz, Stava, Beck, & Vassilopoulou-Sellin, 2003). It puts information and power into the hands of consumers, especially those with chronic diseases. Half of clients with a chronic disease or disability go online. Of this number, 86% have searched for information about health topics (Fox, 2007). Millard and Fintak (2002) found that clients with chronic illnesses frequently accessed websites to get information about their illness and engaged in self-care and self-diagnosis. In a large study, they found that users were skeptical about health care in general. Some users were not satisfied or had experienced problems with access to the healthcare system. Others lacked insurance coverage or found it difficult to obtain healthcare services. Favored health websites were those designed specifically for health topics, medical journals, advocacy groups, and academic websites.

Other ways that clients can access health-related information is through YouTube, podcasts, and streaming video. A difficulty with websites is that clients do not know if the information is reliable.

Evaluating Website Information

Almost anything can be found on the Web, so it is important to evaluate each site for accuracy and reliability. Although websites can be a source of excellent information, they also can be misleading and provide misinformation. It is your responsibility to thoroughly evaluate each website that you recommended to clients. Monsivais and Reynolds (2003) and MedlinePlus offer guidelines for evaluating websites:

- What is the source of the information? Is it from an individual or an organization? Examples of reliable sources of information include local, state, and federal government sites, U.S. colleges and universities, professional organizations, and voluntary health organizations. Look at the about us webpage for this information. Is there a way to contact the webmaster?
- What is the quality of the information? The writers of the information should be identified and may be found in the about us webpage or in the mission statement. Who are they? Are they recognized experts in the field about which they are writing? Be skeptical; quackery thrives on the Internet. Look for claims that sound too good to be true, such as promises about new cures and secret ingredients.
- What evidence is offered to support the claims? Is it based on medical research conducted by properly credentialed researchers at known healthcare institutions, scientific laboratories, or universities? Is the evidence based on personal testimony and opinion? If so, are the persons and their credentials identified? Is there a way to contact them? Be skeptical of anonymous testimonials that claim cures and promote treatments.
- How current is the information? Note the date the information was posted and the last time the site was updated. Credible sites provide dates. Does the site provide references and maintain hyperlinks to other credible sites?
- Is the information biased? What is the purpose of the site, and who is sponsoring and funding it? Is it supported by public funds, donations, or commercial advertising? The distinction between health information and advertisements should be clear. Websites can appear to be credible, but a careful observer may discover likewise. The purpose of many websites is to sell a product or recommend a particular treatment (Butler & Foster, 2003). Such a site would not be considered an objective source of information.

When clients search for information on the Web, many options appear, and choosing among them is confusing. Talk with clients about how to find credible websites. Also urge clients to talk with their healthcare providers about the accuracy of health information they are finding on the Web.

Social Networking Websites

Boyd and Ellison define social network sites as "web-based services that allow individuals to (1) construct a public or semi-public profile within a bounded system, (2) articulate a list of other users with whom they share a connection, and (3) view and traverse their list of connections and those made by others within the system. The nature and nomenclature of these connections may vary from site to site" (2007, p. 2). Although social network websites are popular, it is not known how many adults use them to gather or share health information. Most users who access these sites share updates about themselves or their friends (Fox & Jones, 2009). Facebook, Twitter, and Myspace are examples of social networking sites that are used by clients to share information.

Email, short for electronic mail, is used by both healthcare providers and clients, especially in rural areas. It increases the speed of communication and the ability to keep in contact with other clients and providers. Electronic communication also has disadvantages (Sopczyk, 2008). It lacks context, such as facial expression and tone of voice. Email is an efficient way to communicate; service has improved as the networks and speed have expanded. Instant messaging is also effective but more information can be communicated via email than with instant messaging. Response time to email and instant messaging are dependent on the promptness of the intended receiver. With email there is a written record of the information shared or the advice given. It is important that this be accurate and appropriate and a copy of it be placed in the client's record. Although healthcare institutions and agencies take steps to ensure privacy in electronic communications and have guidelines for their use, you can never assume that the communications are private.

Hawn (2009) anticipates that social networking sites will become increasingly used by clients and healthcare providers. Hawn reports that through email, instant messaging, or video chat, some clients can now contact their physicians directly. It is a way for clients to stay in touch with their physicians. Email access to personal physicians and nurse practitioners is now available through some health maintenance organizations, such as Kaiser Permanente and Palo Alto (California) Medical Group. Clients can also make appointments, refill prescriptions, and see their personal test results online. Some physicians are establishing their own Facebook-like profiles and communicating with clients via secure email message networks. Some are writing blogs about common health topics (Hawn, 2009).

Electronic discussion boards have been useful for clients who are experiencing similar health issues and share common concerns. Clients post their experiences and thoughts on the site and gain the support of other clients who are experiencing similar problems. Clients exchange helpful messages with each other. It is an effective, relatively inexpensive way to provide social support to clients. Discussion boards are also a promising health resource (Scharer, 2005; Schultz et al., 2003). HealthBoards.com is an example of a social support site (http://www.healthboards.com/). Clients have access to more than 150 message boards that cover a wide range of health topics. This resource may be especially helpful for clients with disabilities or chronic illnesses.

SELECTING INSTRUCTIONAL MATERIALS

When selecting instructional materials, review the learning objectives, teaching content, and teaching strategies and ask how you can best supplement these. Consider the characteristics of your clients and which media would best help them learn. In **Box 11-3** we have summarized some questions to ask in this process.

BOX 11-3

Choosing a Medium

Questions to ask yourself when choosing a medium:
1. What medium is most appropriate given the learning objectives, teaching content, and teaching strategies?
2. Is sound necessary, or can a silent medium be used?
3. Is motion important, or can still pictures convey the ideas?
4. Is color important, or is black and white more advantageous?
5. Is individual study encouraged?
6. Is the focus on learning as a group?
7. How often is the material likely to need updating?
8. Do you have the technical competence to use this medium?
9. Can you handle common problems with this medium?
10. Do you know where to get help with it?
11. What is realistic for you to accomplish given your budget and time constraints?
12. What resources are necessary in the learning environment to use this equipment, such as a screen, podium, and electrical outlets?

Table 11-1 summarizes the advantages, disadvantages, and helpful hints for using the various types of instructional materials. We hope this is helpful to you in making a selection.

CLIENTS WITH SPECIAL NEEDS

Clients with hearing and visual impairments present special challenges when it comes to the selection of instructional materials and media. Insofar as possible, materials and media should be adapted to the particular needs of each client. It helps to involve the client's family, significant other, or caretaker if that is appropriate and the client is agreeable. They may have suggestions that will facilitate your health teaching.

Depending on the client's degree of impairment, you need to identify the best way to communicate with hearing impaired and visually impaired clients. We offer some practical suggestions here.

Many clients who are hearing impaired are able to benefit from print media and video recordings. If a client is receptive to print media, choose materials that are appropriate in terms of readability and information, such as pamphlets and brochures. If the client knows how to write and has the strength to do it, providing paper and pencil may be an effective way to communicate. If the client is computer literate and a laptop computer is available, this may be helpful. Many health-related videos are commercially available and also available online. You can also custom make videos to suit the special needs of your client.

Visual impairments can be mild, moderate, or severe, or the client may be blind. You need to know each client's specific capabilities to make an appropriate selection of instructional materials and media. Many clients who are visually impaired benefit from auditory media. If the client is not a reader or has poor literacy, Pittman (2009) recommends using audio media.

TABLE 11-1

Features of Instructional Materials

Type	Advantages	Disadvantages	Helpful Hints
Video media	• Good substitute for actual experience • Easily obtainable • Easy to remake and update • Can be stopped and rerun • Familiar to many	• Size of monitor limits audience distance • Technical skill needed • Expensive initial investment	• Need compatible equipment • Can take longer than expected to make a tape or DVD • Store properly
Audio media	• Can be used with individuals or groups • Good for developing listening skills • Accessible • Inexpensive • Can be tailor-made, erased, or remade	• Can be dull if used by itself or for too long a period • Audiocassettes can be damaged easily • Need proper playback equipment	• Store properly • Should be of high audio quality to maintain interest
Computer-assisted instruction	• Client controls the pace • Correct responses reinforced immediately • Incorrect responses retaught immediately • Good for sequential thought processes • Allows client to repeat the lesson if necessary	• Depends on client initiative • Time consuming for client • Time consuming for nurse to monitor • Limited value if nurse is not available for questions • Clients must be visual learners and computer literate • Can be boring	• Select the most user-friendly software available • Spend time with client to ensure comfort with the program
Digital camera and photographs	• Images can be displayed and printed immediately • Images easily stored and deleted • Can be used with taped narration or music	• Expensive initial investment • Single photographs distracting if passed around during presentation • Show no movement	• Synchronize with a presentation
Objects and models	• Depict the real thing as closely as possible • Can be handled and studied at client's pace • Replicas are static • Analogies are dynamic • Appeal to kinesthetic learners	• Can be bulky and heavy • Inconvenient to transport • Require storage space • Time consuming • Expensive and fragile • Analogies require conceptual sophistication	• Require advance planning if borrowed • Work well with several stations around a teaching area • Require a teacher at each station

(continues)

TABLE 11-1

Features of Instructional Materials (Continued)

Type	Advantages	Disadvantages	Helpful Hints
Transparencies	• Versatile, inexpensive, and reusable • Teacher can face learners • Eliminate verbal repetition • Can be used with the lights on • Can be used with overlays • Good backup for PowerPoint	• Overhead projector is bulky and needs to be adjusted to the screen • Use bulbs that often burn out • Transparencies are time consuming to prepare	• Protect transparencies from hand oils and fingerprints • Use multicolor, washable pens
PowerPoint slides or storyboards	• Easy to format, create, use and store on disc or flash drive • Show still images, motion, and sound • Stimulating to audience • Allow audience to follow the presentation	• Require expensive equipment and screen • Slides are time consuming to prepare • Must have operational LCD projector and screen	• Be sure equipment is available and working properly • Important to sequence slides and storyboard
Instructional handouts and education pathways	• Developed for specific clients or healthcare institutions • Easily changed and updated • Clients can review at their pace	• Takes time to prepare and update • Duplicating takes time	• Require storage space • Keep materials organized and handy for use
Pamphlets and brochures	• Portable and attractive • Can be used before, during, and after a presentation • Can be studied at client's pace • Readily available • Often free	• May overwhelm clients if too many • May contain outdated or irrelevant information • May be culturally inappropriate	• Distribute at the most propitious time • Check for currency of information
Bulletin boards	• Clients can process at own pace • Attract browsers	• Can get cluttered and outdated • Unsuitable for long or complex information	• Change often • Keep attractive, lively • Contain a minimal number of messages

(continues)

TABLE 11-1

Features of Instructional Materials (Continued)

Type	Advantages	Disadvantages	Helpful Hints
Posters	• Portable and attractive • Attract browsers • Can be used before, during, and after a presentation • Can be studied at client's pace • Readily available • Often free	• Time consuming to make • Provide limited viewing • Need a prop • Bulky to carry and store • Useful only to readers	• Change often • Keep attractive, lively • Contain a minimal number of messages
Flip charts	• Versatile, portable • Use like a whiteboard or chalkboard • May be prepared before or created spontaneously during presentation	• Require artistic talent and good handwriting • Clients may have a limited view	• Have a good supply of black and colored pens • Use masking tape or adhesive to affix flip charts to wall
Whiteboards or chalkboards	• Widely available • Useful for spontaneous illustration at the time of client's concern • Offer reinforcement to respondents • Erasable • Allow teacher to add to and take away from illustration • Good backup aid	• Two dimensional • Messy • Require pen or chalk and an eraser • Require good lighting • Can be time consuming to use • Require legible writing skills	• May need to supply pens or chalk and eraser • Chalk is messy, especially on dark clothing • Write high on board to avoid writing below clients' line of vision • Divide in half for lengthy lists

Audiocassettes, DVDs, and CDs are commercially available and can be custom made to suit the needs of clients. Clients with visual impairments need special equipment to use these media; however, many clients already have recorders and players in their homes.

Clients with limited visual impairment may benefit from print media if the font size is sufficiently large. The background and font colors can be altered to increase readability. Magnifying lamps and handheld lighted magnifiers are also available to assist these clients.

EVALUATING EFFECTIVENESS OF INSTRUCTIONAL MATERIALS

Evaluate the effectiveness of all instructional materials. Evaluation tools should be specific to the type of materials that you are using to supplement health education. **Box 11-4** provides some criteria for evaluating the effectiveness of instructional materials.

BOX 11-4

Evaluating Effectiveness of Instructional Materials

In the teaching plan, were the instructional materials:
- Appropriate to the learning objectives?
- Appropriate to the teaching content?
- Complementary to the teaching strategies?

For the learners, were the instructional materials:
- Appealing to visual, auditory, and/or kinesthetic learners?
- Appropriate to the client's level of comprehension?
- Age, gender, and culturally appropriate and sensitive?
- Engaging to the client?

Was the selection of learning materials:
- Visually pleasing?
- Suitable to the time constraints of the learning activity?
- Visible in terms of contrast, size, and location?
- Easy to use?
- Accurate and up to date?
- Cost effective and within budget constraints?

COPYRIGHT ISSUES IN USING INSTRUCTIONAL MATERIALS

Copyright laws in the United States protect intellectual property and original works of authorship when they are fixed in a tangible form. This protection exists for both published and unpublished works (U.S. Copyright Office, 2009). Knowing about copyright restrictions is important if you are using certain instructional materials, such as text and images. Instructional materials may be copyrighted or they may be in the public domain. Depending on their source, it is important to know the difference and respond accordingly. If you have any questions about copyright issues, it is best to consult with your employer's legal counsel.

Instructional materials taken from professional journals, magazines, and other published sources always carry a copyright. To make multiple copies, you must seek written permission from the publisher or the owner of the materials. When making the request, allow plenty of time and ask how the copyright owner wants the materials cited. It is important to comply with the copyright owner's citation format (Kisak & Conrad, 2004). Copyright law permits an individual to make one copy of a copyrighted document for own personal use without requesting permission.

Instructional materials in the public domain are not protected by copyright and therefore do not require permission. Examples of materials in the public domain include those first published in a U.S. government document. It also includes commonly used materials in which the ownership is unknown or questionable. Some images are also in the public domain and are available for use. Even though no permission is required, credit should always be given to the source of the information.

If you are downloading information from websites, be sure to check the copyright information provided on that website. Clear guidelines are provided that identify what is and what is not copyrighted and any restrictions on the use of the information (Kisak & Conrad, 2004). For example, on The Joint Commission website, there are no copyright or reprinting permissions required for the Speak Up materials. However, the website stipulates that The Joint Commission must be credited as the source of the materials.

CASE EXAMPLE: MRS. ROSA LOPEZ

In this case example, we are creating a teaching plan for Mrs. Rosa Lopez, and we are ready to add suitable instructional materials (**Table 11-2**). To assist Mrs. Lopez's understanding of hypertension and the importance of limiting sodium intake, we would provide her with culturally appropriate pamphlets, such as *Living with Hypertension*. We would also have a chart available that explains the mechanism of hypertension and its relationship to excess sodium intake. To help her learn about sodium in foods, we would give her two handouts: *Planning a Low Sodium Diet* and *Foods High in Sodium* that acknowledge her cultural food preferences and traditions. We might also assist her with how to read food labels the next time she is at the grocery store to identify the amount of sodium in the food she chooses. If she accesses the Internet, we would show her how to search the Web for information about low-sodium diets to include meal planning, sample menus, recipes, and snacks. If she is a member of a health maintenance organization, it may offer instructional materials and interactive tutorials over the Internet or at an educational site. To learn how to take her blood pressure, Mrs. Lopez would need to purchase a digital blood pressure monitor for home use that is available from the pharmacy. You will need to instruct her ahead of time to purchase this, and perhaps identify sources of funding for the equipment. She will also need paper and a pencil to record the findings.

TABLE 11-2

Sample Teaching Plan for Mrs. Rosa Lopez

Learning Objectives	*Content Outline*	*Strategies and Materials*	*Evaluation*
1. The client will correctly verbally explain how excessive salt intake affects blood pressure to the nurse by memory (cognitive).	Greeting and introductions Hypertension Definition Fluid retention Excess sodium intake Role in fluid retention Sodium and salt relationship Sodium is 40% of table salt (sodium chloride) Fluid retention and C-V system	Talking and discussion Answer questions Discussion question: What is the relationship between sodium intake and hypertension? Video: *Understanding Hypertension* Chart: Hypertension Pamphlet: *Living with Hypertension*	Verbal questions Paper and pencil test

(continues)

TABLE 11-2

Sample Teaching Plan for Mrs. Rosa Lopez (Continued)

Learning Objectives	Content Outline	Strategies and Materials	Evaluation
2. The client will choose to limit sodium intake by working with the nurse to prepare a dietary plan for one week (affective).	Four components of dietary plan: 1. Remove salt shaker from table. 2. Use no salt in cooking. 3. Avoid canned or processed foods that are high in sodium. 4. Use low-sodium seasonings, such as herbs and spices.	Talking and discussion Answer questions Read sample labels for sodium content Discussion question: How can you incorporate these changes into your meal planning and usual diet? Handout: *Planning a Low Sodium Diet* Handout: *Foods High in Sodium* Assignment: Read food labels when grocery shopping Internet search: HMO site or Internet search engines (e.g., Google) for low-sodium diets	Short term: Attitude scale Long term: Implementation of dietary changes
3. The client will demonstrate how to accurately obtain her own blood pressure reading using home digital equipment without any verbal guidance (psychomotor).	Techniques for obtaining blood pressure: 1. Read equipment directions. 2. Locate brachial artery. 3. Place arm in cuff. 4. Inflate cuff. 5. Release air in cuff. 6. Record findings.	Talking and discussion Demonstrate procedure Handout: Have client read the printed directions for using the equipment Handout: *Steps to Taking Your Blood Pressure* Have client demonstrate procedure, answer questions, and develop record-keeping system	Blood pressure Checklist to obtain blood pressure Record of blood pressure readings

BOX 11-5

Evidence-Based Nursing Practice

Wilson, F. L., Mood, D., & Nordstrom, C. K. (2010) The influence of easy-to-read pamphlets about self-care management of radiation side effects on Patients' knowledge. *Oncology Nursing Forum, 37*(6), 774-781.

Purpose: The purpose is to test patients' knowledge of side effects after they review six easy-to-read pamphlets, at the fifth- to seventh-grade reading level, on radiation side effects, including the following: loss of appetite, fatigue, skin problems for men, skin problems for women, infection, and emotional issues.

Method: Using a nonexperimental design, 47 patients receiving radiation treatment were selected and their grade level reading skills were evaluated using the Rapid Estimate of Adult Literacy in Medicine. The patients' knowledge was tested using Knowledge of Radiation Side Effects Test.

Results: The scores for each knowledge test increased with literacy level, with statistically significant correlations for pamphlets on fatigue, skin problems for women, and skin problems for men. Patients with a fourth- to sixth-grade reading level scored better than expected. Those with reading levels at or below the third grade had difficulty with many of the test items, indicating they were unable to comprehend much of the information.

SUMMARY

In this chapter we introduced health literacy and the importance of considering readability and appropriateness when selecting written materials. We discussed instructional materials under three broad headings: printed materials, multimedia, and Internet and World Wide Web. Instructional materials are designed to help you achieve the learning objectives and supplement your teaching strategies. The materials that you select should be appropriate to you as the teacher and to clients as learners. Each type of instructional material has advantages and disadvantages that must be considered when making a selection.

Clients with special needs include those with auditory and visual impairments who need special consideration. Instructional materials and websites need to be evaluated in terms of being reliable and accurate sources of information. Criteria were provided to help in the evaluation process. It is important to remember that some instructional materials are protected by copyright. These implications were discussed.

EXERCISES

Exercise I: Assessing Health Literacy

Purpose: Assess the impact of health literacy on client care.
Directions:

1. Select a client you have cared for and who was confronted with a major health decision. Identify that decision.

2. List the literacy and decision-making skills the client needed to make a good, informed decision.
3. Share your thoughts with the class.

Exercise II: Writing Health Information

Purpose: Prepare health information for distribution to clients.
Directions: Work in pairs and prepare a handout that includes the purpose, description, rationale, benefits, and instructions for clients for one of the following procedures:

1. Mammogram
2. Immunizations
3. Colonoscopy
4. Chest X-ray
5. Blood test

Exercise III: Writing Health Information

Purpose: Increase awareness of client perceptions of medical jargon.
Directions:

1. On paper, draw four columns. List the following words in the left-hand column: ambulate, edema, peristalsis, hypertrophy, jaundice, urinate, biopsy, hypertension, vital signs, and NPO.
2. In the middle column, write what a client might think the words mean. If you cannot think of a possible client meaning for the word, ask friends who do not have medical backgrounds or clients who could use some entertainment.
3. In the third column write the medical meaning.
4. In the last column write an alternative word or phrase that conveys the desired meaning.
5. What words would you add to the list that clients might not know the meaning of?

Exercise IV: Rewriting Health Information

Purpose: Evaluate health information.
Directions:

1. Bring a health-related written advertisement for a product or medication to class.
2. Identify the central message of the advertisement. What is explicit? Implicit?
3. What assumptions does the advertisement make about the client's health literacy?
4. At what reading level is the advertisement?
5. Share your observations with others in your class.

REFERENCES

Bandura, A. (1986). *Social foundations of thought and action: A social cognitive theory.* Englewood Cliffs, NJ: Prentice Hall.

Bandura, A. (2001). Social cognitive theory: An agentic perspective. *Annual Review of Psychology, 52,* 1–26.

Boyd, D. M., & Ellison, N. B. (2007). Social network sites: Definition, history, and scholarship. *Journal of Computer-Mediated Communication, 13*(1), article 11. Retrieved from http://jcmc.indiana.edu/vol13/issue1/boyd.ellison.html

Bryan, C. (2008). Provider and policy response to reverse the consequences of low health literacy. *Journal of Healthcare Management, 53*(4), 230–241.

Butler, L., & Foster, N. E. (2003). Back pain online: A cross-sectional survey of the quality of web-based information on low back pain. *Spine, 28*(4), 395–401.

Clancy, C. M. (2008). Navigating the health care system. What's your health literacy score? Retrieved from http://www.ahrq.gov/CONSUMER/cc/cc052008.htm

Clarke, L. K. (2002). Pathways for head and neck surgery: A patient-education tool. *Clinical Journal of Oncology Nursing, 6*(2), 78–82.

DISCERN, a tool for evaluating the quality of health care information. Retrieved from http://www.discern.org.uk/index.php

Doak, C. C., Doak, L. G., & Root, J. H. (1996). *Teaching patients with low literacy skills* (2nd ed.). Philadelphia, PA: Lippincott.

Donald, H., Franklin, V., & Greene, S. (2009). The use of mobile phones in dietary assessment in young people with type 1 diabetes. *Journal of Human Nutrition and Dietetics, 22*(3), 256–257.

Falvo, D.R. (2011). *Effective patient education: A guide to increased adherence* (4th ed.). Sudbury, MA: Jones and Bartlett.

Flournoy, E., Turner, G., & Combs, D. (2000). Critical care nurses read the writing on the wall: Use interactive bulletin boards to teach your nurses. *Nursing Management, 31*(2), 46–47.

Fox, S. (2007). E-patients with a disability or chronic disease. Retrieved from http://www.pewinternet.org/Reports/2007/Epatients-With-a-Disability-or-Chronic-Disease.aspx

Fox, S., & Jones, S. (2009). The social life of health information. Retrieved from http://www.pewinternet.org/~/media//Files/Reports/2009/PIP_Health_2009.pdf

Franklin, V. L., Waller, A., Pagliari, C., & Greene, S. A. (2006). A randomized controlled trial of sweet talk, a text-messaging system to support young people with diabetes. *Diabetic Medicine, 23*(12), 1332–1338.

Hasselkus, A. (2009, January 20). Health literacy. *The ASHA Leader,* 28–29.

Hawn, C. (2009). Report from the field. Take two aspirin and tweet me in the morning: How Twitter, Facebook, and other social media are reshaping health care. *Health Affairs, 28*(2), 361–368.

HealthyPeople.gov. (2014). Health communication and health information technology. Retrieved from http://healthypeople.gov/2020/topicsobjectives2020/overview.aspx?topicId=18

Jacobi, C., Morris, L., Beckers, C., Bronisch-Holtze, J., Winter, J., Winzelberg, A. J., & Taylor, C. B. (2007). Maintenance of Internet-based prevention: A randomized controlled trial. *International Journal of Eating Disorders, 40*(2), 114–119.

Kisak, A. Z., & Conrad, K. J. (2004). Using technology to develop and distribute patient education storyboards across a health system. *Oncology Nursing Forum, 31*(1), 131–135.

Levy, M., & Royne, M. B. (2009). The impact of consumers' health literacy on public health. *The Journal of Consumer Affairs, 43*(2), 367–372.

Linton, A. D. (2007). Age-related changes in the special senses. In A. D. Linton & H. W. Lach (Eds.), *Matteson and McConnell's gerontological nursing concepts and practice* (3rd ed., pp. 600–627). St. Louis, MO: Saunders Elsevier.

Mark, A. J. (2013). Universal access to essential vital signs monitoring. *Anesthesia & Analgesia, 117*(4), 883–890.

McLaughlin, G. H. (1969). SMOG grading: A new readability formula. *Journal of Reading, 12*(8), 639–646.

Millard, R. W., & Fintak, P. A. (2012). Use of the Internet by patients with chronic illness. *Disease Management and Health Outcomes, 10*(3), 187–194.

Monsivais, D., & Reynolds, A. (2003). Developing and evaluating patient education materials. *The Journal of Continuing Education in Nursing, 34*(4), 172–176.

Mooney, A., & Prins, E. (2013). *Addressing the health literacy needs of adult education students.* Goodling Institute for Research in Family Literacy, PennState College of Education.

National Center for Education Statistics. (2003). National assessment of adult literacy (NAAL). Retrieved from http://nces.ed.gov/naal/health_results.asp

Patient Protection and Affordable Care Act. (2010). Retrieved from http://www.gpo.gov/fdsys/pkg/BILLS-111hr3590enr/pdf/BILLS-111hr3590enr.pdf

Pittman, T. J. (2009). Teaching tools. In A. J. Lowenstein, L. Foord-May, & J. C. Romano (Eds.). *Teaching strategies for health education and health promotion: Working with patients, families, and communities.* Sudbury, MA: Jones and Bartlett.

Plain Language: Improving communication. Retrieved from http://www.plainlanguage.gov/populartopics/health_literacy/index.cfm

Pohl, M. L. (1981). *The teaching function of the nurse practitioner.* Dubuque, IA: Wm. C. Brown.

Roberts, D. (2008). Nursing antidotes for poor health literacy. *MEDSURG Nursing, 17*(2), 75.

Ruhl, T. S. (2009). How to use analogies. Retrieved from http://www.altoonafp.org/how_to_use_analogies.htm

Scharer, K. (2005). An Internet discussion board for parents of mentally ill young children. *Journal of Child and Adolescent Psychiatric Nursing, 18*(1), 17–25.

Schultz, P. N., Stava, C., Beck, M. L., & Vassilopoulou-Sellin, R. (2003). Internet message board use by patients with cancer and their families. *Clinical Journal of Oncology Nursing, 7*(6), 663–667.

Seligman, H. K., Wallace, A. S., DeWalt, D. A., Schillinger, D., Arnold, C. L., Shilliday, B. B., . . . Davis. 2007). Facilitating behavior change with low-literacy patient education materials (Suppl. 1). *American Journal of Health Behavior, 31*, S69–S78.

Sopczyk, D. (2008). Technology in education. In S. B. Bastable (Ed.), *Nurse as educator: Principles of teaching and learning for nursing practice* (pp. 515–552). Sudbury, MA: Jones and Bartlett.

The Joint Commission. (2009). Speak Up Initiative. Brochures and Infographics. Retrieved from http://www.jointcommission.org/topics/speakup_brochures.aspx

Thomas, C. M. (2007). Bulletin boards a teaching strategy for older audiences. *Journal of Gerontological Nursing, 33*(3), 45–52.

U.S. Copyright Office. (2009). Retrieved from http://copyright.gov/help/faq/faq-general.html#what

U.S. National Library of Medicine and National Institutes of Health. (2012). Interactive health tutorials. Retrieved from http://www.nlm.nih.gov/medlineplus/tutorial.html

Webster's All-In-One Dictionary and Thesaurus (2nd ed.). (2013). Springfield, MA: Federal Street Press.

Wikipedia. (2014). History of the Internet. Retrieved from http://en.wikipedia.org/wiki/History_of_the_Internet

Wilson, F. L., Mood, D., & Nordstrom, C. K. (2010). The influence of easy-to-read pamphlets about self-care management of radiation side effects on patients' knowledge. *Oncology Nursing Forum, 37*(6), 774–781.

Winslow, E. H. (2001). Patient education materials: Can patients read them, or are they ending up in the trash? *American Journal of Nursing, 101*(10), 33–38.

Wood, M. R., Kettinger, C. A., & Lessick, M. (2007). Knowledge is power: How nurses can promote health literacy. *Nursing for Women's Health, 11*(2), 180–188.

Zarcadoolas, C., Pleasant, A. F., & Greer, D. S. (2006). *Advancing health literacy: A framework for understanding and action.* San Francisco, CA: Jossey-Bass.

V

Client Education Outcomes

12

Formative Evaluation

INTRODUCTION

The final step of the teaching and learning process is evaluation. Evaluation means to determine the value, significance, worth, or condition of something by careful appraisal and study (Webster's, 2013). Applied to health education, evaluation is the process of judging the effectiveness of your teaching efforts from beginning to end. Everything you have studied to this point has a bearing on evaluation. The Miller–Stoeckel Client Education Model is the conceptual framework for this text, and in this chapter we address the final component of the model, client education outcomes. The model shows two distinct aspects of client education outcomes: formative evaluation and summative evaluation. This chapter describes different forms and purposes of evaluation and how it fits into the Miller–Stoeckel Client Education Model. The main focus of this chapter is to discuss formative evaluation.

EVALUATION

Evaluation is important for nurses as educators, clients as learners, health team members, and educational program managers because it informs them about their progress in learning and the **effectiveness** of the teaching and learning process. Evaluation is feedback that tells clients and educators if their time and effort together have been well spent (Slavin, 2012).

Evaluation is about judging and providing a basis for making those judgments (Morrison, Ross, Kemp, & Kalman, 2007). It tells us the degree to which the learning goals and objectives have been met or not met, and if they were appropriate (Falvo, 2011). Evaluation tells us whether or not the **content** was suitable and the teaching **strategies** and **instructional materials** were effective. Evaluation in health education provides evidence about the following:

- Client learning
- Effectiveness of the teaching and learning process
- Teacher effectiveness
- Cost–benefit of health education programs

Redman (2007) identifies additional purposes of evaluation, noting that it can motivate clients and reinforce their correct behavior as well as reinforce educators for effective teaching. Evaluation is also useful in working with health team members. It helps to determine if health team members are knowledgeable, safe, and competent to deliver nursing care and perform nursing procedures.

Evaluation provides credibility and accountability to individual client education efforts and to health education programs taught to groups of clients. It is vital to the institution's education department to document the importance and effectiveness of teaching and learning. This includes documenting client learning, the time teaching takes, and the positive, cost-effective results of the time investment. In addition to the preceding political and financial factors, nurses as educators need to be aware of the legal responsibilities of documentation.

BOX 12-1

Client Education Outcomes: Formative Evaluation

Evaluation of the teaching plan:
- Concept comprehension
- Motivation

Evaluation of the learning environment:
- Delivery format
- Technology

Evaluation of the nurse–client interaction:
- Engagement
- Communication

Documentation also provides for continuity of teaching efforts because it serves as a **communication** tool among health team members (Rankin, Stallings, & London, 2005).

The process of evaluation has evolved over time and is divided into two broad categories: **formative** and **summative.** Scriven (1967) made the initial distinction between the two types of evaluation. He stated that formative evaluation is intended to promote improvement within an ongoing activity, person, or program, and summative evaluation is used to assess whether the end goals of the activity, person, or program had been met. Scriven placed more emphasis on summative evaluation to determine the appraisal of the final product. Saettler (1990) further defined the two types of evaluation by saying that formative evaluation is used to refine goals and evolve strategies for achieving goals, and summative evaluation is used to determine the impact of educational practice so future efforts can be improved. He pointed out that formative evaluation can give more detailed information, but it takes longer and is labor intensive.

Box 12-1 presents the formative evaluation portion of client education outcomes for the Miller–Stoeckel Client Education Model. It is the framework for this chapter and addresses three areas: evaluation of the teaching plan, evaluation of the learning environment, and evaluation of the nurse–client **interaction.**

FORMATIVE EVALUATION: EVALUATION OF THE TEACHING PLAN

Formative evaluation can be thought of as assessment *for* learning, as opposed to summative evaluation, which is assessment *of* learning. It begins with evaluation of the teaching plan based on the learning objectives. **Learning objectives** inform clients and educators of the criteria for success and are part of a feedback loop designed to provide information about the learning experience. Evaluation strategies help determine the effectiveness of learning objectives on learning experiences (**Figure 12-1**).

FIGURE 12-1

Learning Objectives Feedback Loop

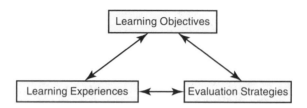

Concept Comprehension

Evaluation of the teaching plan includes determining concept comprehension based on the learning objectives. Tools and techniques exist for both clients and educators to assess how well they are meeting the learning objectives. They are not used to grade or determine the end results of learning. Mastery is not expected when concepts are first introduced. The purpose of formative evaluation strategies is to assess concept comprehension along the way and provide information needed to adjust teaching and learning while they are still occurring. Evaluation of the teaching plan enhances the client's motivation to learn, helps identify gaps in knowledge, fosters self-study, and informs the client of misunderstandings. Examples of formative evaluation tools include quizzes; direct observation; simulations; concept maps; and Classroom Assessment Techniques (CATs), such as the 1-minute paper, think-pair-share, and case-based learning. The construction of a portfolio also serves as formative evaluation. A portfolio is defined as a collection of evidence that is gathered to show a person's learning journey over time and to demonstrate his or her abilities (Butler, 2006). The tools assist the clients in being informed about their progress and help them identify their strengths and weaknesses to target areas that need work.

Formative evaluation of the educator is used to provide information and feedback about his or her teaching for the purpose of learning, developing, and improving. Examples of formative evaluation tools for educators include peer observation, using a checklist or narrative feedback form, one-on-one teaching consultations, and questionnaires. Formative evaluation of the educator is designed to assist in making refinements and adjustments midway through teaching to better meet the learning objectives and needs of clients (Falvo, 2011). It is also helpful in analyzing usefulness of instructional materials. The Suitability Assessment of Materials (SAM) tool measures how well materials fit your clients; it compares different materials and selects those most suitable for your clients. It helps you tailor existing materials to a particular population, sets standards, and guides development and testing of culturally and linguistically appropriate materials.

As you are teaching, it is important to know if you are responding appropriately and effectively to clients. This means monitoring your ability to observe behavior and ask pertinent questions. Observing client behavior in face-to-face encounters includes awareness of verbal and nonverbal cues as you are teaching (O'Brien, 2007). Demonstration and return demonstration is an effective way to observe the client's progress in mastering psychomotor skills. It is an opportunity for you to reinforce what the client is doing right and correct any mistakes that the client is making. Direct questioning is another way to assess client progress in learning. By asking a question, you immediately pick up any gaps or misunderstandings and can clarify the information. Using open-ended questions that require clients to think through an answer is preferred over questions that result in a simple yes or no answer. The educator demonstrates an attitude of openness and willingness to change to improve the quality of client education.

Motivation

While going through the learning process, a client decides whether he or she will pay attention. If the learning objective is judged as important and doable, then the client is motivated to engage in it. If the task is presented as having low relevance or that there is a low probability of success, a negative effect is generated and motivation to complete the learning task is low. Responses to teaching are also influenced by individual experiences, behaviors, and attitudes that influence health behaviors. These influences should be a part of an ongoing formative evaluation of motivation. The Pender Health Promotion Model provides a framework for predicting health-promoting lifestyles and specific behaviors. It seeks to promote healthy behavior of individuals and groups through understanding biophysical processes that motivate them to engage in behaviors directed toward health enhancement (Pender, 2011). The model posits that cognition, action, and environment influence individuals' health-promoting behaviors. It is used extensively as a framework for research and can also be used as a guide for nurses as educators in evaluating teaching plans for client education.

Promoting healthy behavior through education is not isolated to understanding a person's characteristics; it is also interactive with the environment. The environment is not limited to the physical space occupied; it includes the cultural and social influences within the community. Due to this environmental influence, behaviors that may deter the success of health education must be addressed. The nurse as educator uses the concepts of the model to develop, modify, and deliver health promotion education to individuals, families, and groups. The Health Promotion Model provides a lens through which the nurse as educator can evaluate clients' capacity for self-care with the goal to promote, retain, and restore health. The process evaluating motivation and willingness to act is ongoing and implies that nurses as educators will adjust the teaching plan to accommodate changes in the patient's health status, beliefs, and environmental circumstances. **Figure 12-2** shows the adaption of the Pender Health Promotion Model to the nurse–client relationship component of the Miller–Stoeckel Client Education Model.

Kirkpatrick (1994) stated that formative evaluation should include how well the client liked a particular learning process. Results of surveys to determine satisfaction with the learning process give feedback about motivation. It is important that clients and family are satisfied with the health education process. Satisfaction is important when educating clients and families about health (Falvo, 2011; Rankin et al., 2005). Dansky and Miles (1997) suggested that satisfied clients are more likely to maintain relationships with providers. Other important outcomes are that satisfied clients are more likely to keep appointments, comply

FIGURE 12-2

Evaluation of Client Motivation to Act

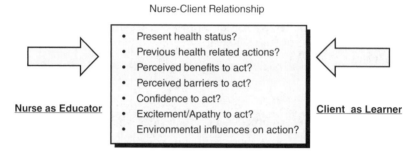

Source: Data from the Health Promotion Model: Pender, 1996. Pender, N.J. (1996) Health promotion in nursing practice. Norwalk, CT: Appleton-Centuy-Crofts

with treatment, and refer other patients to their providers (Chung, Hamill, Kim, Walters, & Wilkins, 1999). If evaluation reveals that the teaching plan is not relevant to the client, it means that more effort has to be put into the design and presentation of the learning process. You should be aware that the design of the teaching plan should promote the learning process rather than just making it entertaining. If the teaching plan is built on sound purpose and design, it should motivate the client to learn and support improved performance. Evaluation of motivation and concept comprehension give you information for improving and evaluating the learning process.

FORMATIVE EVALUATION: EVALUATION OF THE LEARNING ENVIRONMENT

Learning environments include the delivery format of the teaching plan and the technology that supports the teaching plan. Formative evaluation assesses the delivery format, which includes one-on-one teaching, the traditional classroom, distance learning, or a blended format. One-on-one teaching and traditional classroom learning involves educators in face-to-face situations, whereas in distance education the vast majority of teaching takes places with the educator and client apart. Distance learning uses teaching methods that deliver education outside the traditional classroom through the computer, Internet, software programs, electronic conferencing, or other approaches. Blended learning combines both classroom and online education so the client may both attend class and independently complete online learning components. Technology resources are all the tools and resources we use in education. Technologies should focus on the needs of the client. When they are combined with the appropriate delivery format, they should create an effective and rich learning environment. Formative evaluation includes assessing comfort and the ease of use of delivery formats and technologies.

Delivery Format

Formative evaluation of the delivery format involves assessing the type of **delivery format**—whether it is face to face, distance learning, or blended—and if it meets the needs of the client and educator. When teaching at a distance you must address different challenges than when teaching in a traditional classroom. Individual preferences for different formats should be acknowledged and efforts should be made to promote a positive learning environment. The classroom evaluation includes both physical and psychological aspects. Questions to ask clients include the following: Does the delivery format support your ability to learn? Do you feel that the physical environment is safe and comfortable? Is there a culture of mutual respect and understanding? What is the comfort level of interacting with the instructor and other clients? Distance learning formats are evaluated with questions such as the following: What is your comfort level with the method of distance instruction? What is the appropriateness of content and assignments? Does the design of learning activities support learning? Are there adequate support services for distance learners?

Technology

Technology includes the resources used during client education. It provides different channels of communication, such as text, audio, visual, and motion, and runs the gamut from slide shows and videotapes to PowerPoint presentations and hyperlinks. Technologies selected for learning should be effective, efficient, and appealing in meeting the needs of clients. An important part of formative evaluation is that the technology should focus on the needs of the client instead of being used because of an expectation for technology integration. Questions to ask clients include the following: Is the technology meeting your needs? Is the technology user friendly? Is the technology the best approach to helping you learn? Questions to ask educators include the following: Are you comfortable using the technology? Is the technology engaging clients and supporting the learning objectives?

FORMATIVE EVALUATION: EVALUATION OF THE NURSE–CLIENT INTERACTION

Positive relationships are the heart of successful teaching and learning, whether they are defined in terms of respect and rapport, therapeutic interactions, or personal relationship building (Danielson, 2007; Saphier, Haley-Speca, & Gower, 2008). The Miller–Stoeckel Client Education Model includes the nurse–client relationship as an interaction between nurses and clients to promote, retain, and restore health. It is a professional and planned relationship between client and nurse that focuses on the client's needs, feelings, problems, and ideas. Formative evaluation examines the interaction as it progresses from inception of the teaching plan to the point of summative evaluation. The level of engagement and communication between the client and nurse are evaluated to determine if changes are needed to make the interaction more supportive of learning.

Engagement

The nurse–client interaction is directed by the nurse and involves engaging clients in their care, providing information and explanations, and answering questions. Engagement is defined as "an agreement to meet or be present at a specified time and place" (Webster's, 2013). This implies that clients and educators take initiative and make the effort to participate. For learning to occur, the client and educator must engage in the learning process. Client engagement can be evaluated by determining if the client is present and showing interest in learning activities. Questions for engagement evaluation include the following: Are clients paying attention? Do clients participate in the teaching sessions? Do clients exhibit interest and curiosity about what is being taught? Taking attendance in a classroom setting or showing up to one-on-one teaching sessions helps reveal who is engaged and who is not. Engaged clients will attend and participate in activities, including asking questions. Online engagement can be determined by the number of times the client views or participates in the learning activities, such as online discussions. Educator engagement can be evaluated in similar ways. Questions to evaluate educator engagement include the following: Is the educator paying attention? Does the educator ask and respond to questions in class or online? Does the educator show enthusiasm and interest in what he or she is teaching? A formative evaluation can assist both clients and educators address ways to increase or maintain engagement as part of the nurse–client interaction.

Communication

Communication is the exchange of meanings between individuals through a common system of symbols (Webster's, 2013). Clients and educators communicate by speaking and writing, and through body language or nonverbal means. Communication is a two-way process that involves getting your message across and understanding what others have to say. It involves active listening, speaking and writing, and observing. The communication process loop reviews how communication takes place; the sender gives the message to the receiver, and the receiver gives feedback to the sender (**Figure 12-3**).

Clients communicate feedback about learning, and educators communicate clear direction and encouragement for continuous improvement. Both clients and educators are expected to speak with respect, listen for understanding, and speak so others can understand. Both clients and educators should evaluate communication skills by asking the following questions: What are the barriers that keep us from understanding each other's ideas and thoughts? How am I coming across in the way I interact? Am I stating my message clearly?

FIGURE 12-3

Communication Loop

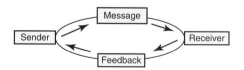

An important type of communication for nurses as educators is giving effective feedback. Nurses should ask themselves if they are giving effective feedback. Feedback should be supportive, behavior specific, and nonjudgmental. **Table 12-1** provides examples of helpful and unhelpful feedback.

TABLE 12-1

Helpful and Unhelpful Feedback

Unhelpful Feedback	Reason	Helpful Feedback	Reason
Your nonverbal behavior was not good as you interacted with the client.	Judgmental	I observed you looking at the computer screen, not at the client, as she was answering your questions.	Identifies a specific behavior
You were not empathetic toward the client.	Nonspecific	To show empathy, acknowledge the problems that the client has in dealing with her husband's illness.	Identifies a different solution to a specific problem
You were very abrupt in your response to the client.	Nonspecific	I noticed that when the client was talking about her family, you interrupted her.	Identifies a specific behavior
It would be better if you did it this way.	Does not support critical thinking	Have you thought about trying it in a different way?	Helps generate alternatives
You did not see how upset the client was.	Judgmental	Did you notice that at one point the client was looking down and appeared upset, but you continued to question her?	Describes specific, detailed behavior to encourage reflection
You did a really good job.	Nonspecific	You started the interaction with open-ended questions and allowed the client time to tell her story by remaining silent and attentive.	Describes positive feedback that is specific and descriptive

Source: Adapted from Wood, D.V. (2007) Formative Assessment, ASME, p. 15.

During the process of formative evaluation, nurses need to be adaptable. If communication is ineffective, consider what would be a better approach and change what you are doing as you are doing it.

CASE EXAMPLE: MRS. ROSA LOPEZ

Formative evaluation of the interaction with Mrs. Rosa Lopez begins with reviewing the learning objectives and critiquing the teaching and learning process as it is ongoing. For example, by the end of the lesson, the cognitive objective is to have Mrs. Lopez correctly verbally explain how excessive salt intake affects blood pressure to the nurse by memory. An example of mid-course correction might be to notice that Mrs. Lopez preferred the videotape instruction to viewing charts and pamphlets. Consequently we would focus on the videotape and reinforce its message.

In evaluating the affective objective—the client will choose to limit sodium intake by working with the nurse to prepare a dietary plan for one week—we would ask, "How do you plan to incorporate these changes into your meal planning and usual diet?" Note the strength of Mrs. Lopez's desire and willingness to limit excessive sodium intake. Depending on her response, we would follow up with suggestions for how she could accomplish this. We would also ask how these dietary changes would help control her high blood pressure. We would reinforce Mrs. Lopez's correct responses and reteach if her responses demonstrate a lack of understanding. It also might be helpful for Mrs. Lopez to talk to clients who have a similar diagnosis to gain practical meal planning suggestions.

The psychomotor objective is to demonstrate how to accurately obtain her own blood pressure reading using home digital equipment without any verbal guidance. We would have Mrs. Lopez read the equipment directions as we demonstrate how to take the blood pressure using her own digital equipment. Mrs. Lopez would then perform a return demonstration and record the findings following the procedure checklist. She would be given a checklist of the steps to follow at home in obtaining her blood pressure, after which she would be given an opportunity to evaluate her own performance. During this time Mrs. Lopez would be given an opportunity to ask questions and be given feedback to guide her learning.

In the formative evaluation process, we would encourage Mrs. Lopez, listen to her concerns, correct misunderstandings, and assure accurate skill performance. When necessary, misinformation would be corrected by reviewing and reteaching any missed or misunderstood content.

SUMMARY

This chapter begins the discussion of the final phase of the teaching and learning process: evaluating client education outcomes. Evaluation of client education has two components: formative and summative. This chapter discussed formative evaluation. Formative evaluation is ongoing during the process of teaching and learning. Clients, educators, health team members, and program managers conduct formative evaluations to improve the learning experience. The Miller–Stoeckel Client Education Model identifies specific aspects of formative evaluation to consider, and they apply to all categories of evaluation. As the educator, you continuously monitor the effectiveness of the teaching plan with attention to concept comprehension and motivation of clients. You also evaluate the learning environment as it relates to the delivery format and technology used for learning. The nurse–client interaction is evaluated by determining the level of engagement and communication. These components of formative evaluation begin at inception of the teaching intervention and conclude at the point of summative evaluation. **Figure 12-4** highlights the key difference between formative and summative evaluation.

The desired outcome of all health education is client learning. Formative evaluation asks, How are we doing in the process of learning? Answering that question and facilitating client learning by making necessary changes during the process of teaching and learning are your responsibilities as educator. **Box 12-2** demonstrates the effectiveness of a multimedia learning program to improve educational effectiveness.

FIGURE 12-4

Formative Summative and Evaluation Continuum

	Formative Evaluation (Ongoing, *for* learning)	**Summative Evaluation** (After instruction, *on* learning
Evaluation of Teaching Plan:	Concept comprehension, Motivation	Measures learning
Evaluation of Environment:	Delivery Format, Technology	Measures effectiveness of programs
Evaluation of Nurse/Client Interaction:	Engagement, Communication	Measures Accountability
Tools for Evaluation:	CATs, Simulation, Surveys, Self-assessments, Portfolio	Testing, surveys, rubrics, exams, checklists
Purpose:	Feedback for improvement	Final Assessments

Intervention Inception ⟶ Midway ⟶ End

Source: Data from McTighe, J and Wiggins, G (1999). The understanding by design handbook. Alexadria, VA: The Association for Supervision and Curriculum Development.

BOX 12-2

Evidence-Based Nursing Practice

Lo, Shu-Fen, Wang, Yun-Tung, Wu, Li-Yue, Hsu, Mei-Yu, Chang, Shu-Chuan, & Hayter, M. (2009). A cost-effectiveness analysis of a multimedia learning education program for stoma patients. Journal of Clinical Nursing, 19, 1844-1854.

Purpose: This study compared the costs and effectiveness of enterostomal education using a multimedia learning education program (MLEP) and a conventional education service program (CESP).

Method: Using an experimental design, 54 stoma patients were randomly assigned to MLEP or CESP nursing care with a follow-up of 1 week. The effectiveness measures were knowledge of self-care (KSC), attitude of self-care (ASC), and behavior of self-care (BSC). The cost measures for each patient were healthcare costs, MLEP cost, and family costs.

Results: Subjects in the MLEP group demonstrated significantly better outcomes in each effectiveness measure. The cost–effectiveness ratio showed that the MLEP program was better than the CESP model after one intervention cycle. The total social costs for each MLEP patient and CESP patient were $7,396 and $8,570, respectively.

EXERCISES

Exercise I: Evaluation of the Teaching Plan

Purpose: Apply formative evaluation to the teaching plan.
Directions: Discuss the following situations and describe, as the educator, how you would handle each one.

1. You are teaching a hospitalized client who is ready for discharge about the importance of taking an antibiotic as prescribed. The learning objectives are for the client to explain the purpose of the antibiotic and how to take the medication. You want to conduct formative evaluation to determine concept comprehension as you teach. Give an example of a tool or other evaluation method that will inform you as to whether the teaching plan is working (such as CAT, quiz, role-play, etc.). Explain why you have chosen this method. What types of feedback would indicate that you need to make changes to your approach?

2. You are teaching a series of classes to a group of older clients about the benefits and types of exercise to improve stamina. You notice at the second class that some clients are not participating and seem to withdraw from the group. Give examples of questions you will ask to determine motivation to act as part of formative evaluation of the teaching plan. What are possible barriers to participation in the teaching plan?

Exercise II: Evaluation of the Learning Environment

Purpose: Apply formative evaluation to the learning environment.
Directions: With a partner, discuss the following situations and describe how, as the educator, you would handle each one:

1. You are teaching about caring for ill toddlers to a group of mothers in the clinic. Many of the mothers bring their children and tend to them during the class. As the class progresses, you wonder if the other mothers are comfortable with the learning environment. What kinds of questions would you ask to determine if the environment is conducive to learning as part of a formative assessment? How would having this information help you make improvements in the class?

2. You are leading a bereavement discussion group in the hospital and have arranged for several films to be shown on the experience of loss. You notice that some clients are leaving in the middle of the films and not returning until the lights are turned on. How will you conduct a formative evaluation to determine how technology is affecting learning in this class? Why is it important to evaluate the learning environment in this class?

Exercise III: Evaluation of the Nurse–Client Interaction

Purpose: Apply formative evaluation to the nurse–client interaction.

Directions: Divide into small groups. Discuss the following situations and describe how, as the educator, you would handle each one:

1. To evaluate the educator–client interaction, have each person share a personal experience about learning new information or a skill. Then identify helpful and unhelpful feedback that you received during the experience. Describe what makes the communication helpful and not helpful.

2. Think of a class in which you did not participate and felt uncomfortable giving feedback. Describe what made you disengage and how things could have been changed to make you want to interact with other students and the instructor.

REFERENCES

Butler, P. (2006). Review of the literature on portfolios and e-portfolios. Retrieved from http://www.eportfoliopractice.qut.edu.au/docs/Butler%20-%20Review%20of%20lit%20on%20ePortfolio%20research%20-%20NZOct%202006.pdf

Chung, K. C., Hamill, J. B., Kim, H. M., Walters, M. R., & Wilkins, E. G. (1999). Predictors of patient satisfaction in an outpatient plastic surgery clinic. *Annals of Plastic Surgery*, *42*(1), 56–60.

Danielson, C. (2007). *Enhancing professional practice: A framework for teaching* (2nd ed.). Alexandria, VA: Association for Supervision and Curriculum Development (ASCD).

Dansky, K. H., & Miles, J. (1997). Patient satisfaction with ambulatory healthcare services: Waiting time and filling time. *Hospital and Health Services Administration*, *42*, 165–176.

Falvo, D. R. (2011). *Effective patient education: A guide to increased compliance* (4th ed.). Sudbury, MA: Jones & Bartlett Learning.

Kirkpatrick, D. L. (1994). *Evaluating training programs*. San Francisco, CA: Berrett-Koehler.

Lo, S. F., Wang, Y. T., Wu, L. Y., Hsu, M. Y., Chang, S. C., & Hayter, M. (2009). A cost-effectiveness analysis of a multimedia learning education program for stoma patients. *Journal of Clinical Nursing*, *19*, 1844–1854.

Morrison, G. R., Ross, S. M., Kemp, J. E., & Kalman, H. K. (2007). *Designing effective instruction* (5th ed.). Hoboken, NJ: John Wiley and Sons.

O'Brien, P. G. (2007). Patient and family teaching. In S. L. Lewis, M. M. Heitkemper, S. R. Dirksen, P. G. O'Brien, & L. Bucher (Eds.), *Medical-surgical nursing* (7th ed., pp. 53–65). St. Louis, MO: Mosby.

Pender, N. (2011). The health promotion manual. Retrieved from *content/uploads/2013/02/HEALTH_PROMOTION_MANUAL_Rev_5-2011.pdf*

Rankin, S. H., Stallings, K. D., & London, F. (2005). *Patient education in health and illness* (5th ed.). Philadelphia, PA: Lippincott Williams & Wilkins.

Redman, B. K. (2007). *The practice of patient education: A case study approach* (10th ed.). St. Louis, MO: Mosby Year Book.

Saettler, P. (1990). *The evolution of American educational technology.* Englewood, CO: Libraries Unlimited.

Saphier, J., Haley-Speca, M. A., & Gower, R. (2008). *The skillful teacher: Building your teaching skills* (6th ed.). Acton, MA: Research for Better Teaching.

Scriven, M. (1967). The methodology of evaluation. In R. W. Tyler, R. M. Gagne, & M. Sciven (Eds.), *Perspectives of curriculum evaluation* (pp. 39–83). Chicago, IL: Rand McNally.

Slavin, R. E. (2012). *Educational psychology theory and practice* (10th ed.). Boston, MA: Pearson.

Webster's All-In-One Dictionary and Thesaurus (2nd ed.). (2013). Springfield, MA: Federal Street Press.

Wood, D. (2007). Understanding medical education: Formative assessment. Edinburgh, Scotland: Association for the Study of Medical Education.

13

Summative Evaluation

OBJECTIVES

Upon completion of this chapter, you will be able to do the following:

- Identify the three components of summative evaluation in the Miller–Stoeckel Client Education Model.
- Distinguish between measurement and evaluation.
- Describe the evaluation of client learning using direct and indirect measurement methods.
- Describe four sources of error in measurement.
- Select measurement methods best suited for cognitive, affective, and psychomotor objectives.
- Describe the evaluation of educational effectiveness as it relates to course and program evaluation.
- Describe the evaluation of the integration of learning into clients' daily living as it relates to adherence and the impact on the community.
- Describe facilitators of client adherence.

KEY TERMS

adherence	evaluation	reinforcement
choice	formative	sources of error
collaboration	measurement	summative

INTRODUCTION

In this chapter we discuss summative evaluation and how it enhances health education. Summative evaluation occurs at the conclusion of teaching and learning. In this chapter you will learn how the nurse as educator uses the results of summative evaluation to improve client

BOX 13-1

Client Education Outcomes: Summative Evaluation

Evaluation of client learning:
■   Measurement
■   Direct measurement methods
■   Indirect measurement methods

Evaluation of educational effectiveness:
■   Course evaluation
■   Program evaluation

Evaluation of integration of learning into daily living:
■   Client adherence
■   Impact on the community

learning, courses, and programs. The ultimate test of our educational efforts is improvement in clients' health and the health of the community.

The Miller–Stoeckel Client Education Model is the conceptual framework for this text. In this chapter we address **summative evaluation**, which is a component of the client education outcomes portion of the model. Summative evaluation focuses on three areas: evaluation of client learning, evaluation of educational effectiveness, and evaluation of integration of learning into daily living (**Box 13-1**). This chapter explores each component of summative evaluation.

SUMMATIVE EVALUATION: EVALUATION OF CLIENT LEARNING

After any teaching effort it is important for nurses as educators to pause, look back, and reflect on what has been accomplished and what they can learn from their efforts. Did clients achieve the knowledge, attitudes, and skills specified in the learning objectives? What evidence do we have of client learning? Were the objectives, content, teaching strategies, and instructional materials suitable and effective for the clients? Would different instructional materials be more effective; for example, would having models and equipment to manipulate be more effective than watching a video? Summative evaluation involves making comparisons between what is effective and what is not. To begin our discussion of summative evaluation, we must first focus on measurement and the difficulties of measuring learning.

Measurement

Evaluation is about judging and determining the value, significance, worth, or condition of something. It is how we support that evaluation, and it establishes the criteria by which to judge something. **Measurement** means gauging the dimensions, quantity, or capacity of something by comparing it with some kind of standard (Webster's, 2013). Measurement ranges from the concrete, such as clients learning to take their own pulse, to the abstract, such as learning better ways to handle stress. Both phenomena are important; however, the former is much easier to

FIGURE 13-1

Direct and Indirect Measurement Continuum

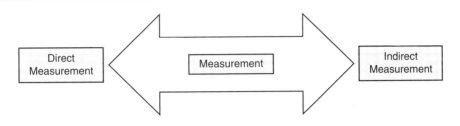

measure than the latter. Methods of measurement are ordered along a continuum from direct to indirect at opposite ends (**Figure 13-1**).

Measurement involves both observation and recording behavior, regardless of whether the measurement is direct or indirect. Direct measurement is the most accurate when it takes place in the actual situation and, ideally, when it occurs over time. It is direct observation of the behavior being measured. For example, nurses make observations at the hospital bedside, in the home, or at the work site. Direct observations are also obtained from equipment and monitors that measure things such as vital signs, oxygen levels, blood glucose, and so forth.

Indirect measurement is not as accurate as direct measurement. It occurs when the educator creates substitute situations or takes incomplete samples of behavior. For example, if you role-play with clients, you create substitute situations that imitate, or substitute for, the real one. When you give clients paper-and-pencil tests, you attempt to measure cognitive processes indirectly. No one knows what thinking is or what it looks like. Therefore, you must infer from what clients write whether or not they have thought about, retained, and gained the knowledge and understanding you hoped they would grasp.

Measurement methods are also categorized as being objective or subjective (Lorig et al., 2001). Examples of objective measures include observable factors such as vital signs, weight, blood glucose, cholesterol levels, wound healing, hospital readmissions, and class attendance. Subjective measures are data from human observers (clients, providers, educators) and are therefore considered biased measures. These measures are less reliable because there are multiple explanations for client behavior. There may be extenuating circumstances that affect whether the client can successfully meet the objectives, and these circumstances may be unknown to the observer. For example, a nurse reports that an overweight client has little interest in weight reduction when in fact the client does not understand how to diet. The nurse assumes the client is not motivated to learn about weight reduction because the client discarded reading material that she was given, when in fact the client has low health literacy skills. The client can also be a subjective observer. For example, the client who chain smokes reports that she stopped smoking, when in fact she cut down to one to two cigarettes per day.

Sources of Error in Measurement

Error is always possible in measurement, and the more indirect the measurement, the more likely errors will occur. Redman (2007) notes the following common **sources of error:** indirect measurement, the complexity of behavior, observer bias, and sampling error. A brief description of each source of error follows.

Indirect Measurement

Indirect measurement provides a false picture of how a client would react unless the nurse observes that person in the actual situation. The saying "he talks a good game" indicates that many people know the difference between talking about a situation and actually handling it. Because your time with clients is limited, your only **choice** may be to measure the learning objectives by indirect means, such as oral quizzes and paper-and-pencil tests. Keep in mind that these methods are indirect and you infer the degree of client learning from them.

Complex Behavior

Behavior, by nature, is complex. The causes of behavior, especially thought patterns, feelings, and attitudes, are difficult to identify for both the observer and the client who exhibits the behavior. As an educator you may not be able to discover what, if any, impact the learning had on clients. A client may act agreeable just to please you, or he or she may choose not to tell you all the variables involved in a failure to learn. Indeed, clients themselves may not be fully aware of all the factors that help or hinder their learning.

Observer Bias

Humans are limited in the amount of stimuli they can notice. Observers draw conclusions based on their own perceptions, culture, and past experiences. This can lead to erroneous inferences and conclusions about client learning. One advantage of working with colleagues is that it can help balance the perceptions of individual clients. How others see a particular client influences your perceptions. When you team teach, you and your colleagues give balanced views of the clients. If a colleague tells you a client, a family, or a team member is difficult to deal with, you are likely to approach that individual in a different manner. This can lead to bias, but it can also lead to a collaborative effort to help the client learn. Approach each individual with openness.

Sampling Error

Sampling is obtaining a small picture of the client's behavior that is representative of all the learning you provided. From this sample you infer that the client has or has not mastered the learning objectives. Sampling error occurs when the sample you choose to measure is not representative of client learning. Clients may have learned A, B, and C; but if you measure D, E, and F, you get a false picture of the client's learning and achievements.

The period of time during which you choose to measure the behavior can also be misleading. For example, you form a different perception of your client's willingness and ability to do range-of-motion exercises if you test him or her early in the morning rather than waiting until later in the day. It is not possible to observe all the required behaviors. Therefore, your task is to select behavioral samples that are as representative as possible and relevant to the variables that are most critical. In general, you can compensate for measurement errors by using a variety of measurement methods.

Direct Measurement Methods

Remember that measurement methods must be consistent with the learning objectives. You cannot test everything you have taught or that clients have learned, so you must select a representative sample to test (Slavin, 2012). Direct measurement of behavior is achieved through observation of behavior, video recordings, rating scales, checklists, evaluation rubrics, and anecdotal notes.

Observation of Behavior

Direct observation occurs when the nurse observes clients demonstrating mastery of psychomotor skills. For example, you observe a client properly using crutches with no axillary pressure and no loss of balance. Another example is observing how skillfully a client removes a dressing, cleans the wound, and applies a fresh dressing without contamination. Both examples are direct observations of client behavior.

Direct observation also involves nurses using the senses. For example, the nurse listens to breath sounds through a stethoscope after a guided session of turning and deep breathing. Or the nurse counts the client's pulse and respiration rate to observe the impact of a relaxation exercise. Direct observations of client responses are documented by using a checklist designed for specific procedures, which is discussed later in this chapter.

Video Recordings

Direct observation of behavior is also achieved through video recordings. Video recordings offer the advantage of accuracy. The video camera observes and records what happened, rather than depending on the nurse's interpretation of what happened. The recording is useful in that the nurse and client get accurate feedback by watching it. This is especially useful when teaching health team members new psychomotor skills. The recording can be studied repeatedly and at length for feedback to improve performance.

Video recordings are helpful when clients role-play new affective behaviors, such as improving interpersonal communications. Families who are puzzled by their communication difficulties can sometimes gain insight into their patterns when viewed from a different perspective. Video recording helps decrease defensiveness and increases objectiveness as they watch themselves.

Video recordings are effective for teaching health team members how to interact with clients who are depressed, anxious, or hostile. They are also effective for nurses who are new in the role of educator and for experienced nurses who want to improve their teaching performance. It is much easier to accept feedback from observing a video recording of one's performance rather than an instructor's critique.

Rating Scales

Rating scales on surveys and questionnaires use a Likert-type scale to rate client responses. For example, one rating scale asks if clients strongly agree, agree, disagree, or strongly disagree with a number of specific items. Another rating scale asks how clients would evaluate items on a scale that ranges from 1 to 5, in which 1 means no confidence and 5 means total confidence. There are a variety of responses for this scale, depending on what you want to know. The meaning of the numbers can also vary but should be clearly identified in the legend. For example, 1 could mean "did not help me" at the low end, and 5 could mean "helped me a great deal" at the high end of the scale.

Rating scales are given to clients to fill out at the conclusion of a teaching session, course, or program to evaluate their satisfaction with the teaching experience. They provide insight into the clients' perceptions of learning effectiveness. They also provide helpful feedback to improve the teacher's performance. Rating scales are used for statistical purposes. Collating the results and determining the mean and standard deviation for each item on the rating scale provides instructive information. These data collected over time provide useful feedback to evaluate clients' perceptions of teaching and learning effectiveness. **Figures 13-2 and 13-3** are sample rating scales that are used to evaluate learning objectives and teacher evaluations.

Checklists

Checklists are more precise than rating scales because they identify each of the desired behaviors and provide space for recording the presence or absence of each behavior. When you create a checklist, identify the critical elements of the desired behaviors and exclude nonessential ones. For example, when you measure a mother's bonding behavior, include observations such as whether she looks at, touches, and talks to the infant rather than whether she has the most updated equipment. Another example is teaching a client to give a self-injection. It is not critical how the client arranges the placement of equipment on a tray. It is critical, however, that the sterility of the equipment is maintained. **Figure 13-4** is a sample checklist of critical requirements for giving an injection. The learning domain is psychomotor and the learning objective is as follows: the client will perform an injection accurately according to the steps of the procedure.

Assistance from colleagues is valuable in developing a checklist. They can try out the checklist to refine the items and wording. Because clients do not pass until they can do every step correctly, it is important to establish the number of times clients must exhibit the correct behaviors to ensure they have mastered the task.

FIGURE 13-2

Sample Form to Evaluate Learning Objectives

List each learning objective here	0	1	2	3	4	5
1.						
2.						
3.						
4.						

Descriptors for the key can vary.
For example, the stem can read "To what degree did this course help you achieve the learning objective?" and the key could be a 3-point rating scale: not at all, somewhat, and a lot.

Key:
0 = not applicable
1 = did not help me achieve this objective
2 = helped me less than I expected
3 = helped me about what I expected
4 = helped me more than I expected
5 = definitely helped me achieve this objective

FIGURE 13-3

Teacher Evaluation Form

Teacher Evaluation Form

Key:
0 = not applicable
1 = definitely below average
2 = slightly below average
3 = average
4 = slightly above average
5 = definitely above average

Speaker:_____

Evaluator: _____

Objectives — Were the objectives:

    Clearly presented to the clients?

    Evident throughout the presentation?

        0 1 2 3 4 5

Content — Was the content:

    Clearly explained?

    Accurate?

    At the right vocabulary level?

    Appropriate to the audience's background?

Strategies — Were the strategies:

    Appropriate for the content?

    Appropriate for the audience?

Teaching aids — Were the materials:

    Appropriate to the context?

    Appropriate to the objectives?

    At the client's level of comprehension?

    Pleasing to the eye?

    Visible (contrast, size, and location)?

    Used in a practiced manner?

Performance — Did the teacher:

    Dress appropriately to the clients and topic?

    Maintain eye contact with the audience?

    Speak in a clear audible voice?

    Use a pace appropriate to the audience?

    Stay attuned to the audience?

    Give recognition for contributions?

    Allow time for questions?

    Seek feedback periodically?

    Show preparation by smooth performance?

Comments:

Source: Data from Babcock and Miller. (1994). Client education: Theory & practice. St. Louis: Mosby.

FIGURE 13-4

Checklist for Giving an Injection

Name of Client: _____					
Behavior	**Dates**				**Comments**
1. Selects appropriate equipment.					
2. Identifies action, use, side effects, and dosage range of medication.					

3. Maintains sterility:
   a. of equipment.
   b. in administration.					

4. Prepares accurate dosage:
   a. verifies dosage prescribed.
   b. draws up correct dose.
5. Selects acceptable injection site.					

6. Injects at appropriate angle:
   a. 30-to 60-degree angle for SQ
   b. 90-degree angle for IM
7. Aspirates plunger before injecting.					

8. Injects medication.					
9. Disposes of needle safely.					

Evaluation Rubrics

An evaluation rubric combines features of the rating scale and checklist that are useful for evaluating team members' performance when a team member is your client (**Figure 13-5**). The example uses Benner's (1984) five levels of proficiency (novice, advanced beginner, competent, proficient, and expert) to evaluate nurses in their role as educators. The evaluator notes the level of proficiency at which the team member is performing each criterion. The evaluator then writes an anecdotal note in the space provided. An alternative rating scale that could be used instead of Benner's levels is beginning, developing, proficient, and independent. Whichever rating scale is used, a committee of nurses in the healthcare institution should define the rating levels. There should be broad agreement of the definition of the scope of skills and responsibilities for each level. The criteria in the example are samples of what could be included in the rubric.

Anecdotal Notes

An anecdotal note is a brief vignette of a client's behavior at a particular moment in time. This type of note is used in psychiatric facilities because it helps observers detect changes in clients' behaviors over time and the circumstances under which changes occurred. For example, an adolescent client hospitalized for severe behavior problems was cooperative with her therapist

FIGURE 13-5

Evaluation Rubric

Criterion	Novice	Advanced beginner	Competent	Proficient	Expert	Notes
Communicates learning objectives				Yes		Clearly stated at outset
Presents accurate information		Yes				Much improved over previous session
Uses appropriate teaching strategies		Yes				Tried another strategy when the first was ineffective
Uses appropriate handouts			Yes			Distributed two handouts written in client's native language
Answers questions	No					Needs to take the time to answer questions
Seeks feedback periodically	No					Needs to pause and seek feedback
Maintains eye contact		Yes				Fairly consistent eye contact

Definitions of these terms should be created by a committee of professional nurses in the healthcare institution/agency using the tool: Novice, Advanced beginner, Competent, Proficient, and Expert.

away from the hospital, but she was obstinate and defiant with caregivers on the psychiatric unit. The nurse must determine the following:

- What is the client's behavior with her family and friends?
- What is the gender of the therapist and other caregivers? Does the gender of the caregiver make a difference?
- How are the therapist's interactions with the client different from that of the staff?

It is crucial for various caregivers on the unit to use the observations as important data for evaluation. They should not automatically jump to a conclusion like, the client always acts fine for me. The hidden implication is, what are the rest of you doing wrong?

Anecdotal notes must be recorded consistently over time for the caregivers to pick up client behavior patterns and changes. They should be pertinent to the learning objectives with related comments. They should also clearly and specifically describe client behavior and be free of bias or derogatory terms.

The following example illustrates an inappropriate comment: the client is obnoxious and uncooperative. It would be better to restate such an observation as follows:

- The client refuses to get out of bed until …
- When client is reminded about the importance of exercise to his recovery, he avoids eye contact and does not respond.

The latter example may create a climate of investigation rather than disapproval. If nurses are curious rather than judgmental, they will more likely discover clues that help create a learning environment that is conducive to success. If they maintain an attitude of curiosity, they are more likely to discover if there are disparities between the client's and nurses' goals.

Indirect Measurement Methods

Indirect measurement methods must be consistent with the learning objectives. Develop questions that provide evidence of how well clients achieved the learning objectives. Indirect measurement of behavior includes direct questioning and written measurement.

Direct Questioning

Direct questioning is an effective way to determine a client's level of understanding of what you taught. It is useful in both **formative** and summative evaluation; however, it is more often used in formative evaluation when teaching is ongoing. Its use in summative evaluation is limited to oral quizzes, which have little application in health education. Direct questioning is also used to obtain oral feedback from clients at the conclusion of a teaching session or program to learn what was most and least helpful.

Written Measurement

So far we have considered measurement involving direct transactions with clients in which you have observed the learning directly or asked clients for their perceptions of the learning that took place. A more indirect way to gather evidence of learning is written measurement; however, there are prerequisites to using this method for evaluation. For example, to use written measurement, clients must be able to read and have the ability to see. A well-educated client who is taking medications that cause double vision cannot participate in written measurement, nor can clients whose reading glasses are unavailable. Clients who are bilingual but read only in another language, or clients who are so weak they cannot write, are inappropriate subjects for written evaluations.

One of the main advantages of written measurement is its efficiency in terms of time and energy. One person (not necessarily the nurse educator) can distribute a written measurement tool to many people at once. The data can be analyzed at the evaluator's convenience and can be easily stored along with the conclusions. In this computer age, written measurements for evaluation are part of software educational programs.

Test Construction

To construct an effective test, you need to keep many variables in mind. A good test covers all of the relevant material and relates directly to the learning objectives. Because you cannot ask everything on a test, the test should include a representative sample of what was taught (Gronlund & Brookhart, 2009). Testing is sampling what clients have learned.

Any test should be relevant to the clients in terms of their life experience and health literacy level. If the clients' reading skills are limited, use very simple words and supplement them with pictures. If they are unable to understand written directions, give the directions orally. Reviewing a couple of sample items with clients helps them to understand your expectations.

Many clients are more confident if you show them what you want them to do. Be aware that clients may read directions only as a last resort.

A good test uses different types of items, such as true or false, multiple choice, matching, fill in the blank, and short-answer essay to test learning in a variety of ways. True-or-false and fill-in-the-blank questions are good for testing knowledge of facts. Matching questions are good for testing recall of related concepts. Multiple-choice questions are good for distinguishing myths from reality and for measuring some levels of problem solving, inference, and making generalizations. Short-answer essay questions reveal the clients' thinking process. They also provide clues to the clients' use of the information you taught. See **Box 13-2** for guidelines to help you write test questions.

When preparing test questions, avoid using the exact words you used while teaching so you measure understanding rather than memory. The use of giveaway words should also be avoided, although they can be used as distracters in the questions. The words *never, always*, and *all* usually indicate that the answer is false. The words *generally, mostly*, and *usually* commonly indicate that the answer is true. If words such as these are used, the test may measure the test-taking skills of clients rather than their attainment of the learning objectives. Be clear about what you want to measure.

True-or-false questions are good for testing common misperceptions about health and illness. These questions test recognition of information rather than recall. The advantage is that they are easy to write. The disadvantage is that clients have a 50% chance of selecting the correct answer regardless of their knowledge. If you use true-or-false questions, write out *T or true* and *F or false* in front of the question and instruct clients to circle the correct answer. When clients have to write either T or F, sometimes it is difficult to decipher their handwriting.

Each multiple-choice question has three parts: the stem, the correct answer, and the distracters. The stem is the lead-in sentence or question to which the client must then fit the correct answer. Distracters are other possible but incorrect answers. Myths and plausible answers are

BOX 13-2

Guidelines for Writing Test Questions

- Group questions according to type: true or false, matching, multiple choice, fill in the blank, and short-answer essay.
- State general directions at the beginning of the test; for example, "This test is designed to measure what you know about how to take care of yourself. It will help us plan further teaching." (For clients with low literacy say, "Please take this test. The results will tell us what else we need to teach you.")
- State specific directions before each group of questions.
- Indicate where to record the answer and provide a place for the clients' answers.
- Use vocabulary that fits the reading level of the clients.
- Make the directions as clear and as short as possible.
- Underline or bold the directions and special words.
- Make all multiple-choice options similar in length.
- Put the multiple-choice question and answer options on the same page.
- Make all multiple-choice options grammatically parallel.

BOX 13-3

Examples of Multiple-Choice Questions

---

1. Which of the following statements is true about parenthood? It is a/an:
   a. Impossible role for most couples
   b. Demanding but growth-enhancing experience
   c. Essential element of a healthy marriage
   d. Necessary for a well-rounded, fulfilled life
2. Effective crutch walking includes all the following <u>except</u>:
   a. Avoiding slippery surfaces so you remain stable
   b. Keeping the crutches snug in your armpits by leaning on them
   c. Practicing until you have developed a smooth rhythm
   d. Placing your most important items in a fanny pack

---

good distracters. A good test question is grammatically consistent with all the possible answers. All answer options should be about the same length. Inconsistencies in length can give clues to the correct answer. Clients guess the right answer by looking for the best grammatical fit in matching or multiple-choice questions. If all of the options begin with the same word or phrase, that word or phrase should be stated only once at the end of the stem (**Box 13-3**). Try to avoid negatively stated items. If you use negative items, be sure to underline the negative. An example of this is test question 2 in Box 13-3. A table of random numbers helps you list answers and distracters inconsistently; it is easy to slip into a predictable pattern for listing correct answers. Another way to randomize the sequence of choices in multiple-choice questions is to arrange answers alphabetically.

Matching questions have two columns. The first column gives a list of words that must be matched to the words or phrases in the second column. It is preferable to use phrases in the second column to discourage guessing, and it also makes the test a better measure of the client's knowledge. There should be more words or phrases listed in the second column than in the first column. The words or phrases in the second column will be a combination of correct answers and distracters. The goal is to test the client's knowledge, not their guessing ability.

Fill-in-the-blank questions should contain blanks that are all the same size. If the blanks vary in size, clients will try to guess what word you had in mind when you constructed the test. If you choose to provide a list of correct words, it should contain distracters.

Short-answer essay questions are good because clients can answer them in their own words. When you read the answers, you learn about the clients' perceptions about the health issue and gain insight into their thinking. For health education purposes, the answer to the question should take only a few sentences.

When preparing a test, group questions according to type because clients must switch mental processes to answer each type. For example, all true-or-false questions should be grouped together, and all multiple-choice questions should be together. If the test is likely to produce some anxiety, it may help to start it with some easy items. This helps to measure clients' learning rather than how they think when they are stressed.

Making test directions clear is a challenging task. A good way to clarify the directions is to have them critiqued by someone who knows the subject. Sometimes clients need help and hints. This is especially true when a written tool is used to test children. Include a grading scale if clients are to grade themselves; a key can be provided on the back of the page or upside down at the bottom of the page.

Pretests and Posttests

A pretest is useful for assessing the clients' current knowledge about a subject and their learning needs. The results of the pretest allow nurses to construct the knowledge base for teaching and avoid repeating what clients already know. Pretests are also good for piquing the curiosity of clients. One possible disadvantage of pretests is that they are often perceived as threatening. This threat may be outweighed by the fact that pretests are helpful as self-diagnostic feedback.

At the conclusion of the teaching session, administer a posttest. The posttest should be the same as the pretest to determine the gains made as a result of the teaching session. The results of both pre- and posttests are compared to measure client learning. Some test services design equivalent pretests and posttests. This means that although the tests are not exactly alike, they test the same knowledge or skills. The process for developing equivalent tests is lengthy, expensive, and must be done with populations of significant size. This involves sophisticated statistical analysis that is beyond the scope of this text.

Choosing Appropriate Measurement Methods

Cognitive, affective, and psychomotor learning objectives require different measurement methods. To determine which are best, ask which are most appropriate for the learning objective you are measuring. For example, which are most appropriate to measure cognitive learning? The most appropriate methods to use here are oral questions and written measurement. These methods are indirect because you cannot measure cognition (thinking) directly.

How do you measure changes in clients' attitudes or feelings? You may be able to question them directly if they trust you. Their willingness to share is affected by the quality of the nurse–client relationship. Direct observation is also an excellent method because you can infer much from clients' behavior. Clients are not always fully aware of or willing to admit their attitudes and feelings. However, a client's behavior may give clues if you are an astute observer. Video recordings done with a client's permission and anecdotal notes are two good ways to gather the needed data. Written measurement in the form of an attitude scale or opinion survey may also be useful. The use of open-ended questions is yet another way to measure attitudes and feelings. Many factors influence a person's willingness to admit attitudinal change or lack of change.

How do you decide whether or not clients can perform a psychomotor skill at a satisfactory level? Direct observation is the main method for evaluating the attainment of psychomotor skills. If performance is being evaluated, a video recording is excellent. Checklists and rating scales are also useful because they enable you to remain objective with a previously constructed and carefully formulated list. Checklists also reduce the likelihood that crucial elements of the desired performance will be neglected.

Evaluation of Health Team Members

Evaluating health team members is similar to evaluating clients, but the outcome for health team members is more consequential. Clients can choose to learn, partially learn, or ignore learning your health message to promote, retain, and restore health. Evaluation is different for health team members because they are required to learn what you are teaching and will be evaluated accordingly. It is important that the behavior and practice of health team members is aligned with the best practices of the profession and the employing healthcare facility.

The purpose of evaluating health team members is to ensure that each member is fully prepared, competent, safe, and knowledgeable to deliver health care to clients. The evaluation should be consistent with each state's statutes that govern nursing practice and the policies of the employing healthcare facility. The outcome of the evaluation ensures that clinical skills and knowledge are current. Team members must be skillful and have the latest understanding of nursing and health care actions and rationales.

It is important to have conducted a thorough assessment of the health team member's knowledge and skills prior to evaluation. Although teaching can be done individually or in a group, evaluation of learning is based on each individual's performance. Health team members should be fully aware of what they are expected to know, the level at which they are expected to know it, and the knowledge and skills they must demonstrate prior to evaluation. Evaluation follows your teaching; you are evaluating what you taught and what you are expecting team members to learn.

Health team members' knowledge and skills are evaluated using many of the same measurement methods described in this chapter for clients. Direct measurement methods are used to evaluate skills and include direct observation of behavior while performing a skill on a client, a simulation manikin, or simulation models. Evaluation may include videotaping performance. Skill evaluation uses rating scales, checklists of critical steps, evaluation rubrics, and anecdotal notes. Indirect measurement methods are used to evaluate knowledge and include direct questioning and written methods such as quizzes and tests.

The level of knowledge and skill that health team members must demonstrate is higher and more consequential than expected of clients. Do team members need to perform all steps of a skill correctly and answer all questions on a knowledge test correctly? Or do they need to correctly answer most of them? Do they need to achieve a given percentage correctly, such as 90%? Are some skill steps or knowledge items more critical than others, so those items must be answered at 100% accuracy? These are questions that must be addressed in evaluating health team members.

SUMMATIVE EVALUATION: EVALUATION OF EDUCATIONAL EFFECTIVENESS

Evaluating educational effectiveness has two aspects: course evaluation and program evaluation. These are discussed in the following section.

Course Evaluation

The focus of course evaluation is limited to the specific teaching you did with a client or a group of clients. It is concerned with the learning objectives, subject matter content that was taught, teaching strategies used, and instructional materials used to supplement your teaching. You will also want to know how the clients viewed your effectiveness as a teacher. Some of this information is gathered using course evaluations, and some information is what you noted in your own evaluation of the course.

Evaluating learning objectives is done in one of several ways. Figure 13-2 illustrates a typical rating scale for evaluating learning objectives. The form is customized by listing each learning objective to be evaluated. Each learning objective is then rated on a 3- or 5-point scale. When you use a form like this, include open-ended questions and leave ample space for clients to provide written responses. A similar form could be created to have clients evaluate the teaching strategies and instructional materials.

Another evaluation method is comprised of open-ended questions. Such questions require clients to provide more thoughtful responses than on a rating scale or checklist. For example, to gain additional evaluative information from the clients, ask questions like these:

■ What content was most helpful for you? (Variations: What was the most important thing you learned? Name the two most important things you learned.)
■ What content was the least helpful for you? (Variations: What was the least important thing you learned? Name the two least important things that were taught.)
■ What content was not covered that you think should have been? (Variation: What content would you like to see covered in this course in the future?)
■ What would be helpful for us to know that would make the course better?

To evaluate your own performance as a teacher, see Figure 13-3. It covers how effectively you addressed learning objectives, the subject matter content, your teaching strategies, the teaching and instructional aids, and your performance. At the bottom of the evaluation form is an opportunity for clients to write their own impressions and comments. It should be administered at the same time as the form to evaluate learning objectives. We have used this form on numerous occasions and found it very helpful for nurses as educators. Administer both evaluation forms at the last class while everyone is still present. The forms should be administered by the department secretary or someone other than the nurse who taught the course. The nurse should leave the room when the forms are distributed. The responses are confidential, and clients should not be asked to provide their names on the forms. After clients have completed the forms, the responses can be tabulated and then shared with the nurse who taught the course and the head of the health education department.

Program Evaluation

Health teaching is often delivered through structured programs. A program is any group of related, complementary activities intended to achieve specific outcomes. The process of program evaluation includes the systematic gathering, analysis, and reporting of data about a program to assist in decision making. Program evaluation is usually broad in scope, covering an entire department or a specific program; however, it can also refer to a single course (Worral, 2014).

The purpose, scope, and context of evaluating a program must be clearly defined. In contemplating program evaluation, consider the questions you want answered (Lorig et al., 2001). Do you want to know about a program's overall effectiveness or the clients' perceptions of the degree to which the learning objectives were taught? Do you want to know the clients' level of satisfaction with the program or whether the cost of the program was worth the outcomes? Is the purpose of the evaluation to justify the expenditures of time and money by the health education department, or is it to identify the program's strengths and weaknesses?

Also consider the intended audience for the evaluation and how the evaluation report will be used. The report may be intended for the healthcare institution or agency management accreditation bodies, or it may be for internal use by the health education staff. The intended use of the program evaluation may be to improve services or justify additional funding.

The data you gather must be consistent with the questions the program evaluation is designed to answer (Lorig et al., 2001). For example, if a health education course was designed for staff to reduce hospital-acquired infections, you would collect data about the infection rate before and after the teaching intervention to determine its impact. If a program was designed to reduce hypertension in clients, you would collect blood pressure readings and medication usage before and after the teaching session to determine its impact.

Table 13-1 introduces you to a variety of program evaluation models. These models have been selected as the most useful approaches to program evaluation. It is not an exhaustive list of models; rather, we have selected ones that we think are most applicable. The table identifies the name of the model, its purpose, and a summary of the unique application components to program evaluation.

To conduct a program evaluation, identify the purpose for the evaluation by identifying the goals and answering the questions we identified earlier in this section. Since resources for program evaluation are always limited, decision criteria are needed to help you determine who will use the results and what information will be most useful to them. Carefully consider how much time and how many resources are available for the evaluation. Then look at the choice of models in **Table 13-1** and select the one that best helps you achieve that goal.

SUMMATIVE EVALUATION: EVALUATION OF INTEGRATION OF LEARNING INTO DAILY LIVING

Client Adherence

Of great importance to health education programs is whether or not clients have benefitted from what they have learned. Have they incorporated their new learning into their daily lives? Are they living more healthfully as a result of your teaching? This area of summative evaluation is known as client **adherence**, formerly known as compliance. Adherence refers to the degree to which clients are following the agreed-upon recommendations of nurses and other healthcare providers (Chisholm-Burns & Spivey, 2008). The word *adherence* suggests a collaborative relationship between nurses and clients, whereas the word *compliance* suggests an obedient relationship. When clients are called noncompliant, it implies that nurses and healthcare providers know what is best for clients and expect them to follow orders. When clients do not comply, they are at fault. Adherence implies a cooperative relationship that is based on shared responsibility. A cooperative relationship respects clients as independent, intelligent, and autonomous individuals who are active participants in promoting, retaining, and restoring their health (Falvo, 2011; Lutfey & Wishner, 1999).

Adherence refers to all health-related behaviors that both clients and healthcare providers agree are necessary to promote, retain, and restore client health. It covers behaviors such as keeping follow-up appointments, obtaining immunizations, and properly self-managing chronic diseases such as asthma and diabetes. It is following recommended health-promoting behaviors, such as regular exercise, a healthful diet, and smoking cessation.

TABLE 13-1	

Program Evaluation Models

Models for Program Evaluation	*Application*
Roberta Straessle Abruzzese (RSA) Education Model (1996)	■ Process evaluation ■ Content evaluation ■ Outcome evaluation ■ Impact ■ Total program evaluation
Alspach's Evaluation Model (1995)	■ Satisfaction ■ Learning ■ Application ■ Impact
Consumer-Oriented Evaluation Model (Scriven, 1967)	■ Formative: Improve development ■ Summative: Assess value, costs, merits, worth
Stake's Countenance Model (1967)	■ Antecedents ■ Transactions ■ Outcomes ■ Unexpected outcomes
Developmental Model for the Evaluation of Health Education Programs (Nutbeam, Smith, & Catford, 1990)	■ Does it work? ■ Can it be repeated and refined? ■ Can it be widely implemented?
Improvement-Oriented Evaluation Model (CIPP) (Stufflebeam, 1971)	■ Context: The environment ■ Input: System capabilities ■ Process: Implementation ■ Products: Worth and merit
International Association of Continuing Education and Training's 10-Level Model (1991)	■ Assessment of learning outcomes ■ Program evaluation
Kirkpatrick's Four-Level Model (1994)	■ Reaction ■ Learning ■ Behavior ■ Results
Logic Model (Frye & Hemmer, 2012)	■ Inputs ■ Activities ■ Outputs ■ Outcomes
Haggard's Three Dimensions in Evaluating Teaching Effectiveness (1989)	■ Assimilation during teaching ■ Information retention after teaching ■ Use of information in day-to-day life
Object-Based Model (Tyler, 1967)	■ Satisfaction or dissatisfaction ■ Effectiveness of planning and actions ■ Fit between student performance and objectives ■ Methodology dependent on the evaluator's definition of *measurement*

(continues)

TABLE 13-1

Program Evaluation Models (Continued)

Models for Program Evaluation	Application
Program Evaluation for Public Health (Centers for Disease Control and Prevention, 1999)	■ Engage stakeholders ■ Describe program ■ Focus the evaluation design ■ Gather credible evidence ■ Justify conclusion ■ Ensure use and share lessons learned
Rankin and Stallings's Five Levels of Evaluation of Patient Learning (Rankin, Stallings, & London, 2005)	■ Assessment of learning needs and influencing factors ■ Diagnosis of learning needs ■ Goal setting ■ Implementation of patient teaching ■ Evaluation of learning
Zhang and Cheng's Planning Development Process and Product Model (PDPP) (2012)	■ Planning ■ Development ■ Process ■ Product evaluation

Adherence is not an either/or situation. For example, nonadherence to medication may include not taking a medication as prescribed or missing doses, or discontinuing or lowering the dose because of undesirable side effects or financial concerns. Nonadherence to a diet includes failure to consistently follow dietary guidelines, not changing bandages as frequently as recommended, or using hot and cold therapeutic applications incorrectly. Nonadherence can result in worsening of the client's health problem, and it impacts the family, increases healthcare costs, and even results in preventable death (Osterberg & Blaschke, 2005; Rolnick, Pawloski, Hedblom, Asche, & Bruzek, 2013; Wells, 2011).

Scope of Nonadherence

Statistics on nonadherence vary widely and differ in reference to specific health problems. No demographic variable has been consistently correlated with nonadherence. Demographic variables include age, sex, race, ethnicity, marital status, educational level, socioeconomic status, and religion (DiMatteo, 2004; Falvo, 2011; Magai, Consedine, Neugut, & Hershman, 2007; Miaskowski, Shockney, & Chlebowski, 2008; Rolnick et al., 2013; Vermeire, Hearnshaw, Van Royen, & Denekens, 2001; Wells, 2011). Nonadherence has also been studied from the perspective of psychological factors, social factors, and client–provider interaction factors, and no clear patterns have emerged (Lutfey & Wishner, 1999). Nor was the level of health literacy a factor in adherence (Mosher, Lund, Kripalani, & Kaboli, 2012); older veterans with low health literacy followed their medication regimens, as did their counterparts who had adequate health literacy, even though the former group had less knowledge about their medications. Adherence to long-term therapy for chronic illnesses in developed countries averages 50%, according to the World Health Organization (2014).

The fact that adherence does not consistently correlate with any studied variables may seem confusing because education does appear to be correlated with health-promoting behaviors. However, we know that knowledge of health and illness is not enough to motivate lasting change and relinquish addictions. For example, some nurses smoke, abuse substances, suffer from eating disorders, and avoid getting flu vaccines, even though they know the risks of such behaviors.

Barriers to Adherence

Clients who are nonadherent are so for a variety of reasons. Clients choose the health behaviors in which they will engage. Generally the choice is a trade-off among a variety of influences in their lives. For example, dietary modifications may be difficult to follow if there is insufficient money to buy food. Or it may be impractical to prepare the food as instructed. Perhaps the rationale for behavior change does not make sense to the client. It is also possible that a client's social network does not offer enough **reinforcement** to sustain a behavioral change, such as quitting smoking. It may be that the client does not like the side effects of a medication and does not understand the reason to continue taking it. This is especially true when the disease does not cause noticeable symptoms, such as hypertension and hyperlipidemia. The client may be overwhelmed with the complexities of his or her treatment plan, medication schedule, and cost in terms of dollars and time. Consider, for example, the challenges of HIV clients who must adhere to antiretroviral therapy to suppress viral replication and avoid developing resistance. The treatment involves expensive medications with complex dosing schedules that may cause food interactions and side effects (Osterberg & Blaschke, 2005).

Psychological barriers related to nonadherence include forgetting, not wanting to use medications, unpleasant side effects of medications, lack of motivation, inability to understand instructions, being uncooperative, or psychiatric illness such as depression. Clients may not see themselves as susceptible to disease or understand the severity of a disease. Social barriers include the lack of family member and peer support, poor family cohesiveness, stigma of the disease, different approaches to treatment, difficulty navigating the healthcare system, living conditions, and financial limitations. Finally, nurse–client interaction factors may be related to nonadherence. For example, the nurse may be rushed, does not clearly explain the rationale for the treatment, directs rather than collaborates with clients, or fails to understand and address the client's needs. Why clients do not adhere is an individual matter.

Predictors of Nonadherence

Nurses as educators can anticipate nonadherence from clients under certain circumstances. Knowing who is likely to nonadhere to a treatment regimen alerts nurses to assess clients more carefully and provide additional education if indicated. Predictors of nonadherence include clients with chronic diseases that require long-term treatment, clients who are not responding as expected to therapy, and clients who have a history of not adhering. Other predictors include clients who do not believe the treatment will be helpful, lack of support from family and friends, unpleasant side effects, and complex medication regimens. Less likely to adhere are clients who

FIGURE 13-6

Factors That Deter Adherence

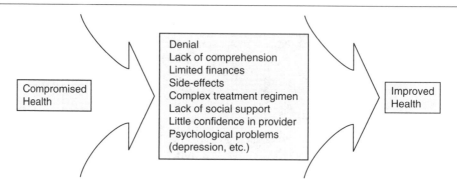

have psychological problems such as depression or those who have poor communication with the nurse (Miaskowski et al., 2008) (**Figure 13-6**).

Facilitators of Adherence

This section looks at strategies to foster adherence through a discussion of health education, the nurse–client interaction, stages of behavioral change, locus of control, and follow-up strategies.

Health Education

Our basic assumption is that if we as educators provide relevant, culturally appropriate health education, clients will adhere to the recommendations. Nurses are obligated to provide accurate, relevant, and timely health information. Information is the basis for making positive behavioral and lifestyle changes. This is what the role of nurses as educators is all about.

If clients are motivated to learn and you have their attention, teach them about the nature of their health problem and the purpose of the treatment regimen. Teach them about the importance of following the treatment regimen and its rationale. Point out the positive signs of progress and the side effects of treatment. Reinforce the physician's directions. Often clients ask nurses questions they do not want to bother the physician with. Select the major points you wish to communicate using concrete, nonmedical jargon. Use pictures or models to facilitate learning along with written instructions. Ask clients to restate your major points and reinforce the clients when they have done so successfully. Repetition of the message aids learning and emphasizes the points you make. We believe that clients who are informed and active participants in their health care are more likely to adhere to recommendations to promote, retain, and restore their health.

If appropriate, involve and educate family members about the client's needs. For example, teaching a male client about a low-sodium diet does little good if his wife, who does all the cooking, does not participate in learning. Be sensitive to roles and responsibilities in families and use clinical judgment in working with them. When conflicting roles and responsibilities occur, family members may not be available to help (Miaskowski et al., 2008). For example, people in the sandwich generation include parents who are attempting to meet the needs of their children and those of their aging parents. Many factors influence family involvement in the care of a family member.

Nurse–Client Interaction

The nurse–client interaction is important in fostering adherence. A communication style that allows clients to verbalize their feelings and concerns is desirable. This collaborative style encourages clients to make behavioral changes to retain, promote, or restore health. It is a relationship of equals who mutually respect each other and work together to achieve the common goal of adherence. This shared decision making and open communication are effective strategies in fostering adherence (Robinson, Callister, Berry, & Dearing, 2008).

Remember to listen to the client's perspective. It is by listening and being nonjudgmental that nurses gain insight into how clients view the necessary changes and adjustments they must make. Based on these insights, nurses can offer suggestions for clients to consider. Be persuasive in helping clients see the importance of making a behavioral change. Notify the physician if you determine that clients are having trouble with the treatment regimen and are unwilling or unlikely to adhere to it. There may be good reasons why clients do not adhere, and nurses need to know the client's perspective (DiGiacomo, 2008).

Stages of Behavioral Change

When clients are confronted with the need to change their behavior or adhere to a treatment regimen, they have decisions to make. Behavioral and lifestyle changes usually do not happen instantly; rather, change is a process that occurs over time. Prochaska, Redding, and Evers (2008) proposed a model of behavioral change that is useful in health education. They posit that behavior change occurs in a series of stages: precontemplation, contemplation, preparation, action, maintenance, and termination (Prochaska & Norcross, 2001; Prochaska et al., 2008). Actions to support behavioral changes are included in **Table 13-2**.

Locus of Control

As you work with clients, assess how they see their role in promoting, retaining, or restoring their health. The concepts of locus of control and self-efficacy are interrelated and are important to adherence. Self-efficacy is a person's belief that he or she is capable of performing successfully to attain specific goals (Bandura, 1986). Before clients can adhere to any treatment regimen, they must have confidence that they are capable of doing what is required of them. Locus of control refers to beliefs about the source of control over one's life, whether it is within or external to the individual (Slavin, 2012). Clients who have an internal locus of control believe that success or failure results from their own efforts and abilities. They believe they have some control over their health and are more likely to adhere to the treatment regimen and health recommendations. Clients who have an external locus of control believe that success or failure is beyond their control; that is, it is caused by fate, luck, or other people's actions. These clients are less likely to have confidence in their ability to control their state of health. Clients with an internal locus of control and a high sense of self-efficacy are more likely to be receptive to health education and adhere to health recommendations.

TABLE 13-2

Prochaska and Colleagues' Stages of Behavioral Change

Stage	Characteristics	Nurse as Educator Role
Precontemplation	The client is unaware of the problem, but others are aware of it.	Supports and nurtures
Contemplation	The client is aware of the problem and thinks about changing within the next 6 months. The client contemplates the pros and cons.	Encourages client to examine the problem and gain insight
Preparation	The client intends to change soon, within the next month. The client has a plan of action but has not yet made a decision.	Serves as a coach as the client makes plans to change; suggests programs, such as weight loss, smoking cessation, etc.
Action	The client takes the time and makes an effort to modify the behavior. This stage lasts up to 6 months.	Serves as a consultant, providing advice and guidance
Maintenance	The client maintains the change and prevents relapse. This stage lasts longer than 6 months.	Serves as a consultant, providing advice and guidance
Termination	The client is fully committed to behavioral change and is 100% confident of his or her ability to maintain the change.	Reinforces success

Follow-Up Strategies

The degree to which clients have integrated what they learned into their daily living activities is the true test of adherence. We are interested in the behavior and lifestyle changes that persist long after the completion of the health education intervention. In other words, do clients maintain these changes when they return to their homes and usual routines? The best way to determine adherence is to observe clients in their homes when they are unaware of your presence. This is unrealistic, so we have to employ other methods to gain this information.

If you are working in a clinic or doctor's office, reinforce health teaching at each visit with the client. Rather than asking if a client has exercised, ask that person to tell you how he or she is working exercise into a daily routine. Instead of answering yes or no, the client will likely give a more thoughtful and accurate response. Provide written information and brochures to supplement your teaching and encourage adherence. Other strategies include postcards or letters reminding clients about appointments and screening tests. Sometimes support staff will telephone clients to remind them about appointments or follow-ups.

Follow-up questionnaires can be sent to clients at different time intervals after discharge. This can be done at 6-month, 1-year, or 2-year intervals depending on the level of follow-up information desired. Questions can be constructed that indicate the level of adherence to the treatment regimen. This same process and data gathering can be done by telephone interviewing. Another option is completing a questionnaire via email if clients have Internet access.

Instruct clients to keep a log of their progress in adhering to a treatment regimen. For example, have clients record their medications, exercise activities, or weight management (DiGiacomo, 2008). This gives clients an active role in the treatment plan and motivates them to assume responsibility for adherence. Contracts between clients and providers based on mutually agreed-upon goals may be used to ensure client commitment to the desired change.

Sometimes clients are referred to support groups of people who are grappling with the same health issues. Support groups are powerful motivators and are a source of encouragement by others who are dealing with the same health issue. Voluntary health organizations can be a source of information and support if the client needs more information (Miaskowski et al., 2008).

If clients are not following the recommended changes, you need to find out why (Rankin et al., 2005). Nonadherence could be for good reasons instead of unwillingness. It may be caused by financial factors, such as a medication regimen that is too expensive or inflexible. It may be that clients do not know how to substitute recommended foods for locally available foods they can afford. It may be that clients simply misread or misunderstood the discharge directions. The only way nurses will know is to ask and then listen to what clients say. When you know the reasons for nonadherence, you can make suggestions that are appropriate and acceptable to clients.

In summary, as you teach clients, stress the importance of their role in promoting, retaining, and restoring health. Remember that adherence requires **collaboration** among nurses, other healthcare providers, and clients. Clients make the final decision about whether or not to implement health recommendations. Do your best to empower clients and support their role in assuming responsibility for their health. Nurses should respect the decisions clients make.

Impact on the Community

As clients improve their health behavior, one person at a time, it changes the health of the community. This is why we engage in health education to promote, retain, and restore health. Health is emphasized by government at all levels and multiple voluntary health organizations. The health department in each state is charged with monitoring health conditions and specific health parameters. These state health departments cooperate and coordinate with the Centers for Disease Control and Prevention (CDC) at the federal level. The state health departments and the CDC monitor many variables that impact health—from the food we eat and the air we breathe, to health trends, disease outbreaks, and morbidity and mortality statistics. They also identify groups at risk for health problems, develop programs to address health problems, and evaluate the effectiveness of strategies designed to promote health.

Many community health issues are important today, such as access to healthy food, healthy nutrition in schools, tobacco use, substance abuse, obesity, and promotion of exercise and activities for all ages, including the elderly. For example, decreasing the rate of obesity is an important state and national goal. While adult obesity rates have remained level in every state except one in the past year, they are expected to increase in the future (Trust for America's Health, 2013). Obesity contributes to the development of cardiovascular disease and diabetes, resulting in increased healthcare costs and early mortality. Nurses as educators work with many different groups to provide age-specific and culturally appropriate health education.

A healthy community is everyone's concern, and health education is one of the most important strategies we have to achieve this goal. When clients engage in healthful practices, the community benefits; when clients do not, it impacts not only them but also the larger community. The consequences of nonadherence to the community are individual, societal, and economic (Falvo, 2011). Individual consequences refer to the prevention, development, and progression of disease states. Examples include failure to obtain immunizations, failure to change unhealthy lifestyles, and failure to follow self-management recommendations to control the progression of chronic disease. These consequences are especially important because chronic diseases are expected to increase in the aging U.S. population. Societal consequences occur when individuals fail to effectively self-manage chronic diseases, which results in decreased workplace productivity, increased insurance rates, and overutilization of healthcare services. It impacts public health and the control and eradication of infectious diseases. Economic consequences occur when individuals require repeated hospitalizations for treatment of complications. Other consequences include additional visits to primary care providers, increased use of home care services, and increased cost of providing healthcare services at a time when there are limited financial resources and the aging population requires those services. Nonadherence is estimated to cost $100 billion each year in the United States, and it is responsible for 10% of hospital admissions and 23% of nursing home admissions (Aliotta, Vlasnik, & Delor, 2004; Dezii, 2000; Vermeire et al., 2001). The largest proportion of this cost (70%) appears to be a result of decreased productivity and premature death, with direct medical costs accounting for the remaining 30% (Dezii, 2000).

A significant barrier to promoting, retaining, and restoring health is the healthcare system's focus on caring for people after they have become sick or harmed. Focusing on prevention addresses this barrier. Prevention is an essential aspect of a community approach and is supported by a report released by the Trust for America's Health in July 2008. This report found that a small investment in disease prevention could result in significant savings in U.S. healthcare costs. The report concluded that an investment of $10 per person per year in proven community-based programs to increase physical activity, improve nutrition, and prevent smoking and other tobacco use could save the country more than $16 billion annually within 5 years. The report supports a continued focus on health education.

CASE EXAMPLE: MRS. ROSA LOPEZ

We now illustrate how to measure each of the learning objectives for Mrs. Lopez. The cognitive objective—the client will correctly verbally explain to the nurse, from memory, how excessive salt intake affects blood pressure—can be measured in several ways. We would ask Mrs. Lopez to verbalize the relationship or give her a brief paper-and-pencil test. The test questions could be true or false, multiple choice, short-answer essay, or fill in the blank (**Table 13-3**).

The affective objective—the client will choose to limit sodium intake by working with the nurse to prepare a dietary plan for one week—would be evaluated in several ways. A short-term measure would be to have Mrs. Lopez fill out an attitude scale, as seen in **Box 13-4**. Another approach would be to have her construct a meal plan from a list of foods to determine her choices. The long-term measure would be whether or not she makes the dietary changes resulting in lower blood pressure. To determine this she records her blood pressure on a chart.

TABLE 13-3

Sample Test Questions for Mrs. Rosa Lopez

Sample True-or-False Questions

Directions: Circle T if the statement is true. Circle F if any part of the statement is false.

T F 1. It is OK to add a small amount of salt to my food at the dinner table.

T F 2. Processed and canned foods are low in sodium.

T F 3. Excess sodium intake can cause body fluid retention.

T F 4. Excess fluid retention can result in the elevation of blood pressure.

Sample Multiple-Choice Question

Directions: Put an X in front of the one best answer.

1. A sodium-restricted diet is important in the treatment of hypertension because it:

_____ a. minimizes excess fluid retention.

_____ b. results in fluid accumulation.

_____ c. expands the blood capillaries.

_____ d. increases urinary output.

Sample Short-Answer Essay and Fill-in-the-Blank Questions

Directions: Fill in the blanks to make the statement correct. The missing words are listed at the bottom.

1. Although _____ sodium in your_____ is important to make a regular part of your _____ routine, it may not _____ the need for medication. Dietary changes will help you to control _____ accumulation and may help you _____ your blood _____.

Possible missing words:
  daily
  pressure
  diet
  limiting
  style of life
  eliminate
  rate
  fluid
  reduce

2. In 25 words or less, describe the relationship among sodium, fluid retention, and hypertension.

Dietary changes should result in lowered blood pressure readings. The ability to take her own blood pressure is a psychomotor skill, so the chart measures her success in the affective domain.

The psychomotor objective—demonstrate how to accurately obtain your own blood pressure reading using home digital equipment without any verbal guidance—can be evaluated by observing Mrs. Lopez's performance. The steps of the procedure are shown in the checklist in **Box 13-5.**

Mrs. Lopez would be considered successful when we observe her complete each step of the procedure correctly. We would have her perform the procedure once initially to check her familiarity with the procedure. She would be tested once. If she does not perform correctly, then we would repeat the procedure until she is accurate and is comfortable with the procedure.

BOX 13-4

Sample Attitude Scale for Mrs. Rosa Lopez

Directions: Place an X in the column that most closely describes your feelings toward each of the statements. Be as honest as you can; this information is for you.

Statement	Agree	Neutral	Disagree
1. I am too busy to worry about meal planning.			
2. Altering my diet requires making too many changes.			
3. I can tell when my blood pressure is up.			
4. I am worried about stroke or heart disease.			
5. Everyone must die of something sometime.			
6. Proper diet can have a positive effect on my life.			
7. My children are cooperating with my dietary changes.			
8. I like salty snacks when I watch television.			

Mrs. Lopez would use the chart shown in **Box 13-6** to record her daily blood pressure readings. Each time she comes in for a weekly checkup, her readings would be reviewed and her blood pressure would be checked to assess her progress. We would expect to find similar readings to our own. If they are similar, we would consider her performance successful. Because some digital blood pressure equipment also calculates the pulse rate, we have included a row on the chart to record the pulse.

Adherence for Mrs. Lopez

If Mrs. Lopez adheres to the teaching plan, she would incorporate the dietary changes into her meal planning and daily diet. She would also be taking her blood pressure and recording it daily. At her clinic visits, we would take her blood pressure and compare our readings with hers.

BOX 13-5

Sample Checklist for Taking the Blood Pressure

_____ Reads digital blood pressure equipment directions.

_____ Arranges the digital blood pressure equipment on a table by a chair.

_____ Locates the brachial artery.

_____ Places arm in the cuff.

_____ Inflates the cuff according to equipment directions.

_____ Releases air in the cuff according to equipment directions.

_____ Records the systolic and diastolic pressure, the pulse, and the date.

BOX 13-6

Sample Chart for Recording Blood Pressure

Systolic reading												
Diastolic reading												
Pulse												
Date												

If Mrs. Lopez tells us she is not adhering, our first response would be to reinforce her honesty and talk about the perceived barriers. After listening to her story, we would help her identify options to surmount the problems. As we identify these options, we might preface them with a question such as, Have you thought about ..., or, How would ... work for you?

For illustrative purposes, we have created a problem that interferes with Mrs. Lopez's adherence. She says she is too busy with her employment, her children, and volunteering to implement all of the dietary changes. She removed the salt shaker from the table, adds no salt in cooking, avoids canned or processed foods that are high in sodium, and uses low-sodium seasonings such as herbs and spices in her cooking, but she enjoys munching on salty snacks in the evening as she watches television. We would focus on her enjoyment of salty snacks. Some options include finding snacks that are satisfying but devoid of the sodium content. We would do this by giving her a handout that lists low-sodium snacks or showing her how to search the Internet for such listings. For example, we would suggest unsalted nuts, crackers, rice cakes, granola bars, and fresh and dried fruits. We might also suggest keeping her mind and hands busy with a craft as she watches television, such as knitting or embroidery, or by taking a walk every evening. **Box 13-7** demonstrates the effectiveness of a telephone follow-up intervention to reinforce client education and encourage client adherence to the health treatment plan.

BOX 13-7

Evidence-Based Nursing Practice

Inman, D. M., Maxson, P. M., Johnson, K. M., Myers, R. P., & Holland, D. E. (2011). The impact of follow-up educational telephone calls on patients after radical prostatectomy: Finding value in low-maargin activities. Urologic Nursing. March–April, 31(2), 83–91.

Purpose: Determine if patients who receive an additional telephone follow-up educational intervention after radical prostatectomy surgery have an increased understanding of how to manage their care at home and use fewer healthcare resources.

Method: Sixty patients were randomly assigned to either a control or an intervention group. Both groups received preoperative education; the intervention group received a telephone follow-up 3–5 days following discharge.

Results: Timely follow-up may be an effective way to assist patients in recalling information. The phone call was individually tailored reinforcement of education and came when it was most relevant. Patients reported it as helpful, and it reduced their need to use other resources.

SUMMARY

Summative evaluation is the final step in the teaching and learning process. Summative evaluation focuses on evaluation of client learning, evaluation of educational effectiveness, and evaluation of the integration of learning into daily living. It is important to use the results of evaluation to improve health education and your effectiveness as an educator. This chapter has covered the details of the evaluation of client learning to include measurement and a variety of direct and indirect measurement methods. Selecting specific measurement methods is based on the domain (cognitive, affective, and psychomotor) of the learning objectives. A variety of methods is available to choose from. The evaluation of health team members is more consequential than evaluating clients, and those differences were discussed. Course and program evaluations are important aspects of summative evaluation, and each has a unique focus and features to evaluate.

We believe effective client education will lead to behavioral and lifestyle changes. Clients who want to promote, retain, and restore their health may need to modify what they are doing and adopt healthier ways of living. The challenges you face as an educator are influenced by client assessment data that you have collected and how you use that data to provide meaningful, interesting, and motivating health education.

We urge you to keep in mind the power of warmth and caring as motivating forces to help clients change. Remember that clients are in charge of their own behavior and live with the consequences of their choices. You can provide interesting, stimulating, and timely health messages, but you cannot enforce adherence. Your role is that of teacher and guide, not health enforcer.

EXERCISES

Exercise I: Evaluate a Test by Finding the Flaws

Purposes:

- Make an inference about the purpose of this test.
- Apply guidelines for proper test construction.

Directions:

1. Find all the flaws in this test and state your rationale for each.
2. Rewrite the test to improve the form, clarify questions, and maintain the purpose of the test.
3. Share your perceptions of the test's purpose with your peers.
4. State the rationale for your conclusion.

Critical Care Unit in the Hospital of St. Anywhere
Directions: Circle the statements you think are true:

1. The damage of a heart attack is caused by:
   a. Too much fat in the blood.
   b. Too much blood in the heart chambers.
   c. Too little blood to the heart muscles.
   d. There is no heart damage; the only damage is a clot in a blood vessel.

2. The pain involved in a heart attack is from:
   a. Heart irritability.
   b. Too little oxygen to the heart muscle.
   c. Too little blood to the heart chambers.
   d. Damaged heart muscle.

3. The damage to the heart muscle from a heart attack is:
   a. Similar to a deep cut.
   b. Similar to a muscle sprain.
   c. Similar to a bruise.

4. The healing of the heart following an attack is:
   a. Never really complete, there is always a scar that is subsequently weaker than the natural heart muscle.
   b. Totally complete, leaving no trace or damage.
   c. Shown by a scar.

Directions: Mark T for true or F for false:

_____ 5. After a heart attack a client will not return to his or her previous level of physical activity.
_____ 6. After a heart attack one's sex life always has to be reduced (in future years).
_____ 7. It was my last meal that led to my heart attack.
_____ 8. Even an occasional cocktail is bad for your heart.
_____ 9. High blood cholesterol signals a proneness to heart attack.
_____ 10. About medication:

   a. You should not become dependent on them as a crutch.
   b. It may help to carry nitroglycerin tablets in your pocket.
   c. After you leave the hospital, medications you are given in the hospital are not to be changed in the future by your doctor.

Exercise II: Program Evaluation

Purpose: Investigate program evaluation in a healthcare institution or agency.
Directions:

1. Working in pairs, interview the head of the education department in a local healthcare institution or agency.
2. Prepare interview questions that are consistent with the content discussed in this chapter. Some sample questions you can ask are as follows:
   a. How do they conduct program evaluation?
   b. Do they have a program evaluation model that they frequently use?
   c. What common indicators do they track?
   d. Describe the health education program being evaluated. What is the purpose of this particular evaluation? What do they hope to learn by the report? Who will read the evaluation report? What types of decisions will be based on the report?
3. Report your findings in class.

Exercise III: Client Adherence

Purpose: Gain insight into client adherence issues.

Directions:

1. Working with your instructor, identify a client for whom you have provided nursing care and health education.
2. Obtain permission to do a follow-up interview with the client either by telephone or by visiting the client at home.
3. Prepare interview questions that are directly related to the health education that you provided.
4. Interview the client.
5. Report in class your findings about the client's adherence to the health education recommendations that you provided. Was the client adhering to the recommendations? If not, why? If not, did the reasons surprise you? Were the reasons different from those described in this chapter?

REFERENCES

Abruzzese, R. S. (1996). *Nursing staff development: Strategies for success* (2nd ed.). St. Louis, MO: Mosby.

Aliotta, S. L., Vlasnik, J. J., & Delor, B. (2004). Enhancing adherence to long-term medical therapy: A new approach to assessing and treating patients. *Advanced Therapy, 21*(4), 214–231.

Alspach, J. G. (1995). *The educational process in nursing staff development.* St. Louis, MO: Mosby.

Bandura, A. (1986). *Social foundations of thought and action: A social cognitive theory.* Englewood Cliffs, NJ: Prentice Hall.

Benner, P. (1984). *From novice to expert.* Menlo Park, CA: Addison-Wesley.

Centers for Disease Control and Prevention. (1999). Framework for program evaluation in public health. *Morbidity and Mortality Weekly Report, 48*(No. RR-11).

Chisholm-Burns, M. A., & Spivey, C. A. (2008, April 1). Pharmacoadherence: A new term for a significant problem. *American Journal Health-Systems Pharmacists, 65,* 661–667.

Dezii, C. M. (2000). Medication noncompliance: What is the problem? *Managed Care, 9* (Suppl. 9), 9–12.

DiGiacomo, M. (2008). Patient adherence: Sharing the responsibility. *PT Magazine, 16*(7), 28–30.

DiMatteo, M. R. (2004). Variations in patients' adherence to medical recommendations: A quantitative review of 50 years of research. *Medical Care, 42*(3), 200–209.

Falvo, D. R. (2011). *Effective patient education: A guide to increased compliance* (4th ed.). Sudbury, MA: Jones & Bartlett Learning.

Frye, A. W., & Hemmer, P. A. (2012). Program evaluation models and related theories: AMEE guide no. 67. *Medical Teacher, 34,* e288–e299.

Gronlund, N. E., & Brookhart, S. M. (2009). *Gronlund's writing instructional objectives* (8th ed.). Upper Saddle River, NJ: Pearson Education.

Haggard, A. (1989). Evaluating patient education. In A. Haggard (Ed.), *Handbook of patient education* (pp. 159–186). Rockville, MD: Aspen.

Inman, D. M., Maxson, P. M., Johnson, K. M., Myers, R. P., & Holland, D. E. (2011). The impact of follow-up educational telephone calls on patients after radical prostatectomy: Finding value in low-margin activities. *Urologic Nursing, 31*(2), 83–91.

International Association of Continuing Education and Training. (1991). *A practical handbook for assessing learning outcomes in continuing education and training*. Washington, DC: Author.

Kirkpatrick, D. L. (1994). *Evaluating training programs*. San Francisco, CA: Berrett-Koehler.

Lorig, K., & Associates (2001). *Patient education: A practical approach* (3rd ed.). Thousand Oaks, CA: Sage.

Lutfey, K. E., & Wishner, W. J. (1999). Beyond "compliance" is "adherence." *Diabetes Care, 22*(4), 635–639.

Magai, C., Consedine, N., Neugut, A. I., & Hershman, D. L. (2007). Common psychosocial factors underlying breast cancer screening and breast cancer treatment adherence: A conceptual review and synthesis. *Journal of Women's Health, 16*(1), 11–23.

Miaskowski, C., Shockney, L., & Chlebowski, R. T. (2008). Adherence to oral endocrine therapy for breast cancer: A nursing perspective. *Clinical Journal of Oncology Nursing, 12*(2), 213–221.

Mosher, H. J., Lund, B. C., Kripalani, S., & Kaboli, P. J. (2012). Association of health literacy with medication knowledge, adherence, and adverse drug events among elderly veterans. *Journal of Health Communication, 17*, 241–251.

Nutbeam, D., Smith, C., & Catford, J. (1990). Evaluation in health education. A review of progress, possibilities and problems. *Journal of Epidemiology and Community Health, 44*, 83–89.

Osterberg, L., & Blaschke, T. (2005). Adherence to medication. *New England Journal of Medicine, 353*, 487–497.

Prochaska, J. O., & Norcross, J. C. (2001). Stages of change. *Psychotherapy, 38*(4), 443–448.

Prochaska, J. O., Redding, C. A., & Evers, K. E. (2008). The transtheoretical model and stages of change. In K. Glanz, B. K. Rimer, & K. Viswanath, (Eds.), *Health behavior and health education: Theory, research, and practice* (4th ed., pp. 97–122). San Francisco, CA: Jossey-Bass.

Rankin, S. H., Stallings, K. D., & London, F. (2005). *Patient education in health and illness* (5th ed.). Philadelphia, PA: Lippincott Williams & Wilkins.

Redman, B. K. (2007). *The practice of patient education: A case study approach* (10th ed.). St. Louis, MO: Mosby Year Book.

Robinson, J. H., Callister, L. C., Berry, J. A., & Dearing, K. A. (2008). Patient-centered care and adherence: Definitions and applications to improve outcomes. *Journal of the American Academy of Nurse Practitioners, 20*, 600–607.

Rolnick, S. J., Pawloski, P. A., Hedblom, B. D., Asche, S. E., & Bruzek, R. J. (2013). Patient characteristics associated with medication adherence. *Clinical Medicine & Research, 11*(2), 54–65.

Scriven, M. (1967). The methodology of evaluation. In R. Tyler (Ed.), *Perspectives of curriculum evaluation*. Chicago, IL: Rand McNally.

Slavin, R. E. (2012). *Educational psychology: Theory and practice* (10th ed.). Boston, MA: Pearson Education.

Stake, R. E. (1967). The countenance of educational evaluation. *Teachers College Record, 68*(7), 523–540.

Stufflebeam, D. L. (1971). *Education evaluation and decision making*. Itasca, IL: F. E. Peacock.

Trust for America's Health. (2008). *Prevention for a healthier America*. Retrieved from http://healthyamericans.org/reports/prevention08/

Trust for America's Health. (2013). *F as in fat: How obesity threatens America's future*. Retrieved from http://healthyamericans.org/report/108/

Tyler, R. (1967). *Perspectives of curriculum evaluation*. Chicago, IL: Rand McNally.

Vermeire, E., Hearnshaw, H., Van Royen, P., & Denekens, J. (2001). Patient adherence to treatment: Three decades of research. A comprehensive review. *Journal of Clinical Pharmacy and Therapeutics, 26*, 331–342.

Webster's All-In-One Dictionary and Thesaurus (2nd ed.). (2013). Springfield, MA: Federal Street Press.

Wells, J. R. (2011). Hemodialysis knowledge and medical adherence in African Americans diagnosed with end stage renal disease: Results of an educational intervention. *Nephrology Nursing Journal, 38*(2), 155–162.

World Health Organization. (2014). *Adherence to long-term therapies: Evidence for action.* Retrieved from http://apps.who.int/medicinedocs/en/d/Js4883e/6.html#Js4883e.6.1.1

Worral, P. S. (2014). Evaluation in healthcare education. In S. B. Bastable (Ed.), *Nurse as educator: Principles of teaching and learning for nursing practice* (4th ed., pp. 601–636). Burlington, MA: Jones & Bartlett Learning.

Zhang, W., & Cheng, Y. L. (2012). Assurance in e-learning: PDPP evaluation model and its application. *International Review of Research in Open and Distance Learning, 13*(3), 66–82.

Appendix A

Psychosocial Vital Signs (PVS)

Psychosocial Vital Signs (PVS) |Spade, 2013|
Patient's Scale: 1–10

	Date:

Perception (P)–Person's thinking about a situation.

10 "What are your thoughts about your health situation and all it involves?"

| "On a scale from 1–10, how would you rate this health situation? One is positive/best & 10 is negative/worst."

1 Pt. Scale:_____

Support (S)–Person's sense of support from people who care.

10 "Who is there for you right now?" "Who can you depend on to give you some support during this?"

| "How would you rate your sense of support? Is it a 1, everyone you need: is it a 10, meaning you have *no one*?"

1 Pt. Scale:_____

Coping (C)–Person's sense of being able to cope with the situation.

10 "How are you dealing with this?" Or, "How are you able to cope with this?"

| "From easiest to most difficult (1-10), how would you rate this health situation?"

1 Pt. Scale:_____

Anxiety (A)–Person's feelings about the situation.

10 How are you feeling about all this?" Or, "How is this situation affecting you?"

| "From feeling calm to terrified, how would you rate yourself on a scale with calm being 1 and terrified being 10?"

1 Pt. Scale:_____

*Clinician's Observation of Anxiety Level [1 – 4]

Anxiety Level	Thinking	*Focus*	*Speech*	Behavior	Physiology
4 Panic	• Impaired thinking	• Cannot be directed	• Incoherent • Shouting or Mute	• Aggressive or very withdrawn • Poor coordination • Terrified expression	• Hyperventilating • Dizziness • Heart palpitations • Hypotension
3 Severe	• Cannot concentrate	• Focus on *specific* detail(s) • Cannot be redirected to *bigger* picture	• Rapid, loud or mute	• Persistent foot/finger tapping/leg swinging • Cannot relax • Startles easily	• Short of breath • Diaphoretic • Urinary urgency • Rapid heart rate
2 Moderate	• Poor concentration	• Easily directed & focused • May be in denial	• States is "nervous" and/or "upset"	• Fidgeting • Trembling lips	• Dry mouth • Pulse increasing
1 Mild	• Alert • Concentrates • Motivated		▪ Speaks clearly, normal rate/volume		• Heart rate & blood pressure slightly elevated

$$PVS:P\_\_\_\_S\_\_\_\_C\_\_\_\_A x\_\_\_\_*[\quad]$$

Clinician's Observation of Human Responses (Narrative Descriptors)

Cognitive/Thinking: Logical, goal-directed, clear, realistic understanding of situation, poor concentration, confused, denial, illogical, loose associations, hallucinations, "worried" suicidal or homicidal thoughts

Affective/Emotions: Feels calm, feeling capable or confident ("I think I can get though this."), uneasy, "nervous", labile, "upset", flat affect, guilt, shame, numb, sad, frustrated, angry, helpless, fearful, terror

Spiritual: Hopeful, "at peace", agony or anguish, speaks of losing purpose/meaning ("no reason to live"), hopeless, "abandoned/alone"

Behavioral: Sociable, calm, cooperative, fidgeting, restless, startles easily, vigilant, pacing, rapid speech, loud, hostile, aggressive, withdrawn

Physical: Vital signs WNL, adequate sleep, elevated VS. dilated pupils, SOB. N/V. diarrhea, insomnia, hypersomnia, loss of appetite, urinary urgency/frequency

Reproduced from Spade, C. M. Nurse Educator: July/August 2008—Volume 33—Issue 4—pp 181–186.

Appendix B
Physical Changes Associated with Aging by System

System	Change
Skin	■ Decreased elasticity with wrinkling ■ Scaly texture ■ Less pigmentation; pale ■ Dry ■ Decreased turgor; tenting
Cardiac	■ Left ventricle thickening, less compliant ■ Tachycardia and bradycardia poorly tolerated ■ Heart tendency to irritability, arrhythmias, and ischemia ■ Changes in conduction system and valves ■ Blood vessels; decreased elasticity, calcified, increased blood pressure ■ Decreased cardiac reserve ■ Increased risk of postural hypotension ■ Increased risk of varicosities, dependency edema, or both
Respiratory	■ Lung expansion decreased ■ Weakened respiratory muscles ■ Calcification of rib articulations leading to stiffness of chest wall ■ Increased anterior–posterior (AP) diameter of the chest ■ Reduced pulmonary reserve ■ Decreased cough reflex with increased risk of aspiration pneumonia ■ Increased risk of infection and bronchospasm with airway obstruction

(continues)

System	Change
Neurological	■ Decreased velocity of nerve impulse conduction ■ Decreased response and sensitivity to outside stimuli ■ Brain weight may be reduced by as much as 10% ■ Decreased blood flow to the brain ■ Slowed speed of cognitive processing ■ Increased risk of sleep disorders, neurologic diseases, and delirium ■ Increased risk of sensory overload or deprivation
Gastrointestinal	■ Teeth loosen, saliva decreases ■ Decreased strength of muscles of mastication ■ Decreased changes in taste ■ Dry mouth, decreased salivation ■ Decreased gastric motility with delayed emptying ■ Decreased secretion of digestive enzymes ■ Atrophy of protective mucosa ■ Malabsorption of carbohydrates, vitamins B_{12} and D, folic acid, calcium ■ Decreased peristalsis, impaired sensation to defecate ■ Reduced hepatic reserve ■ Decreased metabolism of drugs
Musculoskeletal	■ Narrowed intervertebral disks ■ Decreased bone mass ■ Lean body mass replaced by fat with redistribution of fat ■ Decreased muscle mass and regeneration of muscle fibers ■ Increased latency and contraction time of muscle ■ Increased hip and knee flexion ■ Tendon and ligament stiffening ■ Articular cartilage erosion; increased bone overgrowth and calcium deposits
Urinary	■ Nocturnal polyuria ■ Increased risk for dehydration ■ Decreased renal blood flow, decreased GFR ■ Decreased urinary concentration ■ Limitations in excretion of water, Na+, K+, and acid
Endocrine	■ Decreased hormone production and secretion ■ Decreased hormone metabolism ■ Changes in the rhythms in the body, such as the menstrual cycle ■ Increased development of type 2 diabetes ■ Decreased growth hormone levels leading to decreased lean muscle, decreased heart function, and osteoporosis ■ Menopause between 50 and 55 years of age; menstrual periods stop

(continues)

System	Change
Sensory	■ Pupils become smaller; decreased light reaching the retina, resulting in decreased visual acuity
	■ Decreased lens elasticity resulting in decreased accommodation to distance (presbyopia)
	■ Lid laxity, senile ptosis (excess skin)
	■ Dry eye (decreased tear production)
	■ Arcus senilis (lipid deposit in the cornea)
	■ Cataracts; thickening, clouding, and yellowing of lens
	■ Glaucoma; increased intraocular pressure
	■ Decreased hearing due to natural or mechanical means
	■ Presbycusis; degeneration of the inner ear
	■ Cerumen impaction
	■ Increase in dry, flaky cerumen
	■ Decreased sense of taste and thirst perception

Note: Page numbers followed by *b, f,* and *t* indicate materials in boxes, figures, and tables respectively.